AF364669

Pharmaceutical Research Methodology and Bio-statistics

Theory and Practice

Second Edition

Pharmaceutical Research Methodology and Bio-statistics

Theory and Practice

Second Edition

Bayya Subba Rao

M. Pharm, FAGE (MAN),
P.G. Diploma in Patent Laws (NALSAR), IAO, Ph.D
Faculty (Formerly – Patent Analyst at
IPR & Regulatory Centre, Pharmexcil, Hyderabad).

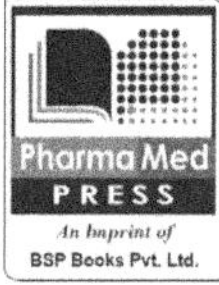

PharmaMed Press
An imprint of BSP Books Pvt. Ltd.
4-4-309/316, Giriraj Lane,
Sultan Bazar, Hyderabad - 500 095.

Published by

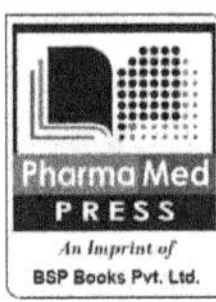

PharmaMed Press

An imprint of BSP Books Pvt. Ltd.

4-4-309/316, Giriraj Lane, Sultan Bazar, Hyderabad - 500 095.

Phone: 040-23445688; Fax: 91+40-23445611

E-mail: info@pharmamedpress.net

www.bspbooks.net/www.pharmamedpress.net

ISBN: 978-93-95039-34-5 (Hardback)

Dedicated to the Pharmaceutical Fraternity,
my parents and family members

PREFACE

With the blessings of Goddess "Kanakadurga, Mookambika", I take this opportunity in presenting the book titled "Pharmaceutical Research Methodology and Bio-Statistics: Theory and Practice". Research is a process of identification of a problem existing in the society and questing for solution leading to implementation for the well-being of the society. A researcher has to inculcate a habit of identifying a problem which is a tedious job of several surveys, thorough literature search.

A researcher has to develop a method suitable and this needs understanding of fundamental concepts so that one can use the appropriate method for the plan of study. Logical bent of mind has to be developed by a researcher so that the plan made earlier and executed does not lead to go back and re-initiate new methodology for a mistake made in the past and over ruled or over looked.

Research is expensive, time consuming and needs patience. Research is a part of execution of an idea developed. Ideas are many for an individual and the same individual needs to filter the ideas and come up with the best idea out of all. The best idea is proposed as a research proposal for funding agency and always need not be successful for funds. Hence an idea should be realistic, practical, a need of a solution for an existing problem. Research always does not lead to business immediately but after subsequent further research may lead to.

A research activity lead to compilation of several numerical data collected and such data collected has to be ensured for the confidence level of the researcher in presenting. This is nothing but the statistical analysis. Statistics are compilation of numerical data collected during execution of a research and this data is analysed with appropriate test either as parametric or non-parametric. Upon analysis, at a defined and accepted probability and significance the data is ensured for researcher confidence level of the data collected. Upon fulfilling significance of the data and statistical analysis, the research is accepted. Hence ideas, data compilation and its statistical analysis have equal role in research.

The objective of the current book titled "Pharmaceutical Research Methodology and Bio-Statistics: Theory and Practice" is to enlighten the fundamentals for the students, researchers at the industry. At the academic level the book is useful for Bachelor, Doctor, Master and Philosophy of Pharmacy students and scholars.

The concepts are precise relating to pharmaceuticals with a practical approach in understanding. The structure of the book is so planned that the researcher develops a habit of presenting his research as research papers, patent documents for the fraternity. Yet another high light of the book is in comparing and contrasting various research documents such as research proposal, project report, research paper, synopsis and patent document.

Last but not the least, the book is well planned in such a way that it is suitable to pharmaceutical and non-pharmaceutical fraternity involved in pharmaceutical profession either as students, post-graduates, researchers, scholars, teaching faculty, policy makers, regulators etc. An attempt is made without any flaws, but it is natural that a few errors may occur during the process of bringingout this book and un-noticed. The author invites the readers for their valuable comments, suggestions and corrections if any felt necessary.

Dr. Bayya Subba Rao
M. Pharm (MAN), P. G. Dip in Patent Laws (NALSAR), IAO, Ph. D

ACKNOWLEDGEMENTS

First of all I thank the almighty for giving all the strengths in bringing out this book.

I thank all the fraternity in well accepting our earlier books titled "Practical Pharmaceutical In-Organic Chemistry, Second Edition" and "Intellectual Property Rights in Pharmaceutical Industry: Theory and Practice, Second Edition".

I thank the Government Authorities, Pharmaceutical Industry, University Authorities, College Managements, Colleagues, Research scholars and students in giving all the moral support and strengths in bringing out this book.

I have to thank IICT, Hyderabad authority for allowing me and using the library facility. I have to extremely thank the trial software providers such as SPSS, SAS, Minitab, Epi info.

I have to thank the president, editor Pharma Times for forwarding and publishing the reviewer comments.

I have to thank the reviewer for his comments which led me to include new chapter on Probability, Permutations and combinations.

Last but not the least, I thank all my family members whose co-operation with, I am able to bring my thoughts into the book.

Dr. Bayya Subba Rao

CONTENTS

CHAPTER 1

Introduction to Research and Bio-statistics in Pharmaceuticals.. 1

CHAPTER 2

Information Sources

CHAPTER 3

Literature Search

CHAPTER 4

Meta-Analysis

CHAPTER 5

Distinguishing Research Proposal, Research Report, Research Paper, Patent Document and Synopsis

CHAPTER 6

Detailed Contents of a Research Paper

CHAPTER 7

Clinical Trials and Clinical Study Design

CHAPTER 8

Principles of Experimental Designs

CHAPTER 9

Need of Sampling and Sampling Techniques

CHAPTER 10

Measurement and Scaling

CHAPTER 11

Scaling Techniques

CHAPTER 12

Introduction to Presentation of Data and Missing Data

CHAPTER 13

Probability, Permutations and Combinations

CHAPTER 14

Statistics, Bio-statistics and their Relation to Distribution Trends

CHAPTER 15

Measures of Central Tendency and Variability

CHAPTER 16

Standard Error, Confidence Level/Confidence Interval/Confidence Limits, Statistical Errors, Hypothesis

CHAPTER 17

Student 't' Distribution and its Applications

CHAPTER 18

Chi-square Distribution 147

CHAPTER 19

F-Distribution (Variance Ratio) and ANOVA

CHAPTER 20

Non-Parametric Statistical Tests

CHAPTER 21

Sample Size Determination

CHAPTER 22

Introduction to Epidemiology

CHAPTER 23

Introduction to SAS, SPSS, Epi Info and Minitab

CHAPTER 24

Applications of SPSS, Epi Info and Minitab Softwares (Screen Shots) 225

CHAPTER 25

Linear Regression, Correlation and Correlation Coefficient

CHAPTER 26

Inventory Control

CHAPTER 27

Accountancy and Book Keeping

CHAPTER 28

Management Report

CHAPTER 29

Role of Computers in Healthcare System

1 Introduction to Research and Bio-statistics in Pharmaceuticals

Research in pharmaceuticals starts from study of etiology of a disease to the study of post marketing surveillance of a drug product in the market. When a disease is identified as an outbreak or for an existing disease, a study at the molecular level of the causative organism of the disease is conducted. In this process, the entire life cycle of the organism is established with the molecular mechanism of its growth. Such study is expected to identify all possible targets to inhibit the growth of the organism. Such targets usually include inhibition of cell wall synthesis, inhibition of enzymes that are responsible for growth of the organism etc. As a lead, scientists initiate research for possible natural herbs or new chemical entities (synthetic or molecular modeling) that can inhibit the growth of the organism. A promising natural herb is phyto-chemically/pharmacognically studied for the active constituents from different parts of the plant by collecting in various seasons, if necessary. Several times a naturally available chemical constituent, that is promising, further acts as a lead for chemical synthesis or on pure chemical synthesis basis, further new molecules are synthesized to minimize side effects and maximize beneficial effects that are established through pharmacological studies on animals. A promising molecule is established through animal studies (pre-clinical) for their pharmacological activity, safety, toxicity and proceeds further for human studies (clinical) as an investigational new drug. Once the investigational drug is through, the new chemical entity has transformed to new drug after scrutiny and approval by drug regulatory at each stage. It is necessary to understand that pre-clinical and clinical studies in most of the times overlap. During clinical studies (phases I to IV), pharmacodynamic and pharmacokinetic studies, route of administration, dosage form, strength, possible combinations are established. Contrary to innovator's drug, generic manufacturer establishes bio-equivalence studies for identical drug product or establish entire pharmacodynamic and pharmacokinetic data for a similar drug product. After the drug regulators review of the drug products for their safety, efficacy and reliability, the drug product is approved for release into the market with simultaneous monitoring of drug products for their therapeutic efficacy during long term by monitoring as pharmacovigilance or post-marketing studies.

Statistics are a compilation of a data and is generated through experimental or available retrospectively (data that is already available, but compiled for analysis). Statistics are derived from a huge population, but such compilations may not be feasible and data is collected from a sample size of a population which itself is derived from statistical calculations. Statistics play a critical role right from individual growth to the economic growth of a country. In pharmaceuticals, bio-statistics are more prominent and have to be interpreted carefully so as to ensure that there is biological significance rather than mathematical significance/insignificance.

In pharmaceuticals, at every stage statistics apply. Any research study is aimed with a statistical planning and the end results are statistically concluded. In research, a problem is identified and is solved through experiments, validated through statistics for drawing final conclusions.

Several questions lead to research activity. For an initiator, the different questions that arise are what disease condition requires new treatments? What is the causative micro-organism or conditions for the disease? What are the molecular mechanisms for growth of the disease causative organism? What are the possible targets for inhibiting the growth of the micro-organism? What are the existing natural herbs, new chemical entities that have required inhibitory activity? How to identify past research conducted for a problem? How to identify the literature as review or research articles? How to compile the findings? How to draw conclusions from the findings for continuing research? How to isolate active ingredients from natural herbs? How to synthesize new chemical entities? How to design new chemical entities through molecular modeling? How to select animals and conduct pre-clinical studies? How to plan for clinical studies? What are the national/international guidelines for clinical studies? How to estimate a population of a disease in a country? How to draw a sample size from a population? What statistical methods to be used to draw conclusions for the studies? What dosage form, route of administration, strength to be planned? What kind of analytical techniques have to be established for biological fluids, for formulations? How to develop a similar, identical drug product? How to establish bio-equivalence studies for the generic drug product? How to file an IND, NDA, ANDA application for drug approval so as to market within a country?

Forth coming chapters are expected to empower the reader to acquire the various kinds of mental approaches to be followed to finally execute research activity, conduct some statistical calculations to achieve final conclusions.

2 Information Sources

2.0 Introduction

Relating to health, information sources can be broadly classified into primary and secondary. Primary information is the one where a researcher has reported his laboratory work in a specified format to a journal publisher and upon acceptance being published as research article/paper in the journal. A research article usually comprises of a title, abstract, author/s name/s, place of work, keywords, introduction, past evidenced work as a basis to take up current work, methodology, materials and methods, description of the experimental work with all the established data in the laboratory, results, discussion, conclusions, acknowledgements and finally with references. Secondary information is the one obtained from books, review articles, association publications, trade publications, from pharmacopoeia, internet, conferences, media etc. In most of the cases information is available in both electronic and printable formats.

2.1 Primary Sources

Primary sources can be further considered as research articles in journals and databases. Reaching the research article of our interest and compiling from different journals is cumbersome and it is through databases one can achieve the information. Some of the globally established databases are Medline, Embase, Evidence Based Medicine database (EBM), International Pharmaceutical Abstracts (IPA), Iowa Drug Information Service (IDIS), BIOSIS, Chemical Abstracts etc.

Medline is a database developed by US Library of Medicine and it is believed that it has over 4500 medical related journals as access. The database is an indication of reported research and published in various renowned journals. Pubmed is a search engine that helps to make the search of the medline database bit faster. US Government initiative of subsidizing Pubmed/Medline has made access of information on free basis on the internet. Such engines work on key words resulting in retrieving several research articles published in various journals. For a precise and required hits of the desired work of interest several commercial service providers such as Dialog, Ovid makes the filtering process of required desired articles still easier.

Embase is a database developed by Elsevier, The Netherlands. The database covers mainly the medical information of the European Union and it has been observed in a study that when a data was retrieved on a subject of interest on both Medline and on Embase, it has been observed that about 35 percent of the data is common and the remaining are unique.

Evidence Based Medicine Database (EBM) is a database relating to evidence established randomized clinical trial study. Such databases helps to understand more prominently clinical research worked in various countries across the globe. Several times, a meta-analysis (analysis of analysis) using such database helps to resolve issues that have ambiguity with respect to conclusions. Yet another database called as Cochrane library was established by Great Britain by assigning interested scholars to compile all the reported and non-reported randomized clinical trial data. Such library has overcome the barrier of research that was not reported or published.

Iowa Drug Information Service (IDIS) is a database established by College of Pharmacy, University of Iowa, US wherein about 200 clinical journal information were provided with an access so that health professionals and public can acquire knowledge of drug, drug interactions, drug combinations etc. The information is especially useful for drug information centers.

Chemical Abstracts is a database established by American Chemical Society (ACS) as Chemical Abstract Service (CAS). The database is mainly useful to pharmaceutical professionals in knowing more about new chemical entities, drug molecules, their physicochemical parameters, synthesis, pharmacological activity, spectral analysis etc. The uniqueness of this database is that every chemical entity being assigned with a unique CAS registry number. The database can be accessed with respect to molecular formula, molecular name, subject name, patent number, CAS number etc. Online version and CD Rom version of the database is available and the commercial versions available to industry are STN, Sci-Finder and as an academic version as Sci-Finder Scholar. The unique feature with the online version of the database is that one can retrieve data based on chemical structure.

BIOSIS Previews is a Biological Abstract and Bio Research Index database, where in information relating to preclinical toxicity and carcinogenicity studies data can be retrieved.

International Pharmaceutical Abstracts (IPA) is a pharmaceutical related database where information relating to research and from associations can be retrieved. Even though several data can be retrieved from various other databases, it has its unique identity. The database is exclusive relating to pharmacy periodicals. The database is established by American Society of Health System Pharmacists (ASHP).

2.2   Secondary Sources

Literature derived from primary sources (also called as primary literature) as a compilation, commentaries or digest is called as secondary source. A review is also considered as a compilation of information from primary sources relating to a particular subject matter. A review article is written upon invitation. There are various secondary sources such as text books, trade literature, pharmacopoeias, formularies, drug compendia, internet sources, electronic mail, discussion groups, search engines like google, MSN, pharmacy websites, various libraries, government websites, electronic publications, online community pharmacies etc.

The combined book of United States Pharmacopoeia and National Formulary (commonly represented as USP/NF) does not include all the drugs approved for use in United States, rather includes drugs and excipients whose standards were established and approved by United Stated Pharmacopoeial Convention, a representation of physicians, pharmacists and other relating health care communities. USP contains monographs of drugs, other substance with therapeutic uses, for some dietary supplements from botanical sources, whereas a national formulary consists of monographs for excipients, non-therapeutic additives used in pharmaceuticals. Several other secondary sources of importance are the British Pharmacopoeia (UK), European Pharmacopoeia (Council of Europe), WHO's International Pharmacopoeia etc.

Earlier a formulary was a recipe book but now it is a list of drug products that are approved by a hospital, health plan or a government for use. A hospital formulary is established and approved by Pharmacy and Therapeutic Committee of a hospital. Likewise yet some other secondary sources are Index Nominum edited by Swiss Pharmaceutical Society, The Merck Index comprising of over 10, 000 monographs on drugs, common organic chemicals.

US Compendia is categorized into prescription, non-prescription, parenterals, catalogs, physical identification, and consumer drug information as individual books. The book usually include information relating to dosage, contraindications, adverse effects and pharmacokinetics, pictures of tablets and capsules for aiding in identification. Especially relating to consumer drug information it may be as a book, pamphlet, newspaper, magazine or internet. Martindale, the extra pharmacopoeia is yet another compendium of drugs and includes medicines covering around the world with list of proprietary products, manufacturers. The book helps in identifying foreign drug products.

The Review of Natural Product, is a monthly loose-leaf service that covers both herbal and other natural products. The monographs include overview of chemistry, pharmacology and toxicology of the product. Several other sources such as Drug Interaction Facts, Meyler's side effects of drugs, Poisindex are some sources for information relating to drug-drug interaction and procedures to treat during drug poisoning conditions.

3 Literature Search

3.0 Introduction

To initiate a research activity, it is necessary to select a subject of interest and identify the current existing problems. In the quest, several problems can be identified in the society. For instance in pharmaceuticals, in therapeutics several problems like multiple drugs are administered individually on the same day or same time, regular puncturing of skin as parenterals, drug combinations not available, highly expensive drug products where competition is minimum and requires generics, several pediatric dosage forms not well accepted by children leading to reflux arc of vomiting when the drug product is orally administered, need of new route of administration, new dosage form, new combination, several individual drugs taken at the same time may be administered in combination form, identification of product patented drugs and release as generics, developing analytical methods for off-product patented drugs/combinations drugs, quest for new combination therapies, practitioners of medicine need for possible combinations, problems of drug in-compatibilities etc. For instance, Botox is widely used for cosmetic purpose, but requires several injections on the face.

Once a problem is identified, the immediate doubt that arise is that what was the research conducted already for the problem and to proceed further. In this process, several hindrances arise to make the review of the literature in the form of organized and un-organized literature search. It is believed that there exists over 40, 000 journals where in every 30 seconds a research article is in the process of consideration for publication (Mohoney, 1985).

In the past, several research activities were not organized initially and later became organized. In the current day scenario of globalization, information resources have become reachable in most of the circumstances through internet, but the information several times is not to the mindset of the researcher and leads to a compromise by the researcher. To overcome this, the researcher needs to set his mind for an organized thinking process several times making a meta-analysis.

In every country in the world, majority of the basic research is invested by the Government where as innovative research is invested by private organisations as business activity. Basic research is most widely initiated by academic institutions, government funded autonomous organisations or government organisations. For instance, Indian CSIR, DST, CCMB, NIN, Government Universities, IICT, AYUSH are granting finance for basic and innovative research activity. For instance, academic institutions in pharmaceuticals are more prone for basic research rather than process research. Handling dangerous chemicals by the students/scholars, lack of facility are some of the reasons that inhibit research.

Some of the Indian inventions that are promising or products available in the market are a breakthrough invention for oral administration of insulin, Centchroman (already available in market), several analytical methods that are available in Indian Pharmacopoeia etc. In several cases, innovative research at the academic levels is limited, for instance, several Active Pharmaceutical Ingredients (APIs) are process developed by the pharmaceutical industry and establishment of the limit tests for in-organic or organic impurities depends on the starting materials, catalyst, reagents used, bi-products formed, impurities formed, type of reactors used and problems rose by the nature and level of impurity can be known by the formulation industry who develop formulation products and hence, it is necessary that inputs for Pharmacopoeial monographs are more valuable from industry rather than the academic organisations. In the same way, a lead for a process may be from the fundamental reactions learnt at the academic levels or so. Several logics learnt from the academic organisations led to innovative products.

Hence, a solution for a problem may be simple, but several times becomes a complex process to reach the solution. In several cases, a research was initiated assuming such research was not earlier reported or patented but, at a later stage being identified as already reported. Such setbacks may be due to improper literature search.

Even though internet is a big global library, searching with keywords is still not precise or accurate. Internet source has become ambiguous in taking decisions. American Chemical Society is providing a rich source of research compilations as Chemical Abstract Services (CAS). The society is currently providing various collective volumes (5 years) to conduct a systematic research. Such collective volumes are being published from end of eighteen century. Hence, a systematic search provides a better clarity of information. The following is an attempt in making the reader to inculcate the habit of conducting systematic literature search chronologically. A systematic literature search using Chemical Abstract Service or from other sources, can be as follows:

3.1   Type of Index as Volumes

A. Dictionary of Organic Compounds:

i. **Name Index:** In these volumes, for a chemical name 2-Bromo-4, 6 – dinitroaniline see B-02330 and upon further referring under B-02330 it is observed 2-Bromo-4, 6 – dinitroaniline, 8CI or 2-Bromo-4, 6 – dinitrobenzenamine [1817-73-8]

   $C_6H_4BrN_3O_4$ M 262

   Yellow needles (AcOH or EtOH) Mp 153-4°, sublimes

BX 9275000

N-Me: Yell cryst (AcOH or EtOH). Mp 153° (147°), N-Ac: Cryst. (EtOH). Mp 235°

D.R.Pat., 610613 (1935); CA, 29, 5860 (Synth); Schouten, A.E., Recl. Trav. Chim.

Pays-Bas, 1937, 56, 541 (Synth)

Wasylishen, R. et. Al, Can. J. Chem, 1970, 48, 1263 (pmr)

Venturella, V.S et al. J. Chromtogr. Sci, 1973, 11, 379 (Chromatog)

ii. CAS Registry Number Index, 6th Edition Vol. 9

2143-88-6: 4-Methyl-4'-nitrobiphenyl-M-0-03105

2144-41-4: Tetrahydro-2,5-dimethyl furan; (2RS,5SR)-from, in T-0-01074

iii. Molecular Formula Index, 5th Edition

    a. $C_{14}H_{17}N_3O_3$

        N-Alanyltryptophan, A-00700

        N-Tryptophylalanine, T-04526

    b. $C_{14}H_{17}N_3O_6$

        3,6-Dinitrophenantraquinone; Monoxime, in D-07580

B. Chemical Abstract Services (CAS):

i. Name Index:

Earlier chemical names are not uniform throughout the World. The chemical names provided in dictionary of organic compounds may be different from chemical names provided in chemical abstract services. Several times, there may be more than two names. Hence, it is necessary to search literature in both the names and it is common that the chemical abstract service provides an indication that if you are referring to one name, it indicates see for the other name mentioned.

For instance: When you are searching the Chemical Abstract Index guide, A-M, 1982-86, it indicates

    a. Albendazole

        seeCarbamic acid, [5-(propylthio)-1H-benzimidazol-2-yl]-methyl ester [54965-21-8]

    b. Alcoholmetry

        See Alcohols, analysis

        Ethanol [64-17-5], analysis

    c. Alcohols, reactions,

        Esterification of-see Esterification

ii. Chemical Substance Index:

In a collective volume of Chemical Substance Index, generic names (International Non-Proprietary-INN names) are observed in alphabetical order.

Under each name, the research conducted as well as abstract number is provided.

For instance:

Chemical Substance 9th collective index, A-Ames, Vol. 76-85, 1972-76 indicates

Acetic acid [64-19-7], analysis

- acetic acid derivs. and formaldehyde detn. In aq. Solns. Of, 78:52379
- acetic anhydride detn. In, 76:107685 y
- chromatog. Detn of in molasses, 77:103604u in molasses and sugar juices, 85:7569f in sugar juices and sirups, 83: 207816e
- chromatography of, 78:66658n
- detn. of 76:67959g, 78:26011q

iii. Molecular Formula Index:

As the name indicates, molecular formulas of compounds are listed in the collective of molecular formula index. It is necessary to know the chemical structure and its molecular formula prior referring for the details.

For instance:

Chemical Abstract, 5th Decennial Formula Index, C_{13}-C_{19}, Vol:41-50, 1947-56 indicates

a. C_7H_8ClN

Aniline, Chloro-N-methyl- 27:74; 32:911

Benzylamine, chloro., 26:2437; 28:4378; 29:7717; 34:997, 998

HCl, 32:4149; 39:4318; and –HCl, 21:54

2,3-Lutidine, 6-chloro-, 35:2517

b. $C_7H_8N_2$

Benzaldehyde, hydrazone, 14:3647; 33:622; 39:1395

Benzamidine, 15:535; 16:3078; 24:5732; 31:5797; 36:6538; 39:P3544, 4073, 40:4367; and –HNO_3, 20: 2320; salts, 24:3013; 30:8156; 36:1917

Formaldehyde, phenylhydrazone, 29:6217; 39:917

iv. Patent Index:

Whether a molecule is having a patent or not is known through "P" indicated along with the abstract number. When the abstract is referred in the abstract index, the patent number is identified. When we proceed further with the patent number in the patent index, the list of family patents etc., can be identified.

For instance:

Chemical Abstract, Patent Index

a. Vol 94, 1981 indicates

   i. 2122655 A, 78:55127n

     FR 2139303 A5

GB 1386872 A

JP 56/010583 B4

US 3825342 A

ii. 2122804 A, 76:73998 k

FI 56713 B

FR 2093716 A5

JP 56/003477 B4

SE 375566 B

US 3716448 A

iii. 2123027 A, see DE 1958608A

b. WO-WO, Vol. 151, No:5, 2009 indicates

i. 2004/020555 A1 (Designated States: AU, BR, CN, IN, RU, ZA), 140:2205064

AU 2003/228122 A1(B2) (Related)

BR 2003/06210 A (Related)

BR 2003/06210 A (Related)

CN 1596293 A (1328358 C) (Related)

IN 2004DN01324 A (Related)

KR 2003/0052954 A (905581 B1) (Related)

RU 2264435 C2 (Related)

ZA 2004/03265 A (Related)

v. General Subject Index:

This is a collective volume of research published and is listed in terms of general subject. For instance: To identify plant/herbal resources that are reported for anti-fertility activity, the information cannot be available in molecular formula or chemical name index. This can be obtained from "General Subject Index". Let us imagine that we are searching for anti-fertility activity of "Achyranthesaspera (Telugu regional names: antisha, uttareni).

The below mentioned table provides a systematic search of the collective volumes of chemical abstracts published by Chemical Abstract Services, American Chemical Society, USA.

Index Vol	Year/s	Name: Achyranthesaspera
5th General Subject Index Decennial 41-50	1947-56	A. aspera: constituents of seeds of 47:3324e
6th General Subject Index 51-55	1957-61	A.aspera 51:13317c, control of 51:10815g, oleanolic acid isolation from 53:7513b, sapogenin from seeds of 53:10667c, saponin from 53:9579f

Contd....

Index Vol	Year/s	Name: Achyranthesaspera
7th General Subject Index 56-65	1962-66	A.aspera compn. and essential amino acids of seeds of 62:13768e
8th General Subject Index 66-75	1967-71	A.asperabetaine from 66:35389y, ecdysterone of 75:137476c, ecdysterone of roots of 75:16683j, structure of saponins from seeds of 73:25788h
9th General Subject Index 85-76	1972-76	A.aspera: not related information observed.
10th General Subject Index 86-95	1977-81	A.aspera: ext. of, abortion from 88:11891j, leaf gall of, compn. of 90:3286s
11th General Subject Index 96-105	1982-86	A.aspera: constituents of 103:157396b, as contraceptive 105:108749b, ext. of contraceptive activity of 105:54739c, saponins of 96:40794a
12th General Subject Index 106-115	1987-91	A.aspera: dihydroxyhenpentaconanoneaand tri-triacontanol from, isolation and structure of 115:110622e
13th General Subject Index 116-125	1992-96	A.aspera: chem.investigation of stem and seeds of 120:265781 h, natural products form A.aspera 125:5473r
CD ROM	1997	A.aspera not related/not found
CD ROM	1998	A.aspera not related/not found
CD ROM	1999	A.aspera not related/not found
CD ROM	2000	A.aspera: three steroids, flavanol glycoside from 132:345481
CD ROM	2001	A.aspera phyto chemical investigations of 134:2612
CD ROM	2002	A.aspera phyto chemical study of 137:122252, oleanolic acid saponin from 137:106514
CD ROM	2003	A.aspera not related/not found
CD ROM	2004	A.aspera not related/not found
CD ROM	2005	A.aspera: sterols from the leaves of apang 142:478694, fatty acid composition of, seed oil 142:245778
CD ROM	2006	A.aspera not related/not found
CD ROM	2007	A.aspera: saponins isolated from, anti-microbial activity of 146:180819

As an another example,

Chemical Abstract Subject Index, P-Z, Vol: 11-20, 1917-26 indicates

a. Parachor, chem. Constitution and 19: 197, 2926, 3263, 20: 386

b. Paraffin wax. (see also candles)

Absorption of, 17:1712

adsorption by charcoal, 17:1571

analysis of, 15:2180

bacterialdecompn. of, 15:3552

for both, 19:195

crystn. In manuf. Of, 14:3787

films, 11:1721, 2135

c. Paraformaldehyde, alc. synthesis with, 17: 1420

detn. in tablets, 16:395

formaldehydedetn. in, 17:2544

vi. Abstract Index

Each volume of abstract index is identified and picked based on the starting and ending abstract numbers mentioned in the book. If the number is within the picked volume, under the corresponding abstract number, complete abstract published in the journal, journal name, issue number, year and page numbers are mentioned. Based on this, the corresponding journal is referred in the said volume, issue, page for the entire research article published in the journal.

For instance:

Chemical Abstract Abs No: 40972-57659, Vol. 94, 1981 indicates

a. 94:45358e: Basic principles of antigen-antibody reactions. Kabat, Elvin A. (Cancer Cent., Columbia Univ., New York, NY 10032 USA). Methods Enzymol. 1980, 70 (Immunochem. Tech., Pt. A), 3-49 (Eng). A review with 231 refs. Here, the researcher gets the final information from a book titled "Methods in Enzymology" and he has to identify the book of specific volume from library.

b. 94:45395q: Detection and preliminary characterization of the lectins present in legume seeds. De Navarro, Yolanda; Perez, Gerardo (Dep. Quim, Univ. Nac. Colombia, Bogota, Colombia) Rev. Colomb. Quim. 1978, 8(1), 25-43(Span). Of 23 legume seeds analyzed, bauhinia picta, Tamarindusindica, Dioclealehmannii, and Erythrinarubrinervia contained lectim which agglutinated human erythrocytes without showing specificity for any group of the ABO system. Cassia indecora, Crotalasia species, and Orinosia species selectively agglutinated O-pos erythrocytes. Crotalaria agatifolia agglutinated (weakly). A-pos. erythrocytes from 6 different animal species showed that Cassia fruticosa, C.reticulata, Delonixregia, Poinciana pulquerrima, Abrusfruticulosus, and Mucunamustisiana also possess lectins. Probably, D. lehmannii and E. rubrinervia act on different receptors of the erythrocyte membrane. The erythrocytes of dog and horse showed similar response to all the lectins tested suggesting that they have similar membrane receptors. Here, the researcher has to refer to the jounal Rev. Colomb. Quim of specific year, specific volume and specific issue at the mentioned pages for further study of the research article.

vii. Author Index:

Chemical abstract service also provides an index of research work published as Chemical Abstract Author Index. In this, one can collect the data based on the author name.

For instance:

Chemical Abstracts Decennia Index, Vols: 1-10, 1907-16, Author index: A-K, pp:1-1006 indicates

a. Caren, R. M. Detection and estn. Of halogens in mixed solns. by HNO_3, 3:2278; Systematic Qual. Analysis 9book), 4:290, 5:2793; sepn. of the metals of the Sn group, 647; education of industrial chemist of the future, 9:1976.

b. Dieckmann, W., and Breest, F. Behaviour of carboxylic acid toward phenylisocyanate, 1:54.

viii. Ring Systems:

Standard chemical names denotes for various ring systems can be identified in Chemical Abstracts Index of Ring Systems.

For instance:

Chemical Abstract, 11th Collective Index, Index on Ring Systems, Formulas A-C_5H_8OTe, Vol: 96-105, 1982-86 indicates

a. C_6-C_6-C_6N

7-Azatricyclo $[6.3.1.1^{2,\,6}]$ tridecane

1H-Dibenz[b,d] azepine

Spiro [5H-2-benzazepine-5,1'-cyclohexane]

PubMed, NCBI databases and several other online journals are available on internet and several cases, a search can be done by Boolean operators. Now a days, Google has become one of the most popular search engine but, the drawback with Google is, giving key words retrieve data both related and non-related and searching with precise keywords is absolutely necessary.

4 Meta-Analysis

4.0 Introduction

Meta-analysis in simple terms is called as analysis of analysis. Meta analysis is a procedure for merging data from multiple studies. The analysis helps in identifying the common effects or causes for the variations in two or more studies. The historical roots of meta-analysis can be traced in the 17th century relating to astronomy. In 1904, collated data from several studies of typhoid inoculation was subjected to meta-analysis. In 1976, Gene V. Glass proposed a method to integrate and summarize the findings from a body of research and the method was called as meta-analysis. In this category of analysis, research studies are collected, coded and interpreted using statistical methods. Meta-analysis helps to identify any relation among study features and study outcomes. One can proceed with meta-analysis only if we are able to identify a common statistical measure that is shared among studies, called the effect size, which has a standard error so that we can proceed with computing a weighted average of that common measure. Such weighting usually takes into consideration the sample sizes of the individual studies, although it can also include other factors, such as study quality. Understanding meta-analysis is an understanding of effect sizes. They provide a way to standardize effects across studies using different measures, allowing common analysis. Out of many possible effect sizes, two widely used meta-analysis are

i. Correlation: eg., r (product-moment correlation)

ii. Mean differences: eg., Cohen's *d*, Hedge's *g* etc.

Meta-analysis is expected to increase the power of statistical study as conclusions are drawn from several studies, accumulation of subjects with greater diversity. Different effect sizes are calculated for different constructs of interest, as predetermined by the researchers based on what issues are of interest in the research literature. In meta-analysis, tests of statistical significance can be conducted as well as on the effect sizes (studies having common statistical measures). According to an arbitrary but commonly used interpretation of effect size by Cohen (1988), a standardised mean effect size of '0' means no change, negative effect sizes mean a negative change, with '0.2' a small change, '0.5' a moderate change, and '0.8' a large change. Wolf (1986), on the other hand, suggests that 0.25 is educationally significant and 0.50 is clinically significant. Meta-analysis is usually used when there are conflicting results i.e., a drug does or does not work. A meta-analysis data is represented in a forest plot. A good meta-analysis aims for coverage of all relevant studies, presence of heterogeneity, robustness to achieve a sensitive analysis. For the existence of heterogeneity, Cochrane's Q, a statistical based chi-square test is conducted. Since Cochrane's Q test has less power, a second test 'I^2' statistic test is suggested for testing as inconsistency index, a measure of total variation across studies. I^2 test ranges heterogeneity between 0% and 100%. As a thumb rule, 25% indicates low, 50% for moderate and 75% for high heterogeneity. As I^2 statistical test also have low power, a meta-regression technique is introduced to overcome heterogeneity. A meta-regression analysis helps to explore which types of patient-specific factors or study design factors contribute to the heterogeneity. In addition to this, a funnel plot is expected to assess publication bias. One of the decisions to be made while conducting meta-analysis is that whether to conduct fixed-effects or a random-effects model. In fixed-effects model, the assumption is that the source of variation in outcomes is occurring within the study, that is, the effect expected from each study is the same. Consequently, it is assumed that the models are homogeneous; there are no differences in the underlying study population, no differences in subject selection criteria, and treatments are applied the same way. Fixed-effect methods used for dichotomous data include most often the Mantel-Haenzel method and the Peto method (only for odd ratios). Random-effects models have an underlying assumption that a distribution of effects exists, resulting in heterogeneity among study results, known as τ2. In random-effects model, studies are weighted with the inverse of their variance and the heterogeneity parameter. The most commonly used random-effects method is the DerSimonian and Laird method.

To test heterogeneity, subgroup analysis is one another in addition to meta-regression analysis. In subgroup analysis it is also feasible to estimate the variations (effect size) in group categories such as age, sex etc. In meta-regression approach, use of regression analysis determines the influence of selected variables (independent variable) on the effect size (dependent variable). In meta-analysis, other types of biases i.e., time lag bias (significant study data being published earlier than non-significant data), selective reporting bias (positive results being published sooner than negative results), language bias may exist.

It is necessary to understand the differences between meta-analysis and network meta-analysis. In case of meta-analysis a comparison is made between two treatments, where as in network, multiple treatment regimens, even when direct comparisons are unavailable by indirect comparisons. For instance, a trial compares drug A to drug B. A different trial studying the same patient population compares drug B to drug C. Assume that drug A is found to be superior to drug B in the first trial. Assume drug B is found to be equivalent to drug C in a second trial. Network analysis then, allows one to potentially say statistically that drug A is also superior to drug C for this particular patient population. (Since drug A is better than drug B, and drug B is equivalent to drug C, then drug A is also better to drug C even though it was not directly tested against drug C).

4.1   Limitations of Meta-Analysis

i.   Results of meta-analysis data can be considered significant provided original data is valid.

ii.   Variance in dependent variable and the role of independent variables can be better interpreted provided, the original studies provide data.

iii. "Apples and oranges" effect – i.e., there is a risk/tendency in meta-analysis to average/mash together desperate effects.

iv.   Can lack in qualitative insight.

4.2   Advantages of Meta-Analysis

i.   Greater statistical power.
ii.   Ability to extrapolate to general population affected.
iii. Consideration of evidence based research.
iv.   Results can be projected to population.

4.3   Disadvantages of Meta-Analysis

i.   Difficult to identify appropriate studies i.e., similar studies to be identified (eg: all randomized controlled trials).
ii.   Time consuming studies.
iii. Requires advanced statistical techniques.
iv.   Requires heterogeneity of study population.
v.   Analysis should include all published and un-published results to avoid publication bias.
vi.   File-drawer problem i.e., unpublished paper or data.
vii. Requires more data for significance.
viii. Sources of bias of various studies cannot be controlled.

4.4   Case Studies

1.   Earlier studies have shown conflicting results whether periodontitis (PD) is associated with increased risk of coronary heart disease. Meta-analysis of the 5 prospective cohort studies (86, 092 patients) indicated that individuals with PD had a 1.14 times higher risk of developing CHD than the controls (relative risk 1.14, 95% CI 1.074-1.213, P<0.001), indicating that both the prevalence and incidence of CHD are significantly increased in PD. Hence, it was concluded that PD may be a risk factor for CHD.

2. The concept that venous thrombo embolism (VTE) and atherosclerosis are two completely distinct entities has recently been challenged because patients with VTE have more asymptomatic atherosclerosis and more cardiovascular events than control subjects and by using meta-analysis techniques, it was taken up to assess the association between cardiovascular risk factors and VTE. Twenty-one case-control and cohort studies with a total of 63, 552 patients were included, showing the risk of VTE was 2.33 for obesity (95% CI, 1.68 to 3.24), 1.51 for hypertension (95% CI, 1.23 to 1.85), 1.42 for diabetes mellitus (95% CI, 0.67 to 2.02). This demonstrated that cardiovascular risk factors are associated with VTE, which is clinically relevant with respect to individual screening, risk factor modification, and primary and secondary prevention of VTE. Prospective studies should further investigate the underlying mechanisms of this relationship.

3. Chondroitin is a polysaccharide derived from cartilage. It is commonly used by people with arthritis in the belief that it will reduce pain, but clinical studies of its effectiveness have yielded conflicting results. Reichenbach et al (2007) performed a meta-analysis of studies on chondroitin and arthritis pain of the knee and hip. They identified relevant studies by electronically searching literature databases and clinical trial registries, manual searching of conference proceedings and the reference lists of papers, and contacting various experts in the field. Only trials that involved comparing patients given chondroitin with control patients were used; the control could be either a placebo or no treatment. They obtained the necessary information about the amount of pain and the variation by measuring graphs in the papers, if necessary, or by contacting the authors.

    The initial literature search yielded 291 potentially relevant reports, but after eliminating those that didn't use controls, those that didn't randomly assign patients to the treatment and control groups, those that used other substances in combination with chondroitin, those for which the necessary information wasn't available etc., they were left with 20 trials.

    The statistical analysis of all 20 trials showed a large, significant effect of chondroitin in reducing arthritis pain. However, the authors noted that earlier studies, published in 1987-2001, had large effects, while more recent studies (which you would hope are better) showed little or no effect of chondroitin. In addition, trials with smaller standard errors (due to larger sample sizes or less variation among patients) showed little or no effect. In the end, Reichenbach et al. (2007) analyzed just the three largest studies with what they considered the best designs, and they showed essentially zero effect of chondroitin. They concluded that there's no good evidence that chondroitin is effective for knee and hip arthritis pain. Other researchers disagree with their conclusion (Goldberg et al. 2007, Pelletier 2007); while a careful meta-analysis is a valuable way to summarize the available information, it is unlikely to provide the last word on a question that has been addressed with large numbers of poorly designed studies.

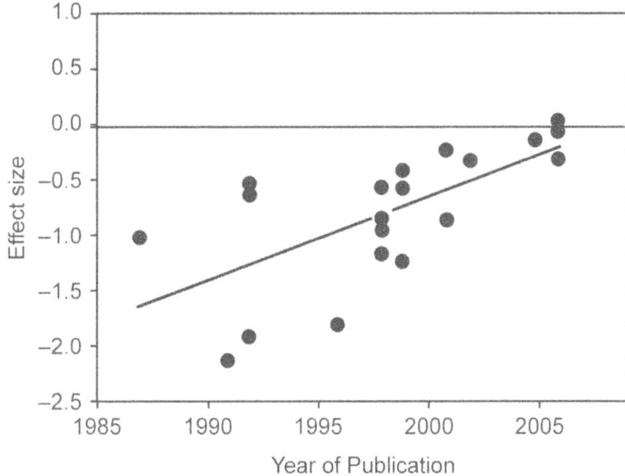

FIGURE 4.1 Effect of chondroitin vs. year of publication of the study

Negative numbers indicate, Figure 4.1, less pain with condroitin than in the control group. The linear regression is significant (r^2=0.45, p=0.001), meaning more recent studies show significantly less effect of chondroitin on pain.

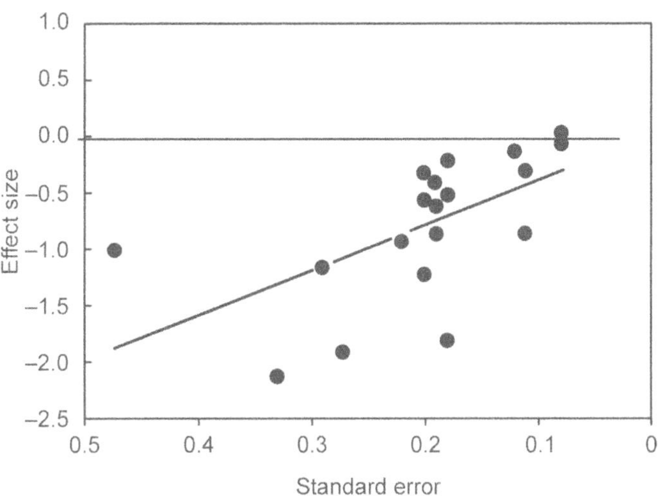

FIGURE 4.2 Effect of chondroitin vs. standard error of the mean effect size

Negative numbers indicate, Figure 4.2, less pain with condroitin than in control group. The linear regression is significant (r^2=0.35, p=0.006), meaning better studies (smaller standard error) show significantly less effect of chondroitin on pain.

4.5 Steps/Criteria for Meta-Analysis

a. Prior collecting studies, the investigator has to decide the inclusion and exclusion criteria of various studies.

b. Should be objective so that a third person should be able to sort the studies that can be included and excluded i.e., when looking for effects of a drug on a disease, we may have to decide that only double-blind, placebo-controlled studies.

c. Sample size should not be a criterion for inclusion and exclusion of a study.

d. One has to find all the studies relating to the subject of interest.

5 Distinguishing Research Proposal, Research Report, Research Paper, Patent Document and Synopsis

5.0 Introduction

For initiating a research, it is necessary to identify a problem and for identifying a problem the lead is either from past work, from public facing an issue, or identification of a new problem from a current research activity done. For the past work, it is necessary to conduct systematic literature review. In case of current problems faced by the public, it can be identified through a survey (from doctors, patients, pharmacists, bureaucrats, pharmaceutical industry, dry laboratory research). In case of the latter condition, a research was conducted to solve a problem and this led to a new problem and needs new research. Once a problem was identified, the first step is to propose the research. The proposal is either made to the ethics committee, to the academic higher authority, to the government funding organisation or to the employer of the pharmaceutical industry. Once a research proposal was accepted, with the funding either from the government, industry or self-financing, necessary planning is made for conducting the research. At various stages of research activity, a research report is submitted to the authority to know the status of the work and this may lead to further release of funding to complete the work. Hence, a research report may be an intermittent or at the final stage of research activity. Usually a research report may lead to a synopsis writing, thesis writing, research paper, patent document which is an outcome to bring an awareness to the evaluators, policy makers, government authority, industry authority and making it available to public (or confidentiality maintained by industry) or to the stake holders. Such awareness is expected to further explore, make the research activity for implementation for real use by the society. Hence, an invention leads to an innovation.

It is necessary to understand role and distinguishing features of research proposal, research report, research paper, synopsis and a patent document.

5.1 Research Proposal

As the word indicates, a proposal is made to the authority for approval, especially the funding organisation (industry, government etc.,). Ideas are many but funding is limited. It is the funding organisation (sponsor), who is very selective and more practical whether the proposal to be accepted or rejected. In several cases, government grants research proposal for basic research where as pharmaceutical industry grants research proposal for innovative research. Proposing a research is the initiative step indicating a problem is identified and needs a study to explore and solve the problem. A research proposal should be short, precise and interesting to the evaluator to further study and approve. A research proposal may be a few pages (say 10 pages or even more). A research proposal comprises of a title, place of work with address, name/s of researchers, introduction, objective, purpose, null hypothesis, methodology, criteria for selection of subjects, criteria for elimination of subjects, rationale of sample size determination, various attributes such as physical or abstract scales being collected as data, procedure of collection of data, type of analytical/statistical analysis being planned, if a clinical study compensation planned if any damages (such as death, organ damages etc.,), how the compilation of all the data as results is made, expected inferences, expected conclusions etc. In case of non-clinical research proposal, an emphasis is made relating to type of formulation, dosage form, route of administration, drug combination, types of analytical method etc, new chemical entity is viewed and a proposal is made.

5.2 Research Report

Several times a research report depends on the objective to be fulfilled. A research report may be an intermittent report during a research project is in progress so as to understand the status of the work. Conversely, a research report is a submission of entire research made to the funding authority or to an educational authority as a fulfillment of academic criteria such as post-graduate study or as a fulfillment of doctorate programme or a research project funded by government or industry funding authority. Depending on the circumstances, a research report may be of 2-3 pages to several hundred pages. A research report contains all the experimental data generated during the study after final processing. A research report is usually submitted to government, industry or academic authority. It is necessary to understand that, a research project is initiated with one objective and the result may be as expected or contrary. In several cases, huge data is generated during the study, but only certain data is included in the report, which the researcher may feel comfortable to be reported. It is also necessary to understand that, the researcher should be mentally ready to disclose the entire data either positive or negative. A research report may be a few pages or a thesis book (for post graduate or PhD work). A research report comprises mainly title, name and address of work place, sponsor name, contents page, acknowledgements, list of tables, list of figures, list of research paper publications, certification of the immediate higher authority under whom the researcher is working, declaration by the researchers, introduction, literature review for identifying the problem, sources of information for supporting your research activity, proposing a null hypothesis, methodology, determination of sample size, procedure followed in collecting samples/subjects, procedure for collecting data using physical or abstract scale, compiling/presentation of all the data as observations/tables/figures, interpretation and inferences drawn from the data indicating the research project is in favour of null hypothesis or not, summary and conclusion drawn, list of appendices, index (if necessary), errata, bibliography.

5.3   Research Paper

A research paper is a document containing an invention sent by the inventor to the journal publisher for acceptance and publication upon scrutiny. A research paper publication is an indication that a research problem identified was solved and is made public as awareness to the fraternity. A research paper may lead to a patent filing and grant, provided the research published as research paper is submitted as a patent application within a stipulated time from the date of publication. If a patent application is not filed for the research published, within a stipulated time, the research loses its patentability criteria and a patent is not granted. Hence, there is a necessity to plan either both or any one. The contents of research paper document comprises of title, name/s of inventors/authors, place of work, abstract, key words, introduction, methodology, observations/results, discussion and/or conclusion, references/bibliography. A research paper is an outcome of several drafts and it is necessary to ensure spell, grammar etc before sending the paper to the editor of the journal. Upon scrutiny by experts in the field, once accepted, the paper is published in the journal. A research paper is a document that may be considered up to 5-10 pages.

5.4   Patent Document

A patent is a document granted by the government to the inventor as an exclusive right to make, sell, use, import for a certain period of time upon disclosure of the invention. A patent grant is a limited time of monopoly. Both in research paper and patent document, the invention is disclosed. All inventions granted with a patent fulfill patentability criteria, but all inventions published as a research paper may not fulfill patentability criteria. In India a patent term is for 20 years from the date of first filing. For an invention to be patentable, it has to fulfill all the patentability criteria i.e., novelty, non-obviousness, useful and enabled whereas, a research paper need not fulfill all the criteria. The contents of a patent document comprises of title, patent number, date of grant, bibliography data, abstract, field of invention, summary of invention/introduction, prior art, detailed description of invention with figures/ tables/graphs, best embodiment or best mode, claims. A bibliography presentation in a patent document is different from bibliography presentation in a research report/paper/proposal. Claims in a patent document provide the boundaries of the invention, the inventor is claiming as exclusivity.

5.5 Synopsis

A synopsis is a document comprising a few limited numbers of pages containing the outcome of a research activity which is usually from a research report (as a thesis for UG/PG or a PhD or a government/industry project) submitted. A synopsis is a document briefing the information provided in the research report. Hence, a synopsis drafting should be well planned in such a way that it gives entire picture of the research conducted and upon reading the contents in the synopsis, an interest should be generated to the reader so as to read the entire research project either to scrutinize for an award of degree or for commercial use etc. A synopsis is circulated not only to the scrutinizers but also to the stake holders (i.e., fellow researchers skilled in the art, industry personnel, academic personal, press, layman etc.,) so that any clarifications/setbacks identified are rectified and a fresh report is made available for reference after the research report is approved. A synopsis contains title, name/s of researchers, place of work, Objective and scope, purpose, already proposed hypothesis, methodology followed with briefing of findings, discussion and conclusions drawn leading to a proposal for implementation by the authority. As a whole, to generate interest, a synopsis reading is expected to lead to reading of the entire research report for approval and/or implementation.

The following Table 5.1 is expected to compare and contrast various research documents:

TABLE 5.1 Comparison and Contrast of Research Proposal, Research Report, Research Paper, Synopsis and Patent Document-Contents Wise

	Research Proposal	Research Report	Research Paper	Synopsis	Patent Document
Stage of Performance	It is a document proposed before conducting the exact research in the laboratory	It is a document which is a final submission to the authority	It is a document that may be a part of the work or after the entire work completion	It is a document to generate interest to read the entire research report	It is document submitted to the government for claiming exclusivity
Number of pages	10-50 pages	2-1000 pages or even more	5-10 pages	10-20 pages	Usually 5 pages and above
Submitted to	Funding authority	Government or academic or industry authority	Editor of a Journal Publisher	All stake holders including the scrutinizers	Intellectual Property Office
Pricing	Nil	Nil	May charge on a nominal basis for publishing and for providing hard copies	Nil	Based on the number of pages and number of claims, corresponding charges have to be paid to the intellectual property authority. Patent has to be maintained for 20 years by paying the prescribed fee every year else, patent becomes invalid and anybody can use the invention.

Table 5.1 *Contd...*

	Research Proposal	Research Report	Research Paper	Synopsis	Patent Document
Legal status	Becomes void after research funding was granted and work submitted.	Lead to award of a degree, making new policies, new product for release into the market	It is available for future research as a journal publication. Anybody can use the invention, provided the invention is not filed/granted with a patent.	Becomes void after approval of the final research report by the authority.	The invention claimed by the inventor has an exclusive right for 20 years (from date of first filing). Once the exclusivity term is complete anybody can use the invention.
Contents	Title, Researcher Name/s, Researcher Place of Work, Abstract, Purpose, Introduction, Literature Review, Methodology, References/ Bibliography, Appendices (research instruments, work plan, budget etc), Bio-sketch/Resumes of the researchers.	Title, Researcher Name/s, Place of Work, Declaration by Research supervisor, Declaration by Researcher, Acknowledgements, List of research paper published, List of figures/graphs/tables, List of contents, Introduction, Purpose, Statement of a problem, Literature Review, Null Hypothesis, Methodology, Observations/ Results, Interpretation/ Discussion/ Conclusion, References/ Bibliography, Appendices (instruments used, entire raw data collected, permissions taken etc), Errata	Title, Researcher Name/s, Place of Work, Abstract, Keywords, Introduction, Null Hypothesis, Methodology, Procedure, Observations/ Results, Interpretation/ Discussion/ Conclusion, Acknowledgements, References/ Bibliography.	Title, Researcher Name/s, Place of Work, Statement of a problem, Why the topic was chosen? Objective and scope, Methodology, Summary of the findings.	Patent Number, Patent date of grant, Title, Bibliography, Abstract, Field of invention, Introduction, Prior art, Summary of the invention, Detailed description of invention with observations (tables/figures/graphs, chemical structures), Best mode or Best Embodiments, Claims (Independent and dependent claims)
Bibliography (well accepted Vancouver Style)	As per international format and contains author names, title, journal name, year of publication, issue number, page numbers	As per international format and contains author names, title, journal name, year of publication, issue number, page numbers	As per international format and contains author names, title, journal name, year of publication, issue number, page numbers	May or may not contain references.	Contains Researcher names, Sponsor name, Date of first filing, Name of country where first filed, Date of filing of the current application, invention classification, Date of Priority, National Phase/International Phase/Paris Convention/PCT application, Patent documents granted, cited, countries designated etc.

Table 5.1 *Contd...*

	Research Proposal	Research Report	Research Paper	Synopsis	Patent Document
Plagiarism (Not to imitate other author's work)	Need to pass plagiarism	Need to pass plagiarism	Need to pass plagiarism	Need to pass plagiarism	Need to pass plagiarism
Commercial Value	No commercial value	May lead to commercial value as innovation	May lead to commercial value as innovation	No commercial value	All the patented inventions are granted based on industrial application (one of the patentability criteria). If no working of the patent or at a later stage if the patented invention is not being used, it may lead to compulsory licensing or revoke of patent grant. May cost upto Rs. 1 Lakh from date of filing to maintenance for 20 years.
Purpose	For a grant of a research project	For an academic award, solving a potential problem that exist and the solution identified being implemented as a new policy, new drug product etc	For gaining the credential of a efficient research activity and bring into the awareness to the stake holders	For creating enthusiasm on the research activity conducted for further study/scrutiny	The invention has commercial value and hence, the inventor claims for exclusivity (a short term monopoly). Moreover, government grants exclusivity to the inventor to get back all his investments so that he will have financial resources for future research projects.
Time limit	If seeking for government funding, the proposal has to be submitted at the right time as suggested.	As per the norms set forth by the authority.	Forever available to the stake holders.	A synopsis is circulated to all stake holders and is expected for their valuable comments while discussing the research report.	If research paper published, a patent application has to be submitted within stipulated time. Exclusivity is for 20 years and later on any interested party can use the invention.
Role of Intellectual Property Rights	Idea is generated and upon approval can be executed.	Intellectual property created is either patent protected or leading to a research paper publication	Intellectual property is dedicated for the wellbeing of the society until unless; it is patent filed/granted.	Intellectual property created is made aware for limited public for final approval of the research report by the authority. May lead to patent filing/granting.	Intellectual property created is protected as an exclusive right so as to get back the investments made.

Table 5.1 *Contd...*

	Research Proposal	Research Report	Research Paper	Synopsis	Patent Document
Limitations	Idea is proposed and it always depends on the financials to execute.	It has become habitual to report positive results avoiding negative results. Several negative results may become positive when a meta-analysis conducted. Several research reports end up at the institutional levels and such work may not be available in public domain as prior art.	A research paper is commonly drafted for positive results. Encourages inventions limiting to lesser innovations. Inventions are made at the institution/governm ent levels where as innovations from inventions are made at the industry level.	The document is meant for creating enthusiasm/mot ivation for further reading of the research report and for accepting for scrutiny of the research report.	There is a mis-conception that, patent applications are not peer reviewed and in the current day scenario a peer reviewing is made by examining of the applications by experts in the field.
Patentability Subject Matter Presence	Idea is proposed and still not executed	The report contains all the information after executing the idea. The experimental subject matter may fulfill patentability criteria.	A research paper may be a single or multiple inventions. The inventions present in the paper may or may not fulfill patentability criteria	The synopsis is a gist of all the entire work of an idea. The subject matter contained may or may not fulfill patentability criteria.	The invention disclosed , only if fulfill patentability criteria of novelty, non-obviousness, useful and enabled, the invention is granted with a patent.
Number of inventions	Idea is not executed	The experimental report may contain one or more inventions.	A research paper may contain one or more inventions. Several times multiple papers are published from one report.	A synopsis may not mention all the inventions and a mention is made with the best conclusions drawn.	A patented document contains only one invention. Hence, it is necessary to get multiple patents if the research report contains multiple inventions.

Hence, the basic objective of identifying a problem and solving a problem is completed not only with experimental activity but also with ample disclosure of the invention to the fraternity so that, duplication of similar research is avoided leading to better innovations and their availability into the market as early as possible. This can be considered similar to ICH guideline, to meet the objective of the drug/drug products reach the market/patients at the earliest possible.

Whenever drafting a research activity, it is necessary to pre-plan, arrange the various aspects in a logical or chronological order and present the information in legible conventional English so that, the activity is well understood not only to professionals but also to non-professionals who have to release the financials. Where ever required, an opinion from the expert in the field has to be taken. However, in several cases, a research report loses its connectivity and one has to ensure in overcoming such issues. It is quite common in receiving comments from scrutinizers relating to lack of good vocabulary and where ever necessary has to be implemented.

6 Detailed Contents of a Research Paper

6.0 Introduction

A research paper is a document comprising of the details of an invention, submitted to a scientific journal publisher (editor) by the inventor as a source of information to the scientific fraternity, up on scrutiny by the experts in the field of invention and acceptance that the invention made is novel, non-obvious, shall be published in the journal to which the inventor has sent the research paper.

Whereas, a patent is a document submitted by the inventor to the Government for an exclusive right to make, sell, use and import for a certain period of time upon disclosure of the invention. Hence, a research paper may lead to a patent grant. It is believed that a research paper is an outcome of a few experiments, whereas a patented invention may be an outcome of hundreds of experiments. It is necessary to understand that several research papers may lead to one patent. For an invention to be patentable, the invention should fulfill patentability criteria i.e., novelty, non-obviousness, useful and enablement. An invention is said to fulfill novelty, provided the invention (believed by the inventor) really has inventive step (judged by persons skilled in the art). An invention is said to be non-obvious provided the said invention does not exist earlier. An invention should have industrial application (use); else the invention loses its patentability criteria. Enabling is an indication that the entire invention should be disclosed including the best method (best mode) of conducting the experiment giving the best result. In India, a patent is granted for an invention on first to file basis. This implies that when two inventors have done the same invention, without knowing to each other, have filed separately patent applications, the patent office shall grant a patent to the inventor who has filed first.

In the current day scenario, several research papers are being published in journals and a question arises to the inventor whether the invention published in journal (obvious) shall fulfill patentability criteria. It is necessary to understand that an invention published in a journal as a research paper, does not lose patentability criteria provided the inventor submits an application for a patent within a stipulated time from date of publication of the research paper in the journal.

A question arises, whether the contents of a research paper and a patent document are same. Well, it varies from one researcher to another based on the strength of past research which was done. In several cases, the contents of the research paper and a patent document have same features but have some features completely distinctive. To the context, a scientific research paper comprises of a title, author/s name, authors place of research work, abstract, keywords, introduction, materials and methodology, details experimental procedures, observations/results, discussion, conclusion, acknowledgements, references etc.

6.1 Title

A title of a research paper must comprise of minimum possible words which on reading should reveal to the reader what is the research about. A broad title may not reveal the details on the invention until and unless the research paper is further read. In several cases, a title should not contain an abbreviation but, in several conditions it may be accepted provided the fraternity is well aware of such abbreviations. For instance, a research paper titled as "Simultaneous estimation of paracetamol and ibuprofen in tablet dosage using UV double beam spectroscopy". Here, the title clearly indicates that the research work is on pharmaceutical quality, pertaining to a solid dosage form tablets, using a UV double beam spectroscopy. The exact method of simultaneous determination of two or more drugs among the UV spectroscopy methods are usually discussed at a later stage in the research paper.

6.2 Author Names

Several journals follow their unique way of presentation of names of authors and currently international standards are maintained for presentation of author names to harmonize at a global perspective. For instance: Alex P, Manoj K, and Subba Rao B*. An indication of asterix is meant for understanding to the readers and publisher that any clarifications and details of the research may be communicated to the person indicated. In several cases, the first author shall have the credit for the research work conducted, while the last author mentioned is the guide or the project leader for the research work (with respect to Indian context). In several cases, while citing or providing cross reference, it is usually mentioned as Alex P et al., (1999) in the text and the complete details being provided about the research paper in references of the current research paper. In several cases, several co-authors are associated because the research project is handled by several departments i.e., department of pharmaceutical chemistry, department of pharmaceutical analysis, department of pharmacology etc.

6.3 Abstract

During literature search, to another researcher, an abstract plays a key role whether he has collected a research article of his interest or not amongst the related well diversified inventions. An abstract comprises of 50 to 100 words providing the researchers rationale or problem existing in a field, experimental conducted to overcome the problem and finally providing his best results that has overcome the problem. For instance, a simultaneous estimation of paracetamol and ibuprofen was taken on the basis that a combination tablet is available in the market, but Indian pharmacopoeia (assumption) provides two separate methods for determining the contents (assay) which is time consuming, expensive. To overcome this, the current research is being conducted for estimation of both the drugs at one single stretch.

6.4   Keywords

Drafting keywords for the research paper needs a complete understanding of the research being conducted and wish to be published. A good key word, helps other scientists interested relating to your research work retrieve the research paper from digital library with the best possible successful probability. For instance, key words: "paracetamol, ibuprofen, tablets, simultaneous estimation, UV double beam spectroscopy" is a precise mention of key words for a research being conducted. Especially when a review is being conducted on digital libraries (say internet etc.,) submission of good keywords (or their combination) provide the research papers that were already published eliminating other research papers not to the readers interest. Currently, Google search is effective but not precise due to several thousands of articles are being retrieved with the same keywords and this can be overcome by using a combination of keywords. Several times Google retrieves articles for a word that have both scientific and English meanings.

6.5   Introduction

An introduction in a research article usually provides the fundamental concepts relating to the research in question and to some extent describes what was the past research conducted along with its benefits and drawbacks and how the current planned research overcome the drawbacks if successful. For instance: Paracetamol[1] and Ibuprofen[2] are widely used over the counter drugs for anti-pyretic, anti-inflammatory and analgesic activity. The drugs are either available as individual tablet[3] or combination tablet dosage forms[4]. Neither of the official pharmacopoeias[5-10] does not mention a single method of estimation of both the drugs and to overcome this problem, the widely available tablet dosage form as combination drugs is chosen for their simultaneous estimation using a selected UV spectroscopy method. The superscript numerical mentioned in the text provides the details of research papers/books etc., referred and the details of the research paper and books are mentioned in the number sequence in the references of the research paper.

6.6 Materials and Methodology

For conducting a research several bulk drugs, formulations, animals, feed for animals, instruments used, climatic conditions maintained, techniques used to collect samples/animals along with source, grade of materials are mentioned. For instance: bulk drugs Paracetamol IP and Ibuprofen IP were procured as complimentary samples from M/s. ABC, Hyderabad and conventional tablet dosage form as combination were procured from local community pharmacies on a random basis. The rationale behind a particular sample size of collection may be mentioned which is by a mathematical statistical calculation or based on similar past work.

6.7 Procedure

Several in-house procedures have to be established or a standard procedure from an official standard book like India Pharmacopoeia are outlined step by step right from weighing to dilutions to final analytical value mentioning the wavelength at which the values were noted. In case of animal experiments, the procedure of dosage calculated, dosage form prepared, route of administration, parameters monitored, time intervals maintained, if any pathology study made, procedure of control, treatment groups, sacrificing and isolating the tissues and finally making pathological slides to take either qualitative or quantitative values are mentioned. In several cases, permission taken from animal ethics committee, institutional ethics committee, local drug regulatory or health authority, hospital authority etc., are mentioned. For new chemical entity synthesis, the procedure followed along with quantities are mentioned.

6.8 Results

The authenticity of conducting an experiment is proved by presenting the results. Results are the numerical values assigned with respect to an observation, where such an observation is made after performing the designed procedures. Results include several mathematical as well as statistical calculations. Results are an aesthetic, systematic presentation of data obtained from observations. Results are either presented as tables, pictorial diagrams as histograms, bar graphs, trend graphs, pi-charts, scattered plots, log plots, stock plots, surface plots, doughnut plots, bubble plots, radar plots, area plots, contour plot, forest plot (for meta-analysis), funnel plot (for meta-analysis) etc. Presentation of results in pictorial formats is found to be less confusing leading to better interpretations. For instance: Presenting data in a tabular form individually for paracetamol and ibuprofen with respect to concentration and absorbance values. Presentation of tabular form of combination of paracetamol with ibuprofen (concentrations) and their individual absorbance values at two different λmax. Presentation of individual and combination standard plots of paracetamol, ibuprofen (i.e., absorbance vs. concentration) etc., For new chemical entities, percentage yield, spectral data such as H^1, C^{13} NMR data, IR spectra data, Mass spectra data, elemental analysis data are mentioned.

6.9 Discussion

In this part of the research paper, a complete description is made relating to the data compiled and an explanation is made with respect to the extremities of variations in the results. The results are ensured for their mathematical or statistical significance and a conclusion is drawn whether the results are in favour or against to a hypothesis framed before starting the experiment.

6.10 Conclusion

Based on the objective with which the research was initiated and the discussion made with respect to the experimental results, a road map for implementation is proposed and put forward to the fraternity and the society.

6.11 Acknowledgements

Several research initiatives are funded by government organizations, industry or the academic institutions and the researcher is expected to acknowledge the funded organizations and the authority at the work place for their moral and facility support. Additionally, ethics committees, hospital authority where work was conducted, the patients who co-operated for the experimental work are acknowledged by thanking. For instance: "The authors thank the XYZ Pharmaceuticals Pvt. Ltd., and Alpha Ltd., for providing gift sample of ACE and PAR respectively"

6.12 References (Bibliography)

A research project is initiated based on past work which was identified from research papers published, books etc. The basis and rationale behind initiating such research activity has to be provided, as a proof how current problem was identified that led to explore and solve the problem. At several places in the text of the research paper, a number is allotted as a superscript and the details of authors, title of research article, name of journal (standard accepted abbreviations), year of publication, volume number, issue number, page numbers are mentioned in the reference part of the paper.

Presentation of references is made uniform globally and several peer journals accept research papers only when the entire research paper along with references are drafted with respect to the standards set forth. Several standard formats are available from PubMed. Vancouver styles, ICMJE guidelines (http://www.icmje.org) of presenting references are commonly used.

It is necessary to understand that a reference writing of one author research paper may vary from two or three authors. Likewise, while mentioning about book, author for the chapter, chapter title, name of the book, name of publisher, year of publication, edition number, page numbers are mentioned.

For instance:

i. Zahra Y, Reza P, Mohammad G. Comparison of Demographic and Clinical Characteristics Influencing Health-Related Quality of Life in Patients with Diabetic Foot Ulcers and Those without Foot Ulcers, Diabetes Metab Syndr Obes [Internet]. 2011 cited [2012 Jul 18]; 4: 393-399. Available from: http:www.ncbi.nlm.nih.gov/pmc/articles/PMC3257967/

ii. Rajnish Kumar R. Battling with TRIPS: Emerging firm strategies of Indian Pharmaceutical Industry Post TRIPS. J Intellec Prop Rights. Jul 2008; 13:301-317.

iii. Kaplan RM, Anderson JP, Ganiats TJ. Quality of Life Assessment: key issues in the 1990s. Dordrecht, Netherlands: Kluwer Academic Publishers: 1993; 65-94.

iv. Joshi M, Leela G. International Treaties and Conventions on IPR Hyderabad: NALSAR Proximate Education, NALSAR University of Law; p.7-13.

v. Hansch C, Fujita, T. P-σ-π Analysis: A method for the correlation of biological activity and chemical structure. J Amer Chem Soc 1964; 86:1616.

vi. Harvey HC. Adrenergic blocking drugs. In:Osol A. editor. Remington's Pharmaceutical Sciences, 16th ed. Easton, PA: Mack Publishing Company; 1980. P.845-6.

vii. Reynolds JE. Martindale; The Extra Pharmacopoeia. 31st ed. London: Published by Direction of The Council of The Royal Pharmaceutical Society of Great Britain and Prepared in The Society's Publication Department; 1996, p. 1062.

viii. British Pharmacopoeial Commission. British Pharmacopoeia. Vol 1. International ed. London: HMSO Publication; 1993, p.483.

ix. WHO, How to investigate drug use in health facilities: Selected drug use indicators. Geneva: World Health Organization; 1993. WHO/DAP1993:1:1-87.

x. Indian Pharmacopoeia, 4th ed. New Delhi: The Controller of Publications, Government of India; 1996, p. 807.

xi. The United States Pharmacopoeia. 24th ed. Rockville, MD: United States Pharmacopoeial Convention Inc; 2000, p. 1208.

xii. ICH guidelines, analytical method validation (Q3). Geneva: July 2000.

xiii. Shimadzu-HPLC User's Manual, LC-10 ATVP, Shimadzu corporation, analytical and measuring instruments division. Kyoto, Japan: p.2-4.

6.13 Errata

In a research paper a separate heading of errata is not seen, but is usually seen in books, thesis books. Errata are usually included as a separate page at the end of a book or a thesis book. As the entire book is published, any spelling or numerical errors are mentioned with respect to a page and corresponding correct spell or numerical is mentioned. Any major changes such as figures, entire paragraph errors cannot be placed in errata and the entire major errors have to be corrected and replaced.

For instance in page 5, replace "Subject" with "subject".

6.14 Spell Check

Every research paper has to be ensured for proper spelling and grammar. Several words are misspelled during typing and drafting of a research paper. In addition to this a research paper is a final draft of several preliminary drafts. Under such circumstances, it is necessary to ensure every word and information is in appropriate and right place. Now a day, computers have made the tedious work easier while typing the final draft of the research paper. Microsoft Word document ensures simultaneous spell and grammar check and the author has to ensure of conducting spell and grammar check before sending the research paper to the editor of the journal publication.

6.15 Foot Notes

Foot notes are widely used in non-laboratory based research papers such as research with respect to mathematics, law etc. In pharmaceuticals, one may come across of usage of foot notes in legal documents, reference books, text books. A foot note is usually indicated with a case study, other possible meanings of a word, the meaning of the word which has to be considered for the current context, the scope of the word for the context etc. In several legal documents, every page is witnessed with a foot note covering the background case decision for the current case decision.

6.16 Plagiarism

A research paper should be drafted with free flow of words constructing sentences. In several cases in the past, research documents were found with fragmented sentences. Whether it is a research paper, research thesis or research proposal, the sentences drafted should not be an imitation of a past work (cut and paste of past work). Every researcher has to ensure that the final draft is free from plagiarism. Currently, several online softwares help to check for plagiarism by cutting text from current article and pasting in the software.

7 Clinical Trials and Clinical Study Design

7.0 Introduction to Clinical Trials

In pharmaceuticals, testing of new chemical entities, new generics, new dosage forms, new strengths, new routes of administration on human beings are called as clinical trials. Especially relating to new chemical entities, it is only after ensuring that the entity is safe on animals enters clinical trials where as remaining were already tested in the past for the new active ingredient but needs some data relating to establishing bio-pharmaceutical data. Clinical trials are categorized in four phase studies as Phase I, Phase II, Phase III and Phase IV. Thus the objective of clinical trials is to ensure the fundamental point of safety, efficacy and reliability.

Phase I Trials: About 20-100 healthy volunteers are selected and the new promising drug candidate is established for desired pharmacological activity, strength, pharmacokinetic and pharmaco-dynamic data. The time period of the trials lasts for a few months to a year.

Phase II Trials: About 100-1000 patients are selected and the drug candidate is ensured for pharmacological activity while monitoring for safety, efficacy and reliability. The trial may last for 1 to 2 years (or even more) and trials may be conducted within the country at various sites or at international levels.

Phase III Trials: About 1000 or above patients are selected for further ensuring the drug candidate for safety, efficacy and reliability. Several new chemical entities fail as new drug candidates at this stage. Once the drug candidate is through, it is approved by the authority for marketing within the country.

Phase IV Trials: The trials are also called as post marketing surveillance trials. The marketed drug is studied to establish the long term effects.

7.1 Classification of Clinical Study Design

For a better understanding the concepts, the design of clinical trials are classified into Type A, Type B and Type C.

7.1.1 Type A Design

In this type, clinical trials are designed as case study design, observational study design and interventional study design.

i.   Case Study Design:

A case study is an analysis of persons, events, decisions, periods, projects, policies, institutions or other systems that are studies holistically by one or more methods. In medical field, an individual enters a hospital when there is a change in physiology from normal condition, which in turn called as disease condition. Hence, every issue of a patient is a case. A case study is conducted by an individual or an organisation. Usually, the output of a case study is both qualitative and quantitative.

Hence, a case study can be considered as a conventional normal or a unique case. The criterion for selection of a case is either as a key case, outlier case or a local knowledge case.

For instance, in a fever hospital, regular out or in-patients are with normal fever conditions, but when a dengue case was first detected, the case has become key case as the symptoms of the disease are not being curing with normal fever treatment.

As an outlier case, when there are several adult out-patients being treated with diabetes, a sudden appearance of child being detected with diabetes becomes an outlier. In the same way, out of several diabetes patients, one or two individuals were diagnosed with kidney complications and such patients fall into outlier whereas the majority falls into one common group.

In case of local knowledge case, a unique case can be identified by the authority only through the passage of information by the local people. For instance, a child has been identified with a liver failure condition and requires an urgent transplantation. Despite the child's parents were regularly providing treatment, a charity oriented doctor or an organisation comes to the rescue only when the case really comes into limelight. When the local people spread the information, the charity oriented doctor took up the case for surgery by transplanting a part of liver from her father. Likewise, several rare diseases are coming into limelight either through local people or through television channels.

Hence in a case study design, the choice of the case is usually unique, evaluative or exploratory and helps in developing theory. A case study is considered as single, multiple, retrospective, snapshot, nested, parallel, theory building, theory evaluation, theory testing case.

ii.   Observational Study Design:

In pharmaceuticals, at the non-clinical level, an observation is a quest for identification of change from a normal condition or reference point. In case of clinical level, an observation is an identification of deviations/changes whether occurred while taking into consideration healthy condition or a stage of disease condition of an individual. Observational studies help in drawing inferences from a sample that can be extrapolated to a population. In observational studies, the investigator does not have a control on the independent variable and he may have to compromise due to logical or ethical issues.

For instance, a study was planned with an objective of identification of association of abortion and breast cancer. The investigator has the options i.e., firstly selecting pregnant women and dividing them into two groups as control (not induced with abortion) and treatment (induced with abortion). The second option is selecting women who had already undergone naturally abortion and conducting the study. As an ethical principle, the investigator has to depend on second study rather than the first.

Classification of Observational Study Design:

Observational Studies are categorized into five types as mentioned below:

a. Case-Control Study Design:

When a wide range of patients are being categorized/sorted with respect to a disease, under a specific disease condition, a unique feature if exist, such case become unique and is different from among the other patients having a same disease (control group), such unique cases are identified using case-control study design.

For instance: In a maternity hospital, daily we come across pregnant ladies giving birth to baby boys or baby girls. As time passed, on one day, one of the mothers has given birth to conjoined babies which is unique and is not regular. Hence, normal babies can be considered as control group and the conjoined baby is considered as unique case, which is not regular.

One another example is, in a hospital daily several diabetic patients visit for treatment, majority of the patients have only variation in their blood glucose levels, but one or few patients have variation in glucose levels as well as kidney issues. Hence, diabetic patients with kidney issues are unique when compared to the control group of patients having only abnormal glucose levels with no other associated organ issues.

Hence case-control study is a type of epidemiological observational study. In general, an observational study is not a randomized study. In a case-control study, the exposure and outcome status are observed over non-randomized exposed and un-exposed groups.

Case control studies were initially analysed by testing whether or not there were significant differences between the proportions of exposed subjects among cases and controls. Subsequently, it was suggested (Cornfield) that when the disease outcome of interest is rare, the odd ratio of exposure can be used to estimate the relative risk (rare disease assumption). Later, it was proposed (Miettinen, 1976) that rare disease assumption is not necessary and that odd ratios of exposure can be used directly to estimate the incidence rate ratio of exposure without the need for rare disease assumption.

Advantages:

i. Inexpensive

ii. The study can be planned in small facilities

iii. Case-control studies are route for discoveries and advancements for a disease.

iv. Case-control studies are helpful to identify rare diseases and their study.

v. Case-control studies help to find association between risk factor and a disease.

vi. The study is of short duration, less expensive when compared to prospective cohort studies.

vii. Case-control study data is of an individual.

Disadvantages:

i. Case-control studies do not provide same level of evidence as randomized controlled trials.

ii. It is difficult to establish time line of exposure of a disease unlike in prospective cohort study.

iii. Case-control studies possess low level evidence relating to individual's exposure.

b. **Cross-Sectional Study Design**

Cross-sectional studies are also called as transversal study or prevalence study. In several cases, a cross-section study is a collection of data from a population and is subjected to analysis. Unlike case control studies, cross sectional studies provide data on the entire population under study, where as in a case-control study an individual with a specific characteristic is considered. Cross-sectional studies are used to assess the prevalence of acute or chronic conditions and helps in answering questions about the causes of disease or the results of intervention.

Advantages:

i. Cross-sectional studies are descriptive (neither longitudinal nor experimental)

ii. Unlike case-control studies, cross-sectional studies describe not only odd ratios, but also absolute risks, relative risks from prevalence.

Disadvantages:

i. The study data which we have to rely is basically a data that was collected for other purposes.

ii. The study is moderately expensive.

iii. The study is not suitable for study of rare diseases.

iv. Difficulty in recalling past events and may also contributes bias.

v. Routinely collected data does not normally describe which variable is the cause and which the effect.

vi. Cross-sectional studies using data originally collected for other purposes are often unable to include data on confounding factors, other variable that affect the relationship between the putative cause and effect.

vii. Cross-sectional study data involves secondary analysis data and individual's records are not available (data from health authorities)

c. **Longitudinal Study Design**

Longitudinal studies are a repeated observational study of a variable over a long period of time (say 10 years). Hence, a longitudinal study helps in recording a series of observations more than once on patients. Longitudinal studies can be structured as longitudinal randomized experiments. As longitudinal studies records observations of the same patients several times, differences observed in those people are less likely to be the result of cultural differences across generations.

Advantages:

i. Longitudinal studies helps in observing changes more accurate.

ii. Longitudinal studies help to uncover predictors of certain diseases.

iii. The studies are observational without any manipulations.

iv. The power of longitudinal study is more than cross-sectional study since observations are taken repeatedly from same individual.

v. A retrospective study may be a longitudinal study that looks back in time i.e., look up of medical records of previous years to look for a trend.

Disadvantages:

i. Longitudinal studies have less power to detect casual relationships than experiments.

ii. Longitudinal studies consume long time and are expensive.

iii. Longitudinal studies are not convenient.

d. **Cohort Study Design**

A cohort is a group of people who have common characteristics within a defined period. Cohort studies are quasi-experimental, observational longitudinal studies. Cohort studies are life histories of defined population. A cohort may start with birth of an individual/s, recording various healthy condition parameters, as time passes with a few identifying with a disease initiation (establishment of baseline for a disease) and continues with further investigations. Several cohort studies are active in various countries of the World and researchers are regularly collecting data from the individuals.

Cohort studies are categorized into two types:

i. **Prospective Cohort Study:**

A prospective study is a study in which right from birth of the individual, various parameters are recorded at different time intervals and are being monitored in future years. In several cases, in a prospective study, the individual is noticed and the study is continued.

Hence a prospective cohort study is a longitudinal study that follows over time on a group of cohort individual who differ with respect to certain factors under study, to determine how these factors affect rates of a certain outcome.

For instance, a group of healthy truck drivers with defined characteristics as cohort were selected and were regularly monitored for their health parameters. The divers were healthy for a period of time and as time passed, several drivers started smoking (attribute) as a habit (establishment of baseline for a disease) and upon continuing (say longitudinal) some of the subjects developed cancer (outcome) over time. This study indicates that, at the initiation of the study the drivers were without any disease, as time passed, certain habits resulted to disease outcomes.

Advantages of Prospective Cohort Studies:

a. Prospective Cohort Studies are helpful to understand the etiology of a disease and disorders.

b. Prospective Cohort Studies are higher in hierarchy of evidence than retrospective.

c. Helps to establish risk factors for being infected with a new disease.

d. Errors can be minimized over time.

Disadvantages of Prospective Cohort Studies:

a. Prospective Cohort Studies are more expensive than a case-control study.

ii. **Retrospective Cohort Study:**

A retrospective cohort study can be considered as a compilation of data which was earlier recorded and further continued as a prospective study. Hence, a retrospective cohort study is a longitudinal cohort study that studies a cohort of individuals that share a common exposure factor to determine its influence on the development of a disease, and are compared to another group of equivalent individuals that were not exposed to that factor.

For instance: A medical and psychological research study in which the records of groups of individuals who are alike in many ways but differ in certain characteristics (for example: female nurses who smoke and those who does not smoke) are compared for a particular outcome.

It is necessary to understand that a retrospective cohort study has existed for approximately as long as prospective cohort studies. In several conditions, in a retrospective cohort study, the researcher collects data from past records and does not follow up patients as in the case of prospective study.

There is a possibility that a starting point of all cohort studies may be the same and groups get established as exposed versus non-exposed and further studied.

Advantages of Retrospective Cohort Study:

a. Retrospective cohort study is performed post-hoc.

b. The study lasts from collection of data to interpretation of data.

c. Retrospective cohort studies are conducted in small scale.

d. Retrospective cohort studies take less time to complete.

e. The studies are helpful to analyze multiple outcomes.

f. Retrospective cohort studies potentially address rare diseases.

g. Retrospective cohort studies are less expensive.

Disadvantages of Retrospective Cohort Study:

a. In retrospective cohort study, all events of exposure, latent period and subsequent outcomes have already occurred in the past.

b. It is only collection of data, unlike in prospective (both groups are initiated).

c. Errors may occur due to confounding and bias (than in prospective).

d. Vital statistics may not be measured.

e. Possibility of occurrence of bias in selecting controls (i.e., selection bias, information bias).

f. Needs to depend on accurate record keeping.

g. Needs large sample size.

Advantages of Cohort Studies (as a whole):

1. Cohort studies can be conducted prospectively or retrospectively from archived records.

2. A cohort study cannot be defined as a group of people who already have a disease.

3. Prospective cohort study data helps to determine the risk factors for contracting a new disease because it is a longitudinal observation of the individual through time and collection of data at regular intervals, so recall error is reduced.

4. Data collected from long term cohort studies (prospective) are of superior quality when compared to retrospective/cross-sectional studies.

5. Prospective cohort studies yield most reliable results.

6. Prospective cohort studies enable a wide range of exposure-disease associations to be studied.

7. Assessment starts with putative cause of disease and observations are made of the occurrence of disease.

Disadvantages of Cohort Studies (as a whole):

1. Cohort studies are expensive.

2. Sensitive to attrition and take a long follow-up time to generate useful data.

3. Rare diseases such as lung cancer are not studied with the use of cohort study, instead studied by case-control study.

e. Ecological Study Design

Study of surroundings is called as ecology. Ecology is the study of the interaction of people with their environment or is a branch of biology dealing with the relations of organisms to one another and to their physical surroundings.

Several ecological studies are being conducted globally and help in identifying the root cause of a problem. For instance, in a particular community, it was identified the death cases are increasing. When an ecological study was conducted, the reason behind the death is due to cholera. On further studies, it was identified the people in the said community were drinking water from a pipeline in a particular street and upon further investigation, it was the tap head of the pipeline, the causative for the cholera disease. Investigators replaced with a new tap head and it was later observed that the death rate decreased.

In yet another case, an ecological study was conducted to identify the association between diet and cancer. Upon investigation, people who are consuming with a non-vegetarian diet or with certain sweeteners are identified with cancer whereas vegetarians were found healthy.

iii. Interventional Study Design:

An intervention can be considered as interference or as a disturbance occurring during a pre-planned process of a study. Interventions can be intentional or un-intentional. In pharmaceutical clinical trials, interventions occur between groups or within a group. Some of the interventions are new drug intervention, change in life style, medical or surgical intervention, food interventions etc.

For instance, an investigator has planned a two group study using a diabetic drug. One of the group is control, whereas the other is treatment group. Food style, time of drug administration etc., were fixed for the study. An intervention may occur if an individual in the treatment group takes diet abnormally than prescribed, administering other drugs, altering time of administering of drugs, consuming alcohol, smoking etc.

7.1.2   Type B Design

i.   Treatment Study Design:

A treatment is a process of identification of a change in physiology as diagnosis and prescribing a medication for the cure of a disease in an individual. A treatment may be surgical, radiation, device or a medicine in nature. For treating cancer, a treatment can be medication, radiation and a surgery or their combinations.

ii.   Preventive Study Design:

A precautionary process of steps taken before hand for a disease not to occur is called prevention. A preventive step may be in the terms of maintaining hygienic conditions, isolation of individuals so that a disease is not spread etc. Several vaccinations act as a prophylactic so that a disease is prevented from occurrence. Globally, biotechnology based vaccines are being developed so as to prevent the occurrence of a disease.

iii.   Diagnostic Study Design:

Despite symptomatic changes being diagnosed by a medical practitioner, several chemical, x-ray, echo, MRI and CT scan techniques are currently playing a key role for confirmation of a disease condition. Development of such techniques and their evaluation is planned by such designs. For instance, identification of glucose levels by normal chemical reactions is superseded by diagnostic strips with detectable electronic sensors.

iv. Screening Study Design:

Drug screening is a widely used term in pharmaceuticals where in, various new chemical entities after separating from unwanted, the wanted are further screened in clinical trials so that a new chemical entity becomes a drug candidate and is available in the market.

v. Quality of Life Study Design (QOL):

A quality of life of an individual is assessed on various parameters like physical health and mental health. Quality of life of an individual depends on poverty, health condition, daily work style etc. Quality of life is assessed based on abstract scaling and a high value of quality of life indicates the individual is having a good quality of life and with a low value indicating bad quality of life. In pharmaceuticals, health related quality of life (HRQOL) instrument is used to assess a patient's quality of life before and after treatment. It is obvious that HRQOL value of the patient improves after treatment. SF 36, (Annexure II) is a globally accepted instrument to assess HRQOL of diabetic patients.

7.1.3   Type C Design

i. Treatment Study Design:

a. Randomized Controlled Trials:

Random indicates devoid from being bias. Such experimental designs minimize errors relating to selection of patients, kind of treatment being provided to patients, preventing from psychological factors that may be responsible in interfering with a treatment. Under such studies, patients are selected fulfilling inclusion and exclusion criteria, grouped randomly and provided with treatment on random among the groups. The groups are mainly divided into control and treatment groups. Such studies are eligible for meta-analysis where in, several studies conducted in several places across the globe are selected and further analysed. Meta-analysis helps in making final decisions where several research conducted on a subject matter is providing with ambiguous results.

i. Blind Trials

In these type of studies, imagine a condition where a generic drug product is compared with innovator drug product to establish a bioequivalence. A researcher (doctor), a pharmacist, a statistician and patients are involved for the task. The patients are screened, selected into four groups say, Control group, Group A, Group B and Group C. Control group does not receive any treatment whereas the other three A, B, C have a treatment. Under such circumstances, in order to minimize the psychological factors that may interfere with the treatment outcomes, blind studies are designed.

Blind studies are usually classified into three types i.e., single, double and triple blind studies.

In the single blind study, it is the doctor only who know to which group A, B, C what treatment was given i.e., innovator drug or generic drug or the placebo and the rest are not aware, including the patients.

In case of double blind studies, neither the doctor nor the patients are aware which group received what kind of treatment. Under such circumstances, the pharmacist plans and maintains the information who received what kind of drug.

In case of triple blind study, all the three that is, the doctor, the patient and the pharmacist are not aware of what kind of treatment was provided. It is the bio-statistician who is aware of what kind of treatment was given to which group. Hence, planning a blind study helps in minimizing errors such as selection of patients on bias, intentionally making the patients aware of what kind of treatment being given etc.

ii. Non-blind Trials:

In these kinds of studies, secrecy is not maintained with the kind of treatment being provided to the different groups undergoing a study. Such studies also help in understanding a treatment when interfered with psychological, bias etc., type of errors. A researcher several times has to accustom to such studies where he/she cannot construct research studies to his wish.

b. Adaptive Clinical Trials:

Such clinical trials are planned where the researcher cannot develop methodologies to his desires. He accustoms to a situation and develops methods accordingly to meet his key objectives with some compromises. For instance, the researcher wishes to study a drug and its interaction with kind of food, alcohol, smoking, working style etc. The researcher adapts his studies in such a way that, he selects patients who are habitual to vegetarian food, non-vegetarian food, alcohol, smoking, different types of work related patients instead going the other way, selecting all the patient who are not-habitual.

c. Non-randomized Trials:

A non-random study is one where researcher has no options of selecting patients into groups on random. This means a bias factor may not be overcome under such circumstances. This bias factor is not intentional but occurred to the circumstances.

ii. Observational Study Design:

a. Case-Control Study

i. Nested Case-Control Study (NCC)

Let us imagine, in a hospital, diabetic patients are being monitored by the physician. Several adult diabetic patients are being examined regularly and when a child patient with diabetes is being identified, the child has to be compared with other children possessing diabetes and not with the adult diabetes patients and this can be considered as Nested case-control study. Likewise, a child with diabetes with other ailments is compared with a child having only diabetes and no other ailments.

Advantages of NCC study:

i. Avoids from conducting new case control studies based on previously collected data for a large cohort study.

ii. About 1 to 4 controls are collected for each case.

iii. Covariates are not measured for all participants.

iv. Less expensive.

Disadvantages of NCC study:

i. Nested case-control study is less efficient than full cohort study design.

ii. Nested case-control study is less efficient due to less controls per case and or stratified sampling.

b. Cross-Sectional Study

   i. Community Survey Study:

The study mainly deals with study of various attributes of individuals living in homes and belongs to an area called as community.

c. Cohort Study

   i. Prospective Cohort Study: As explained earlier

   ii. Retrospective Cohort Study: As explained earlier

   iii. Time Series Study:

Time series can be described as monitoring of an attribute and its variations over a period of time and drawing conclusions with respect to current scenario or based upon the observations, a forecast can be predicted. A time series can be assumed as a trend occurred in the past to the trend that may take place in the future. In pharmaceuticals, a trend of past exports may help in predicting future exports from India to global countries in the World. Time series may be classified into the following categories:

1. **Long Term Time Series (Secular trend/Trend):**

In this type of series, an attribute is observed for a long time for years. Some of the studies include cohort studies, long term studies, export profiles etc.

2. **Short Term Time Series (Short term oscillations):** In this type of series, the monitoring of an attribute may be for a few years or even low for a few months.

Short term oscillations are classified into three types:

a. **Cyclic trend**: In this type of trend, the variations in the attribute are expected to return after a certain period of time. For instance: a global economic recession had occurred about 30-50 years ago and it has occurred in the current decade (i.e., 2010-2020).

b. **Seasonal trend**: A season may be a change in the weather (summer, rainy, spring, winter) or a natural periodic change that is happening for an attribute.

c. **Irregular trend (random trend):** In this type of trend, the variations occurring in the attribute are un-predictable and all of a sudden there is either a positive or negative change in the attribute.

To find out the factors responsible for variations occurring in an attribute, several other methods like free-hand method, semi-average method, moving averages method, least squares method are helpful.

For calculating Overall trend say "Y", the following formulas are applicable based upon the circumstances i.e.,

i. **Additive:**

Y = Trend (a) + Cyclic trend (b) + Seasonal trend (c) + Irregular trend (d)

Or

ii. **Multiplicative:**

Y = Trend (a) x Cyclic trend (b) x Seasonal trend (c) x Irregular trend (d)

A trend analysis is found of great use for fore-casting. In pharmaceuticals, a forecast may be in terms of possible exports in the future years, a disease occurrence, a demand of a drug product into the market, a product expiry date (or shelf life).

Relating to pharmaceutical exports, calculation of Compound Annual Growth Rate (CAGR) needs past years export values and based upon which a CAGR value (percentage) is obtained and based upon the CAGR value, a future possible export of pharmaceuticals can be predicted. The following is the formula used for calculation of CAGR i.e.,

Compound Annual Growth Rate (CAGR) =

$$\{[\text{Ending Year Value/Initial Year Value}]^{1/n} - 1\}$$

Where, n = number of years

As examples, let us suppose that India's export of pharmaceuticals to global countries in World as follows:

Year	Export in Rs. Crore
2001	100
2002	200
2003	300
2004	400
2005	500

Therefore CAGR from 2001 to 2005 = $\{[500/100]^{1/5} - 1\} = 0.4 \equiv 40$ percent

Compound Annual Growth Rate is a widely used parameter at the global and country level not only relating to pharmaceuticals, but also for other disciplines of economics.

As a second example, let us imagine a pharmacy store in a hospital. Observing the past years number of patients visiting the hospital will provide a trend. When a keen observation is made in the trend, one might have observed the maximum number of patients being visiting in the rainy season. This fine observation helps the pharmacist in planning in indenting drug products for the store for the forth coming rainy season. Likewise, a trend analysis of consumption of products in the past in a pharmacy shop may help the pharmacist to order and procure the product that has maximum demand for the coming season.

As a third example, a trend analysis of sale of drug product by manufacturer helps him to plan drug products manufacturing in advance and make available of the product in the market by the season arrives. For such proper planning, the manufacturer has to procure raw materials well before hand, schedule well before for manufacturing in the premises preventing clash with other product manufacturing, supply the product to various parts in the country by the time the season/demand arise. Such planning is imbibed with past data, developing a trend analysis and making the product available in the market well before hand, just the season/demand starts.

As a fourth example, a forecast of when a product patent, process patent, data exclusivity, market exclusivity expires for a drug product helps the generic manufacturer to plan before hand to develop the product, complete bio-equivalence studies, complete drug approval filings and get the drug product approved by the government authority just by the time the product patent/process patent/market exclusivity/data exclusivity of the innovator's expires.

As a fifth example, for every drug product available in the market, the expiry date is mentioned on the product label. The expiry date or the shelf life of the formulation is the time period by which the active drug concentration falls from 100 percent to 90 percent. Hence, when a drug product crosses one day for the expiry date mentioned, it indicates that the concentration (or strength) of the active ingredient has fallen to 90 percent. Calculation of expiry date may also be considered as a forecast since the expiry date has been derived from accelerated stability studies of the drug product.

Table 7.1 to 7.4 and figures 7.1 to 7.3 illustrates sales, export, import and DMF product fillings at USFDA.

TABLE 7.1 Global Pharmaceutical Market (in US $ bn)

Year/Market	2003	2004	2005	2006	2007	2008	2009	2010
Total Global Market in US $ billion (average exchange rate)	561	603	647	692	740	785	840	875
Growth Over Previous Year (average exchange rate)	9.10%	7.60%	7.20%	7.00%	6.90%	6.10%	7.10%	4.10%

TABLE 7.2 Total Size of Pharmaceutical Market by Region

Year	2010	2010	2006-2010	2011	2011-15
	Market Size	% Growth Over Previous Year	CAGR %	Forecast % Growth	CAGR %
US $ in billion	$874.60	4.10%	6.20%	4-5%	3-6%

TABLE 7.3 India's Export-Imports in Drugs, Pharmaceuticals and Fine Chemicals for Financial Year 2004-2011 (in US $ million)

Year/Commodity	Financial Year	2004	2005	2006	2007	2008	2009	2010	2011
Drugs, Pharmaceuticals and Fine Chemicals	Export	3312.99	3972.81	4994.52	5939.75	7644.05	8802.64	8955	10393.53
Medicinal and Pharmaceutical Products	Import	644.17	705.08	1027.75	1292.32	1668.22	1889.11	2100.61	2375.61
Net (Positive Balance)	Net Balance	2668.82	3267.73	3966.77	4647.43	5975.83	6913.53	6854.39	8017.92

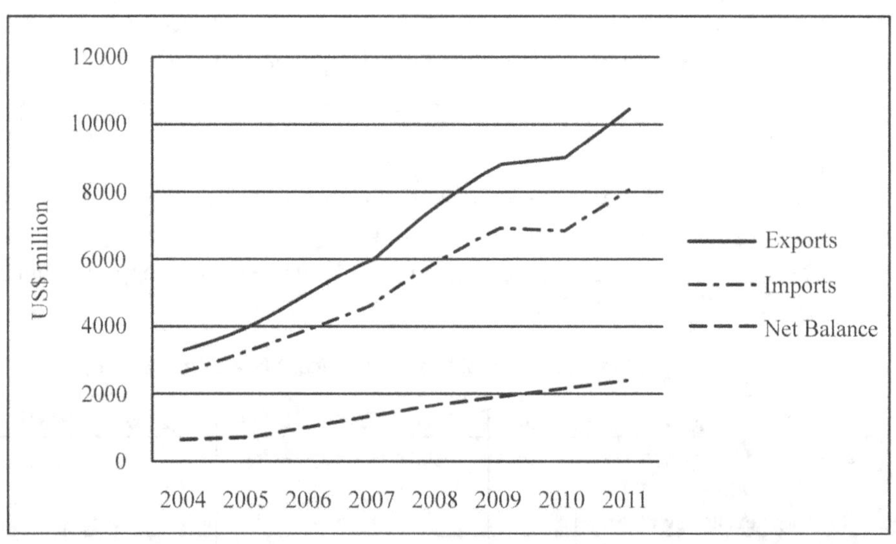

FIGURE 7.1 India's Export-Imports in Drugs, Pharmaceuticals and Fine Chemicals for Financial Year 2004-2011

TABLE 7.4 List of DMF filings at USFDA until 2011-Type Wise

S. No	Type	Type Code	No. of DMFs
1	Manufacturing Sites, Facilities, Operating Procedures and Personnel (no longer applicable)	I	1826
2	Drug Substance, Drug Substance Intermediate, and Material Used in their Preparation or Drug Product	II	15230
3	Packaging Material	III	4511
4	Excipient, Colourant, Flavour, Essence, or material used in their preparation	IV	1749
5	FDA Accepted Reference Information	V	355
6	Blanks	Blanks	1969
	Grand Total		25640

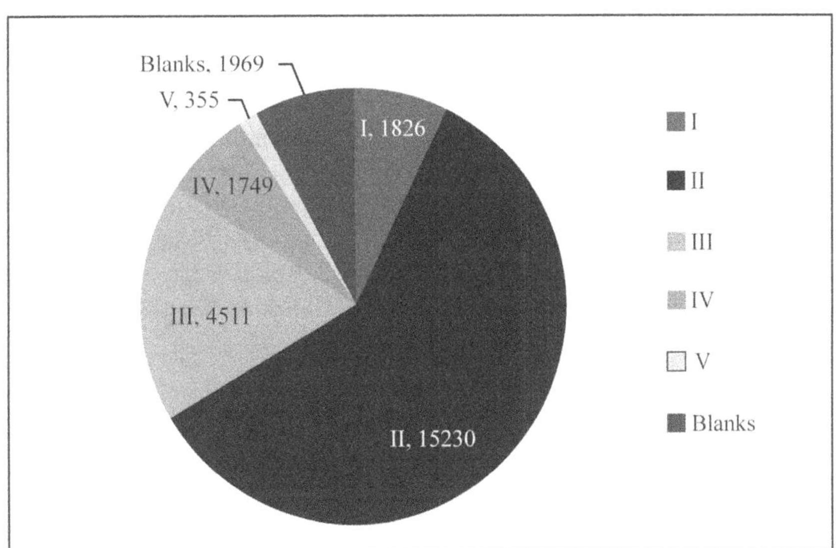

FIGURE 7.2 List of DMFs filed at USFDA until 2011-Type Wise (Global)

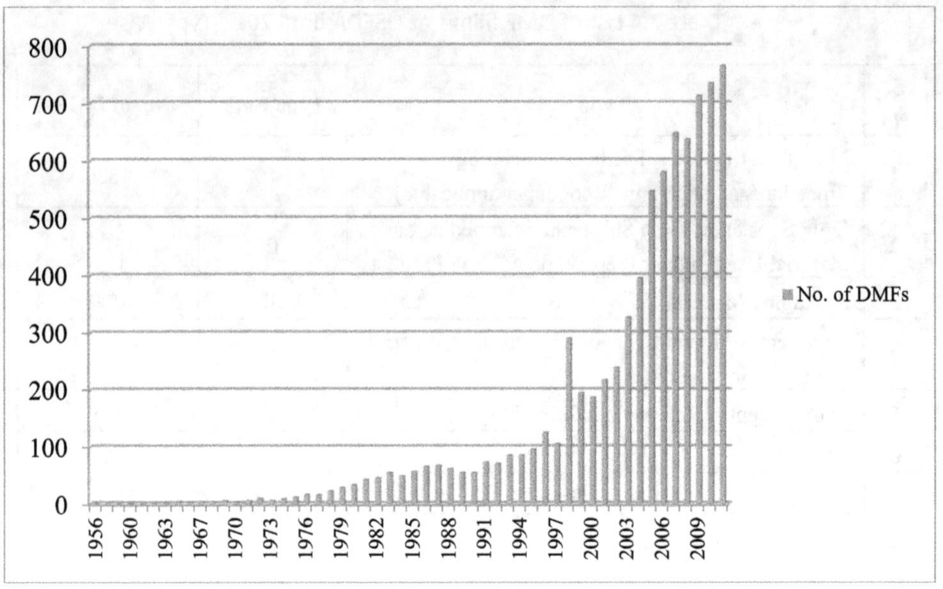

FIGURE 7.3 List of DMFs Type-II Active filed at USFDA (Globally-Year Wise-Until 2011)

iii. Seasonal Study Design

Certain diseases occur in a particular seasonal condition and such study designs are called seasonal. Some of the seasonal diseases are flu, throat infection, dengue fever etc. When a non-clinical study is conducted, imagine in an hospital the number of patients visiting the hospital during rainy season and the current and past statistics of patients visiting will help the hospital administration make necessary arrangements of facilities, key drug products used in the season to predict and make available in the hospital prior hand.

iv. Longitudinal Study: As explained earlier

At the Clinical Trial Registry India (CTRI), the clinical trials are categorized into randomized, parallel group, active controlled; randomized, parallel group, placebo controlled; single arm trial; randomized, parallel group; randomized, parallel group, multiple arm; randomized, cross-over; non-randomized, active controlled; non-randomized, multiple arm; cluster, randomized; randomized factorial; non-randomized, placebo controlled and others.

8 Principles of Experimental Designs

8.0 Introduction

The word principle means a general theorem or law. The three principles of experimental design are principle of replication, principle of randomization and principle of local control.

The objective is to conduct a pharmaceutical non-clinical study or pharmaceutical clinical study with minimal errors and with better precision of results. Hence setting of principles helps the researchers to conduct experiments uniformly.

8.1 Types of Principles

i. Principle of Replication:

In pharmaceutical analysis, for a quantitative method establishment, a drug substance in weighed into a volumetric flask and several dilutions are made with vehicle to get a series of concentrations. The solutions are subjected to UV spectroscopy (double beam spectrometer) to get corresponding absorbance at a specified λ_{max}. The absorbance values are subjected to standard plot against independent variable concentration resulting for a linear plot. Single weighing, single dilutions may result to weighing errors, dilution errors etc. To overcome such possible, the experiment is repeated with at least 6 times so that individual mean absorbance values are taken into consideration.

Likewise, when an investigator is interpreting outcomes of an attribute, there are possibilities of errors and hence, the same experiment is repeated. For instance, Phase II clinical trials are on limited patients and later in Phase III, the studies are extended on a large population at different places. The repetitions of studies are expected to minimize errors.

Yet as one another example, in the determination of LD_{50} of a new chemical entity, say suppose five doses are planned. Hence, six groups containing six animals in each group are planned. Five groups are for different doses, one group as control. The experiment is planned in such a way that every dose group has six animals and each animal receives the same dose in the group. The objective is to minimize the errors (such as dosage error, administration error, accidental death of animal etc.,) that may cause when taken one animal in a group. Hence repetition is expected to minimize the error. A doubt may arise why six animals in a control group. This can be explained that animals naturally have individual variation and various health attributes vary. Collection of data from control group animals will help the researcher to assess the error caused naturally and such variations are taken into consideration while making final judgment of the experiment conducted.

ii. Principle of Randomization:

Randomization is a process of selection of subjects through lottery system, computer generated numbers or through picking a number instantaneously. This is expected to prevent from biasedness in selecting subjects of interest intentionally. Randomization is expected to minimize variations caused by extraneous factors (factors that are irrelevant, external origin).

iii. Principle of Local Control:

For conducting an experiment, a group of diabetic patients were taken into consideration with a selection criterion that the subjects are only having abnormal blood glucose levels with no other associated possible diseases. In the process, the patients visiting the kind of criteria set forth are with blood glucose levels with very high disparity. Considering patients with blood glucose levels with very high disparity is preferable rather than narrow disparity since estimating such wide range disparity that is occurring will result in minimizing errors at a better level. Such considerations are expected to reach the objectives more precisely. Hence, principle of local control is expected to eliminate the variability due to extraneous factors from the experimental error. In simple words, the researcher has to sample from a population in such a way that the sample collected is heterogeneous and not homogeneous to meet the objective that the sample exactly represents the population being studied.

8.2 Types of Experimental Designs

Fulfilling the principles of experimental designs, it is necessary that sampling methods, grouping of subjects, treatment of subjects are not influenced by any unwanted factors. The objective of an experimental design is to ensure better homogeneity is achieved, selection of heterogeneous subjects, so that extraneous factors and other possible errors are minimized. Experimental designs are classified into the following two types:

i. Informal Experimental Designs:

a. Before and after without control design:

In this experimental design an individual (or a group) is checked before a treatment and after the treatment. For instance, an out-patient diabetic has visited for the first time to a hospital and when the doctor counsels the patient, symptoms were identified (either by biochemical tests or by a physical examination) and a medication is prescribed as treatment. The end result is cure from the ailment by checking for normal levels during biochemical tests or by a physical examination. Yet another example is fever condition, where the patient enters the hospital with high fever and after treatment becomes normal.

b.   After only with control design:

In this category of design, a group of patients are divided into two groups (randomly), one as control group (for homogeneity) and other as treatment group. In the control and the treatment groups, the diabetics are tested for blood glucose levels at a specified time. After medication (treatment) to the treatment group, again at a specified time the blood glucose levels of both the groups are checked. The difference in the blood glucose levels between control and treatment groups indicates level of cure of the disease.

c.   Before and after with control design:

In this category of design, two groups are selected (control and treatment group). Dependent variable is measured in both the groups at a specified time. Later, treatment is induced into treatment group and finally, dependent variables are measured at the levels of before treatment (a), without treatment (b) and after treatment (c). The difference between gives the end result of treatment.

ii. Formal Experimental Designs:

a.   Completely randomized design:

The experimental design involves with the principle of replication and the principle of randomization. Uncontrolled extraneous variations can be minimized with complete randomized design technique. The design techniques can be further classified into two i.e.,

i.   Two group sample randomized experimental design:

For instance, 20 subjects were selected as a sample size from a patient population and the patients are equally, randomly assigned into two groups as Control and Treatment groups. The merit of such a design is that it is simple and minimizes the differences among the sample items. But, the demerit is that the individual differences are not eliminated.

ii.   Random replication design:

To overcome the investigators variations in treatments and assessments, a repetition for each treatment is expected to minimize the errors. The design helps to control the differential effects of the extraneous independent variable, randomizes any individual differences among those conducting the treatments.

b.   Randomized block design

In this the experiment, subjects selected for the study are assigned into groups equally, Table 8.1. The subjects in the groups (blocks) are evenly distributed as per the selection criteria. The groups are sub-grouped (sub-blocks) into gender, age etc. Here, a particular group initially considered as control, later as treatment group and further later as placebo group.

TABLE 8.1 Randomized Block Design

Age Group	Group A (Control) Subject No		Group B (Treatment) Subject No		Group C (Placebo) Subject No	
Age 20 to 40 years	1		7		13	
	2		8		14	
Age 41 to 60 years	3		9		15	
	4		10		16	
Above 60 years	5		11		17	
	6		12		18	

c. Latin square design

As the word indicates, when English (Latin) alphabets are arranged in a square manner, the design is called as Latin Square design. For instance, when a four point assay is conducted in the Frog's rectus abdominal muscle for identification of concentration of test sample, the test is compared with standard solution having known concentration. In the experiment, initially, dose response curves with standard solution of different volumes (four volumes) are injected into the tube containing the isolated tissue (connected to kymograph through a lever). Likewise, four response curves are obtained with four volumes of test solution (here concentration of test solution is not known and has to be determined). Out of the four standard responses obtained, two are selected (S_1, S_2) and two test responses (T_1, T_2) are selected. Later, on the same tissue, the solutions are injected as follows, Table 8.2, for recording the responses.

TABLE 8.2 Latin Square Design

S_1	S_2	T_1	T_2
S_2	S_1	T_2	T_1
T_1	T_2	S_1	S_2
T_2	T_1	S_2	S_1

The above design helps in fulfilling the principle of duplication i.e., repeating several experiments on the same tissue helps in understanding the variations that are practically occurring.

d. Factorial design

ICH guidelines insists on Quality by Design (QbD) of experiments with a strong rationale so as to ensure the drug product reach the market at the earliest by doing logical, minimal and effective experiments. Factorial design is one of the approaches for conduct of experiments at the Active Pharmaceutical Ingredient (API) synthesis, formulation development, pre-clinical and the clinical experiments. For optimizing the desired effect, to reach the optimized dependent variable, various independent variables are changed and experiments are conducted to achieve the task to the nearest.

For instance, for achieving the effect of high yield and highly pure API, it is necessary to establish temperature, time of addition and contact of the reactants, kind of catalysts, kind of combination of reactants, sequence of addition of reactants etc., In case of achieving optimal hardness of a tablet formulation, the factors such as pressure, lubricant etc. play a key role. In case of dissolution, the factors such as concentration of lubricant, disintegrating agent etc., play a key role.

A factor is a variable such as concentration of an agent, temperature, drug treatment, diet. In an experiment, the number of factors may be more than one and this depends on the objective and kind of experimental task. A factor can be qualitative assigned with a name and (or) quantitative assigned with a number. It is believed that single factor designs fit for one-way ANOVA. In order to achieve the desired effect, every factor has to be optimized individually and their combinations. In order to achieve optimized factor/s, every factor is studied at various levels, and the levels of various factors that are giving optimized desired effect are considered ideal.

In a factorial design, the number of runs and trials depends on the number of factors and number of levels of the factors. For instance, if there are two factors and two levels, there are four numbers of runs and trials.

For instance, to achieve desired hardness of tablet, two factors such as pressure and lubricant are considered, and then we have the number of runs (or trials) as follows, Table 8.3:

TABLE 8.3 Factorial Design

Desired Effect/Factors	Pressure	Lubricant
Hardness of tablet	High	High Concentration
Hardness of tablet	High	Low Concentration
Hardness of tablet	Low	High Concentration
Hardness of tablet	Low	Low Concentration

When two ingredients such as A, B are taken into consideration, to their highest levels, and their combination as a dosage form resulted in an additive effect, then the effect is biologically synergistic. If the combination resulted into an effect less than the additive, then it is interpreted that there is some interaction (say antagonist activity).

Now let us take into consideration, a lubricant and its effect on drug effect. When the drug effects were measured at low and high lubricant levels and were found to be the same, the system is considered as additive and no interaction exists. In general, during comparisons, additive effects have parallel lines where as interactions have non-parallel lines, in a plotted graph response vs. drug, Figures: 8.1, 8.2.

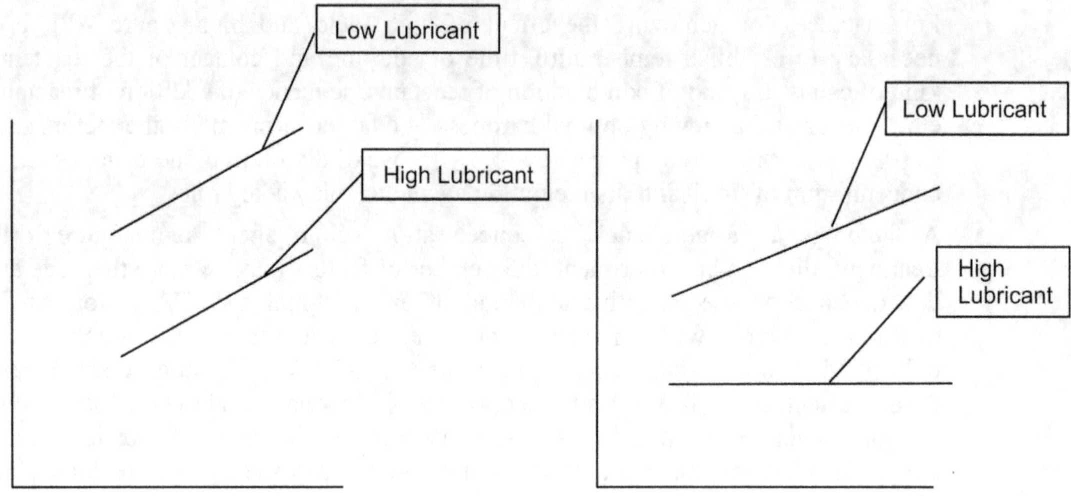

FIGURE 8.1 Response vs. Drug   **FIGURE 8.2** Response vs. Drug

The advantages with factorial design are that, firstly one can estimate maximum efficiency of main effect, when there is no interaction. Secondly, one can identify the type of interactions that exists, thirdly one can draw conclusions of the effects after conducting several runs (or trials) using various levels. Lastly, where factorial designs lead to orthogonal, all estimated effects and interactions are independent of effects of other factors, that is, the main effect is not influenced by other factors of the experiment whereas in non-orthogonal designs, effects are not independent (example of conditions of confounding). This can be explained with an example of two drugs and their comparison being made at two different places. The confounding issues such as difference in patients, difference in treatment, difference in disease state can be minimized by well-planned factorial design.

A factorial design is represented by say "2^3", indicating the base for number of levels and the power for number of factors. Among the factorial designs, the simplest is the "2^2" indicating for four runs (or trails) whereas in case of "2^3", three factors each at two levels, indicating for eight runs (or trials). This indicates, eight experiments are conducted without any duplication of the same experiment. For instance, an experiment is planned to achieve an ideal, uniform thickness of tablet formulation using three factors (components) i.e., stearate, drug and starch. As a thumb rule, the choice of levels in two level experiments is to divide extreme ranges of a factor into four equal parts and take $1/4^{th}$ and $3/4^{th}$ values as the choice of levels. Hence, a factorial design helps in understanding mechanism of experiment system, set practical procedure for manufacture, and is a source of lead for further experimentations. If a response leads to linearity, it is sufficient to have two levels where as in case of non-linear (curved), there is a necessity of at least three levels.

8.3   Experimental Planning of a Factorial Design

Let us imagine to establish thickness of tablet using three components (factors) i.e., stearate, drug and starch. For a three factors, each at two levels, 2 x 2 x 2, eight trials are necessary for a full factorial design. This is called as 2^3 factorial design (i.e., three factors, two levels). Let us image the two levels as high and low levels. In general, let us imagine three factors A, B, C and if all the factors are at their low levels, it is represented by (l), if the factor 'A' is at high level and the remaining factors 'B' and 'C' are at low levels, let us assume the notation as 'a'. If factors 'A' and 'B' are at high levels, and 'C' is at the low levels, let us assume the notation as 'ab'.

It is necessary to understand that a careful and well planned objectives, help in understanding mechanism of experimental system, helps in recommending set of conditions and procedures for manufacturing, and final guidance for further experimentation.

Let us imagine the levels of the factors are as follows:

Factor/Level	Low Level (mg)	High Level (mg)
A: Stearate	0.5	1.5
B: Drug	60.0	120.0
C: Starch	30.0	50.0

If one of the factors is studied at three levels, then 2 x 2 x 3 = 12 formulations have to be tested. As the researcher feels that a two level is sufficient enough to identify the effects, the experiment is so planned. The results without any replications are as follows:

Results of 2^3 Factorial Experiment: Effect of Stearate, Drug and Starch Concentration on Tablet Thickness				
Factor combination	Stearate	Drug	Starch	Reponse (thickness) (cm x 10^{-3})
(1)	-	-	-	475
a	+	-	-	487
b	-	+	-	421
ab	+	+	-	426
c	-	-	+	525
ac	+	-	+	546
bc	-	+	+	472
abc	+	+	+	522

For current two level experiment, to calculate the effects, after assigning the '+ (high level)' or '-(low level)' sign, the arithmetic computation is made. Hence the above mentioned eight experiments (runs) have to be assigned with a sign and are as follows:

Signs to Calculate Effects in a 2^3 Factorial Experiment							
Factor combination	Level of Factor in Experiment			Interaction#			
	A	B	C	AB	AC	BC	ABC
(1)	-	-	-	+	+	+	-
a	+	-	-	-	-	+	+
b	-	+	-	-	+	-	+
ab	+	+	-	+	-	-	-
c	-	-	+	+	-	-	+
ac	+	-	+	-	+	-	-
bc	-	+	+	-	-	+	-
abc	+	+	+	+	+	+	+

Note: '-' factor at low level, '+' factor at high level

= Multiplication of signs of factors to obtain signs for interaction terms in combination

It can be interpreted from the above table that signs in the columns of A, B, C indicate whether in high or low level. In case of columns, AB, AC, BC, ABC, it indicates the multiplication of signs of the individual components. For instance, for interaction of 'AB', we multiply '-' x '-' to get '+' and so on.

To obtain the average effect, multiply the response times the sign for each of the eight runs in a column and divide the result by 2^{n-1}, where n = number of factors.

Hence, the main effect for factor A (Stearate) is as follows:

$$= \frac{\left[-(1) + a - b + ab - c + ac - bc + abc\right]}{4}$$

when the above equation is re-arranged, it can be written as follows:

$$\text{Main effect of A} = \frac{a + ab + ac + abc}{4} - \frac{(1) + b + c + bc}{4}$$

Then above equation can be interpreted as the average of all results at the high level of A minus the average of all results at the low level of A. Upon substituting the values, we get

Main effect of A

$$= \left\{ \left[\left(\frac{[487 + 426 + 546 + 522]}{4} \right) - \left(\frac{[475 + 421 + 525 + 472]}{4} \right) \right] \times 10^{-3} \right\} = 0.022 \text{ cm}$$

From the above equation, it can be interpreted that the net effect by increasing stearate from low level (0.5 mg of stearate) to high level (1.5 mg of stearate), the tablet thickness is increased by 0.022 cm.

For interaction of AC (say), it is defined as one-half the difference between the effect of 'A' when 'C' is at the high level and the effect of 'A' when 'C' is at the low level.

Hence,

$$AC\ int\,eraction = \frac{1}{4}\{(abc + ac - bc - c) - [ab + a - b - (1)]\}$$

Experimentally, it was observed that with starch (factor C) at the high level, 50 mg, increasing the stearate concentration from the low to the high level (from 0.5 mg to 1.5 mg) results in an increased thickness of 0.0355 cm. At the low level of starch, 30 mg, increasing stearate concentration from 0.5 mg to 1.5 mg results in an increased thickness of 0.0085 cm. Thus stearate has a greater effect at the higher starch concentration, a possible starch x stearate interaction.

8.4   Hand Analysis of Factorial Experiments (Method of Yates)

The current method is devised by Yates and is a systematic analysis of data from 2^n factorial experiments and is a simple hand analysis which now a day computer can analyze and give the result. The analysis is with respect to previous section data and is as follows:

Yates Analysis of the Factorial Tableting Experiment for Analysis of Variance						
Combination	Thickness (x 10^{-3} cm)	(1)	(2)	(3)	Effect (x 10^{-3} cm) (3)/4 (say a)	Mean Square (x 10^{-6}) (a)^2/8
(1)	475	962	1809	3874	---	---
a	487	847	2065	88	22.0	968
b	421	1071	17	-192	-48.0	4608
ab	426	994	71	22	5.5	60.5
c	525	12	-115	256	64.0	8192
ac	546	5	-77	54	13.5	364.5
bc	472	21	-7	38	9.5	180.5
abc	522	50	29	36	9.0	162

Step 1: Data (thickness of tablet) are added in pair and placed in first four rows of column (1), later the data are subtracted in pair (second minus first) and placed in the subsequent four rows of the column (1).

Step 2: Data is column (1) are added in pair and placed in first four rows of column (2), later the data are subtracted in pair (second minus first) and placed in the subsequent four rows of the column (2).

Step 3: Data in column (2) are added in pair and placed in first four rows of column (3), later the data are subtracted in pair (second minus first) and placed in the subsequent four rows of the column (3).

Step 4: Data in column (3) is divided by 2^{n-1} (i.e., $2^{3-1}=2^2=4$, where 'n' is no. of factors)

Step 5: Mean square is calculated by taking value in column (3) and squaring it and later dividing by 8.

Step 6: In a 2^n factorial experiment, each effect and interaction has 1 degree of freedom and the error mean square for test can be obtained after running duplicates (i.e., repeating the run right from scratch which means preparing a new mix with the same ingredients, retableting and measuring the thickness of tablets in this new batch). After ANOVA analysis, the data can be seen as follows:

Analysis of Variance for the Factorial Tableting Experiment				
Factor	Source	d. f	Mean Square (x 10^6)	F[a]
A	Stearate	1	968	7.2 (at $p < 0.1$)
B	Drug	1	4608	34.3 (at $p < 0.01$)
C	Starch	1	8192	61.0 (at $p < 0.01$)
AB	Stearate x drug	1	60.5	
AC	Stearate x starch	1	364.5	2.7
BC	Drug x starch	1	180.5	
ABC	Stearate x drug x starch	1	162	
[a]Error mean square based on AB, BC and ABC interactions, 3 d. f				

Taking the mean squares for the effects of interest A, B, C and AC, although not statistically significant, stearate and starch interact to a small extent, and examination of the data is necessary to describe the effect. Since B does not interact with A or C, it is sufficient to calculate the effect of drug (B), averaged over all levels of A and C, to explain the effect. The effect of drug is to decrease the thickness by 0.048 mm (see effect column in above mentioned Table) when the drug concentration is raised from 60 to 120 mg.

9 Need of Sampling and Sampling Techniques

9.0 Introduction

For a statistical study, it is not always possible to compile data from the population. Government spends money for compilation of data from entire population only for Census. Fresh census studies are conducted for every 10 years or so. With the advent of computers, such census studies are being made by compilation of information during birth, death registrations. Where countries does not have any computer facilities, hardcopy of registers are still being maintained. Hence, it is necessary to understand that getting data from entire population is expensive, time consuming, tedious.

Usually scientific studies are initiated on a sample of population. A sample selected from a population must represent all the characteristics of the population. A sample selected should be homogenous keeping in view the heterogeneity of the variables (parameters/attributes) so that end statistical analysis results in precise conclusions.

It is necessary to estimate or calculate errors caused during sampling or non-sampling and at a later stage eliminated from final results for precision. A non-sampling error may not mean that sampling is not being done but means that the investigators are not uniform in conducting same treatment, interpretations, not collecting data from all subjects of the sample etc.

9.1 Types of Sampling Techniques

Sampling techniques are classified into two categories i.e.,

i. Non-probability sampling technique:

Probability is a chance of occurrence of an incident. The maximum value of probability is unity. When a coin is tossed the probability of getting heads is 0.5 and the probability of getting tails is also 0.5.

Non-probability sampling is also called as deliberate sampling, purposive sampling or judgment sampling. In the current technique, the investigator has the independence in selecting subjects of his choice. Hence non-probability sampling technique may yield to a bias in sampling, but investigators ensure that they are impartial; work without bias so that bold judgments can be made to meet the objective of the study. In several cases, in the current technique of sampling, sampling errors may not be estimated and the elements of bias persist. Several investigators are assigned to complete a specific number of data collections per day and are being influenced by some restrictions in filling the data, but are provided with independence in selection of the sample at the investigator's discretion. The advantage with non-probability sampling techniques is convenient and relatively inexpensive.

ii. Probability sampling techniques:

Probability sampling is also called as random sampling, chance sampling. In a population, while selecting subjects for a sample, the chance of each subject of the population being selected is equal. The technique ensures law of statistical regularity which states that a subject drawn on random, the sample has the same characteristics of the population.

Probability sampling is categorised into two types:

i. Simple random sampling:

Let us consider a population of 'N' and from the population, 'n' subjects have to be selected as a sample. The possible combinations of selecting 'n' subjects from the population are given by $^{N}C_n$. The probability (chance) of selection of a subject in the population can be given by $1/^{N}C_n$.

For instance, from a population of 6 (1,2,3,4,5,6) subjects, if a sample of 3 have to be selected means that there are 20 possible combinations of three subjects being selected i.e., $^{6}C_3 \equiv 6 \times 5 \times 4/3 \times 2 \times 1 \equiv 5 \times 4 = 20$. (This implies 123, 456, 124, 125, 126, 234, 235, 236, 345, 346 ......). Finally, the probability of any one of the sample containing 3 subjects being picked is $1/^{6}C_3 \equiv 1/20 = 0.05$.

In several cases, while conducting a random sampling from a population, whether the subject once picked for the sample has to be replaced back in the population? As the chances of the same subject being picked for the second time is also possible, the subject is usually not included back in the population.

ii. Complex random sampling:

In a complex random sampling, the sampling is inherent with both probability and non-probability sampling.

Complex random sampling is classified into six types:

a. Systematic complex random sampling:

Let us consider 100 patients were selected from a population. Out of the 100 patients, the objective is to select a sample size of 10 patients. Let us assume that all the hundred patients are given with 1 to 100 numbers. The first step is out of patients having 1 to 10 numbers, one patient number is randomly selected i.e., say 3. Hence, the ten patients selected for the sample are 3, 13, 23, 33, 43, 53, 63, 73, 83 and 93. It is necessary to ensure that all the hundred patients were assigned with number 1 to 100 on random.

b.   Stratified complex random sampling:

Let us suppose that, the objective of study is to have 10 diabetic patients as sample size without any other complications. Let us image, the population size of diabetic patients is 1000 and they do not have any other complications. The said population are so heterogeneous in their age, blood glucose levels etc. If a random sampling is done, the chance of selecting 10 patients representing the population is less. This means, that all the heterogeneous characteristics of the population are not being available in the sample.

To overcome the situation, the population is divided into strata and each stratum is defined with characteristic features.

TABLE 9.1 Stratification Sampling

Stratum	Age	Population (after sorting)	Proportion with respect to total population (a)	To achieve sample size of 10 patients (10 x a)
Stratum 1	20-40 years	100	100/1000=1/10	10x1/10=1
Stratum 2	40-60 years	300	300/1000=3/10	10x3/10=3
Stratum 3	Above 60 years	600	600/1000=6/10=3/5	10x3/5=6

In the above mentioned Table 9.1, after sorting out the 1000 patients (from population) into the different stratum (here, age wise), the proportions of patients with respect to total population was calculated. The factor is ten multiplied with the required total number of patients for the sample.

Based on the calculation, it is necessary that one patient from stratum 1, three patients from stratum 2 and six patients from stratum 3 are to be included in the sample for further studies.

Now the question is how to select the required number of patients from the stratum. This is achieved by random sampling from the corresponding stratum.

Hence, the current technique gives a route to select samples from different stratum that truly represent the entire heterogeneous population.

Based upon the above exercise, the conditions for this technique are

i.   Defining the characteristics of stratum.

ii.   Achieving required sample size from the stratified population.

iii. Selection of patients on random basis from the corresponding stratified population of the stratum.

c.   Cluster type complex random sampling:

If a sample has to be drawn from a large population area, in this technique, the large population area is sorted into non-overlapping sub-areas called as clusters. Randomly a selected number of clusters are picked from the whole and from those clusters random sampling may be done. The advantage with cluster sampling is that it reduces cost and the disadvantage is that it is less precise than random sampling. If cluster sampling is from a geographical area, it is called as area sampling.

For instance: In a pharmaceutical industry, 10,00,000 tablets were manufactured in one batch. To comply with the pharmacopoeial assay method etc, 20 to 100 tablets are required. In order to ensure the principles of experimental design i.e., principle of replication, principle of randomization and principle of local control, industry develop in-house protocol for sampling at the initial stage while establishing the industry, equipment, manufacturing of the product etc and establish validation procedures (prospective, retrospective, concurrent or revalidation procedures). The entire 10, 00, 000 tablets (population) is divided as clusters (in several containers) and the investigator who wish to collect sample has to selectively pick samples from randomly picked containers (clusters). This may lead to several thousands of tablets. From this he may select at random 100 tablets required for conducting the pharmacopoeial test. As samples selected should represent the population, the investigator has to keep in mind homogeneous factors, heterogeneous factors and also the extraneous factors.

d. Multi-stage sampling:

Multi-stage sampling technique is an advanced technique to cluster sampling technique. In this technique, the sampling is made based on a very large population than in cluster sampling technique. Let us image, the objective of the study is to know the performance of community pharmacies in the entire country. In such a case, a sampling is made similar to cluster design i.e., initially selection of states on a random basis, later selection of districts on random basis, and later selection of towns on random basis and finally studying entire pharmacies in the town or selecting some pharmacies on random basis within the town. If the sample is from all the stages mentioned, the design is called multi-stage sampling.

It is necessary to understand that both in cluster and multi-stage sampling the population number is not the same.

e. Sampling with probability proportional to size:

In this technique, large patient population is divided into non-overlapping clusters and the clusters may or may not contain same number of patients. In this technique, for sampling, clusters are selected on random and the patients in the randomly selected clusters are picked randomly. Here the probability of each cluster being included in the sample is proportional to the size of the cluster.

Let us consider, the objective of the study is to assess the performance of community pharmacies located in 20 cities and the numbers of community pharmacies in each city are 25, 30, 50, 75, 100, 15, 60, 90, 10, 45, 85, 95, 75, 70, 5, 55, 32, 73, 12, and 23. The required sample size of community pharmacies is 30. The question is how to select the cities and how many samples (community pharmacies) have to be collected from the community pharmacies of the cities.

TABLE 9.2 Calculation of Sample Size proportional to Size of Population

City Number	Number of Community Pharmacies in the City	Cumulative total number of community pharmacies	City Number from which samples have to be selected	Total number of samples to be picked from the city and from the community pharmacies
1	25	25	5	1
2	30	55	39	1
3	50	105	73	1
4	75	180	107, 141, 174	3
5	100	280	209, 243, 277	3
6	15	295		
7	60	355	311, 345	2
8	90	445	379, 413	2
9	10	455	447	1
10	45	500	481	1
11	85	585	515, 549, 583	3
12	95	680	617, 651	2
13	75	755	685, 719, 753	3
14	70	825	787, 821	2
15	5	830		
16	55	885	855	1
17	32	917	889	1
18	73	990	923, 957	2
19	12	1002	991	1
20	23	1025		

In the above Table 9.2, initially all the cities are serial numbered and corresponding number of community pharmacies available in the city were mentioned. As a next step, a cumulative total of numbers of community pharmacies available are calculated. It has been observed that a total of 1025 community pharmacies available in the 20 cities. Our objective is to collect 30 pharmacies from a total 1025 cities and 20 cities. The next step is to find the ratio of total number of community pharmacies to number of community pharmacies to be considered as sample size i.e., 1025/30= 34.1666667. Hence, the sample interval can be considered as 34 (factor). Starting with the least number of community pharmacies 5, add cumulatively 34 and from the corresponding city, the pharmacy is randomly selected.

f.   Sequential sampling:

In a sequential sampling technique, the sample design is complex as the investigator is not aware until conducting some sample survey and does some mathematical and statistical decisions. This enhances statistical quality control system. If a particular lot is accepted or rejected based on single sample, it is called as single sampling. If a particular lot is accepted or rejected based two samples, it is called as double sampling. If the acceptance or rejection of the lot depends on more than two sampling but the number of samples is fixed and decided in advance, the sampling technique is named as multiple sampling. If the acceptance or rejection of the lot depends on more than two sampling but the number of samples is neither fixed nor decided in advance, the sampling technique is named as sequential sampling.

For instance, sequential sampling is used to establish sampling procedures, statistical methods for the first time in the pharmaceutical industry where the machines, manufacturing of the tablets are being done for the first time after installation of the machines. This procedure helps in validating the manufacturing processes, sampling procedures etc.

10 Measurement and Scaling

10.0 Introduction

Measurement is defined as an association or an assignment of a number to an experimental observation. A number is assigned for an observation with reference to a physically accepted standard measure (length, weight, height scales, attraction towards colours etc.,) or based on abstract imagination. For instance, weight of the tablet is 500 mg which is based on a comparison with a standard physical weight. In case of assessing level of intelligence, pain, beauty, complexity, odour etc numbers are assigned upon imagination by setting guidelines of number scaling. Hence, measurements can be considered as either qualitative or quantitative.

10.1 Classification of Measurement Scales

Scales in several cases are standard references that are well accepted globally or that are defined for a specific experimentation purpose. Scales are classified into four types i.e., nominal, ordinal, interval and ratio scales.

i. **Nominal Scale:** In case of nominal scaling numbers are assigned for identity purpose. The number does not have any significance for its face and place value. For instance, a population of 30 rats was grouped into six groups and was assigned with group numbers as Group 1, Group 2, Group 3, Group 4, Group 5, and Group 6. The group number helps only in identifying the group. Likewise in a group, six rats were assigned with A, B, C, D, E and F which gives an identity for each rat respectively. Likewise assigning of roll numbers to students in a class. Chi-square test is the most common for such scale for statistical significance.

ii. **Ordinal Scale:** In case of ordinal scale, numbers are assigned in a particular order of priority i.e., 1st rank to student 'A', 2nd rank to student 'Z', 3rd rank to student 'C' etc. Here the rank number assigned is associated to the student 'A' based on the highest marks attained by him in the class, but the rank number itself does not represent the highest marks. Ordinal scale is widely used for non-parametric statistical methods.

iii. **Interval Scale:** In case of interval scale, the difference between two numbers signifies the scale. For instance, while performing pyrogen testing on rabbits, the initial temperature and the final temperature and its difference interval signifies whether there is any elevated temperature or not, signifying the presence or absence of pyrogens. In yet another circumstance, patients are grouped in various strata i.e., age groups (say) 10 to 20 years, 20 to 40 years etc. The interval scale here may or may not be of the same value. For instance, two individuals have fever, one with 100° F and the other with 102° F. The elevation in temperature is signified with the respective difference intervals from the reference temperature of 98.4° F (normal temperature). An interval scale value may be qualitative or quantitative based on the circumstances. The statistical tests for interval scale have significance for "t test" and "F test".

iv. **Ratio Scale**: A mathematical representation of multiplication or division for comparing two individuals leads to a ratio scale. For instance, A (120 kgs) is twice heavier than B (60 kgs) i.e., 120/60=2/1. A ratio scale is a factor several times helpful in stratified sampling technique where the population is so heterogeneous. Geometric and harmonic means are used as a measure of central tendency.

Among the various scales, nominal scale is the least precise and the ratio scale is the most precise.

10.2 Salient Features of Measurement Scales

A measurement scale should fulfill the four criteria of validity, reliability, practicality, accuracy.

i. **Validity:** The scale is expected to fulfill the desired degree of measuring for which it is meant for. Scales are validated based on three categories i.e., a) content validity-covers topic under study, b) criterion related validity-covers and reveals a current condition, c) construct validity-covers predicted correlation with theoretical.

ii. **Reliability:** The scale is said to be reliable provided it gives consistent results. For a research task the instrument should be valid and reliable. It is necessary to understand that a reliable scale is not as valuable as validity, but it is easier to assess reliability rather than validity.

iii. **Practicality:** A scale is said to fulfill practicality in terms of being economical, convenient and provides with good interpretation of results even to a third party. Keeping apart with respect to physical standard scales, in medical and pharmaceutical research it is necessary to design scales (on the spot) and have to be scientifically ensured for validity, reliability and practicality. For instance, several scales are designed as questionnaires for quality of life (QOL) and health related quality of life studies (HRQOL) that includes with abstract questions and answering.

iv. **Accuracy:** A scale is said to be accurate provided it measures the expected value itself and not any value near to the expected value. For instance, a fourth decimal weighing balance gives accurate weighing than second or third decimal weighing balance.

10.3   Designing of Measurement Scales

Especially relating to measurement scales designed for abstract questions and answering, the scale should overcome from errors so that abstract answering becomes a precise outcome. An abstract measurement scale helps to identify the status of a patient before and after treatment. For instance, in a hospital when a patient arrives, a doctor counsels the patient in terms of physical scale parameters as well as abstract scale parameters. In order to measure abstract attributes of a patient, it may be necessary to develop a measurement scale (abstract scale).A researcher should keep in mind the possible errors caused by respondent, circumstances/situation, measurer, instrument itself (questionnaire). Errors are possible from respondent in answering due to lack of knowledge, mood status. In case of circumstances/situation several patients expect comfort and confidentiality of information of the patients.   To overcome this, the patient should be provided with privacy from other patients in answering the instrument. The common errors caused with a measurer are lacking uniformity in questioning, using different languages for the same instrument. Fourthly, improper or ambiguous questioning and answering system in the questionnaire (instrument or scale) itself leads to confusion in answering.

Prior designing a measurement scale, the investigator has to take into consideration the following aspects:

i.   Development of a Concept

ii.   Development of Concept dimensions

iii.   Development of indicators

iv.   Development of Index

The investigator has a concept (i.e., idea) to estimate the Health Related Quality of Life (HRQOL) of diseased patients. Health related quality of life refers to individual's physical, mental and social well being.   The investigator has two options for developing measurement scales i.e., a generic or a disease specific scale.   In the former case, the scale is suitable in any disease condition, but the latter is very specific to a disease condition. With an objective to develop a health related quality of life assessment instrument, the investigator has to identify different attributes (dimensions) that influence the quality of life (health related). For instance, RAND-36 instrument (measurement scale), a health related quality of life (HRQOL) instrument is featured with eight health concepts with multi-item scales (35 items), physical functioning (10 items), role limitations caused by physical health problems (4 items), role limitations caused by emotional problems (3 items), social functioning (2 items), emotional well being (5 items), energy/fatigue (4 items), pain (2 items) and general health perception (5 items).   The entire instrument assesses the patients/subjects physical component as scales. As the name RAND-36 indicates, a total of 36 questions are categorised into eight health concepts. The eight health concepts fulfill for 35 questions and the 36th question is relating to health change.

Each concept comprises of dimensions (called as items) and are as follows:

Question 1. In general, would you say your health is:

Excellent	Very good	Good	Fair	Poor
1	2	3	4	5

Question 2: Compared to one year ago, how would you rate your health in general now?

Much better now than one year ago	Somewhat better now than one year ago	About the same	Somewhat worse now than one year ago	Much worse now than one year ago
1	2	3	4	5

The following items are about activities you might do during a typical day. Does your health now limit you in these activities? If so, how much?

Question 3: Vigorous activities, such as running, lifting heavy objects, participating in strenuous sports

Yes, Limited a Lot	Yes, Limited a Little	No, Not Limited at All
1	2	3

During the past 4 weeks, have you had any of the following problems with your work or other regular daily activities as a result of your physical health?

Question 4: Cut down the amount of time you spent on work or other activities:

Yes	No
1	2

During the past 4 weeks, have you had any of the following problems with your work or other regular daily activities as a result of any emotional problems (such as feeling depressed or anxious?)

Question 5: Cut down the amount of time you spent on work or other activities

Yes	No
1	2

Question 6: How much bodily pain have you had during the past 4 weeks?

None	Very mild	Mild	Moderate	Severe	Very Severe
1	2	3	4	5	6

These questions are about how you feel and how things have been with you during the past 4 weeks. For each question, please give the one answer that comes closest to the way you have been feeling. How much of the time during the past 4 weeks…..

Question 7: Did you feel full of pep?

All of the Time	Most of the Time	A Good Bit of the Time	Some of the Time	A Little of the Time	None of the Time
1	2	3	4	5	6

How true or false is each of the following statements for you.

Question 8: My health is excellent.

Definitely True	Mostly True	Don't Know	Mostly False	Definitely False
1	2	3	4	5

In the above mentioned instrument, several items (questions) were questioned to the patients/subjects. Every question is mentioned with fixed indicators (answers) and based on the patient's condition; he is expected to choose the right one.

The indicator selected is assigned with a score, which is confidential. The researcher is expected to feed the chosen indicator for each item (question) into software that gives the final score under the eight concepts.

The scores can be considered as sub-sub-index leading to sub-index and finally leading to index that finally gives Physical Component and Mental Component Summary Scales and finally as one scale as Health Related Quality of Life (HRQOL) score.

This means that every individual concept (total 8) has a score of 100 and the final HRQOL score is a total of eight concept scores i.e., 100 + 100 + 100 + 100 + 100 + 100 + 100 + 100 = 800. Hence, a HRQOL score of 0 indicates the least quality of life and the score of 800 indicates the highest quality of life relating to health.

10.4   Basis for Design of Measurement Scales

In order to design the concept dimensions, indicators and index, based on the following principles, the scales have to be designed:

i. **Subject Orientation**: Here, subject indicates the patients. A question designed as a dimension/indicator should be either in favour of the subject or in favour of the attribute (stimulus) that is being assessed. In the former case, variations in the subjects are assessed keeping attributes homogenous. Where as in the latter case, variations in the attributes are small and the different stimuli are set for assessment. For instance: subjects and smoking stimulus.

   a. Several subjects being asked whether smoking or not. If smoking, the variation is less and the subjects are analyzed for their variation i.e., how many males, females, age group etc.

    b. Several smoking subjects being asked with no. of cigarettes smoking per day with a scale of 1 to 7.

ii. **Response Form:** A question is framed in such a way that either as rating (categorical scale) or as ranking (comparative scale) formats. In a rating scale, for instance of assessing pungency of a smell, the subject is asked for picking on of the options among 1 to 7 scale. In case of ranking scale, the subject is asked to compare the test smell with a standard reference smell.

iii. **Degree of Subjectivity:** The questions are framed in such a way that the subject selects options from the given large choice or providing options by giving limited choice. For instance, giving more options and picking one is different from giving limited options and asking for picking one option i.e., picking one apple from a basket full is different from picking from a basket having only three apples.

iv. **Scale Properties:** Here the questions are framed based on the type of outcome scale expected i.e., nominal scale, ordinal scale, interval scale or ratio scale.

v. **Number of Dimensions:** Here the question is either single or a single question having several multiple questions for assessing a concept dimension or indicator. In several cases, a multi-dimensional questioning is preferred for precise outcomes. For instance, for assessing patients whether smoking or not, if smoking how many cigarettes per day, age group levels and their smoking status are some of the multi-dimensional scales to explore with respect to patient as well as level of smoking.

vi. **Contribution of Scale Techniques:** Developing a scale can be achieved using various techniques such as

    a. **Arbitrary approach:** In this, the question and scale are developed and checked for its acceptance (adhoc basis) and if identified for changes, necessary are being made.

    b. **Consensus approach:** In this the question and scale are developed initially and with experts suggestions, suitable changes are made, if necessary. The other way is identifying several experts in the field, based on their suggestions, questions and scaling are developed.

    c. **Item analysis approach:** In this the question and scale are developed for several items and analysed by taking feed back with a sample of subjects. Based on the scores, a judgment may be made to incorporate the best suitable questions.

    d. **Cumulative approach:** In this the questions are framed in such a way that a cumulative assessment is made so that several indicators with lower outcome or with higher outcome resulting in precise outcomes.

    e. **Factor approach:** In this the questions are framed in such a way to identify the common factors and their association with other dimensions or indicators.

Here, RAND-36 questionnaire (Annexure III) is a framework of questions keeping in view of all the above mentioned principles of designing a measurement scale.

After a measurement scale has been developed, it is necessary to ensure for validity, reliability and for good interpretations. In case of RAND-36, the questionnaire is ensured for validity in terms of aimed aspect of Health Related Quality of Life (HRQoL), reliability is ensured by subjecting response recorded in the instrument into softwares like SPSS and assessing for Cronbach's alpha. In the third case, a third party can easily administer the instrument and the scores can be assessed and interpreted relating to the outcome of HRQoL of a patient.

11 Scaling Techniques

11.0 Introduction

Developing scale (or questionnaire or instrument) involves development of concept, dimensions, indicators and index. Scaling techniques helps in further precise development of the aspects.

11.1 Classification of Scaling Techniques

Scaling techniques are classified into

i. **Comparison Scaling:** As the word indicates, one is compared with another and a scoring is given. Comparison scaling is classified into three types:

a. **Paired comparison:**

For instance, let us consider ten paracetamol syrups having different colours. Out of the ten colours, the patient is asked to pick one of the colours of his choice. In a scientific manner, the patient has to initially pick one and compare with another one. Out of the one selected, he has to pick another one and compare and select among the two. This process is continued until all the ten colours are compared and finally leading to one colour which he finally decides as his choice.

In order to complete the task, the following formula is the short notation:

No. of Experiments (N) = n(n-1)/2

Where, n= number of objects.

In the above experiment, $10(10 - 1)/2 = (10 \times 9)/2 = 90/2 = 45$ experiments have to be conducted to come to a final judgment.

b. **Rank order:** Let us imagine three products A, B, and C out of which one has to be selected. In a rank order, several persons are asked ranking the three products and a final judgment is made with respect to the product which has the highest number of first rank. For instance:

Product/ Persons	Product A	Product B	Product C
Person 1	I	II	III
Person 2	II	I	III
Person 3	I	III	II
Person 4	I	III	II
Person 5	I	II	III
Person 6	I	III	II

In the above case, Product A has the highest number of first ranks and is considered.

c. **Constant sum:** In this method of choosing, a fixed points (say 100 total) is shared among the products based on person's choice and upon final score for the products, the highest score product is selected.

Products/ Persons	Product A	Product B	Product C	Total
Person 1	100	0	0	100
Person 2	0	0	100	100
Person 3	0	100	0	100
Person 4	90	5	5	100
Person 5	80	15	5	100
Person 6	60	25	15	100

Obviously, Product A has the highest score of 330 and hence, it is selected.

ii. **Non-Comparison Scaling:** As the name indicates, the selections are not based on comparison but on individual considerations. Un-paired comparison are classified into the following:

a. **Continuous rating or graphical rating**

In this scaling, a particular aspect is assessed by a sort of continuous scale within a line and the rater has a choice as per which, the rater has to assess his condition and gives his feedback. The continuous scale is designed in such a way that it covers all the scaling parameters for the corresponding attribute. For instance,

How do you like the branded drug product?				
Like very much	Like some what	Neutral	Dislike some what	Dislike very much

The drawback with this scaling is that the respondent has to carefully assess and select the option. Understanding of the scaling and assessing the product is critical.

b. **Itemized rating**

1. **Likert scale:** The scale was designed by Likert and hence the name Likert scale. In this scale, several degree of description is given for the

respondent to pick the option. Based on the option, a score is assigned and upon total score, a judgment is made with respect to the attribute/s.

Is Indian Pharmacopoeia on par with BP, USP, EP?				
Strongly disagree	Disagree	Neutral	Agree	Strongly agree

2. **Semantic differential scale:** The scaling is helpful to understand the psychological understanding of the word by a respondent. Several English words have more than one meaning and based on the context the word meaning best suits. It is possible for the respondent interpreting a word to his point of view and that meaning may not suit to the context. In other words, whether denotations and connotations are clearly distinguished for an attribute has to be assessed. Here, evaluation, potency and activity of an attribute in adjective pairs are assessed. On the other direction, with respect to respondent, evaluation assesses the positive and negative attitude of a person, potency assesses the depth of understanding, and activity assesses in terms of active and passive directions. For instance, let us take two pharmacists A(*), B(#) are contesting for a leadership in a Pharmacy store. In order to assess, the following semantic differential scale may be planned:

(E) Successful			*			#		**Unsuccessful**
(P) Severe		*			#			**Lenient**
(P) Heavy		*	#					**Light**
(A)Hot		*			#			**Cold**
(E) Progressive		*			#			**Regressive**
(P) Strong			* #					**Weak**
(A)Active			*		#			**Passive**
(A)Fast		*			#			**Slow**
(E) True		*			#			**False**
(E) Social		*			#			**Unsociable**
	3	**2**	**1**	**0**	**-1**	**-2**	**-3**	

Semantic differential scale is a bipolar scale and has a "0" value.

3. **Stapel scale:** The scale is developed by John Stapel. The scale is a unipolar rating scale and has 10 options usually between +5 to -5. The scale does not have 0 or neutral point. Respondents provide their option with reference to an attribute. Positive indicates a positive observation and negative indicates a negative observation. The extremities +5 indicates highest degree of accuracy towards positive reply where as -5 indicates lowest degree of accuracy towards negative reply. For instance: A pharmacy in an hospital can be assessed with the following scale:

Professional Service	Hospitality to patients	Counselling of patients
+5	+5	+5
+4	+4	+4 (√)
+3	+3	+3
+2	+2	+2
+1 (√)	+1	+1
-1	-1	-1
-2	-2 (√)	-2
-3	-3	-3
-4	-4	-4
-5	-5	-5

In case of professional services, the performance of the pharmacy may be considered as 20 percent of the total of 100 percent (on the positive side). In case of hospitality given to the patients by the pharmacy, the performance is weak rating to 40 percent of the total of 100 percent (on the negative side). In case of performance of the pharmacy with respect to counseling of patients, the pharmacy has received a very positive and good feedback of 80 percent of the total of 100 percent (on the positive side). Hence, the scale is assessing the pharmacy either on positive or negative side and the choice of the patient for an attribute is unipolar i.e., selection of the choice is only one side of the scale either on the positive side or the negative side, but not on both the sides for a particular attribute.

c. **Simple/multiple category scale:** The other name for this kind of scale is dichotomous scale. In several cases, the options to the respondent are among the two i.e., true/false, yes/no. In several cases, the respondent has the choice to select one among many options. For instance:

What is the kind of employment?	
Salaried	
Self employment business	
Self employed professional	
Student	
Retired	
Freelancer	

d. **Verbal frequency scale:** In this kind of scale design, the basis for options for a question are with respect to the most frequently answering tendency of the respondent. For instance:

How often you exercise?	
Frequently	
Sometimes	
Rarely	
Never	

iii. **Multi-dimensional Scaling:** In such type of scaling one or more questions are put forward. For example, first question is asked whether the patient smokes or not (stimulus). Later, a second question is asked to the patient, how, many cigarettes per day, provided the patient smokes.

Hence, with the above two questions, the researcher can analyze information for how many patients (male/female) smoke (or do not smoke) and the second question can be used to explore number of cigarettes per day by smoking patients. Here one dimension is exploring patient parameters by keeping stimulus fixed (smoking) and the other dimension is exploring stimulus (no. of cigarettes per day) by keeping patients fixed.

12 Introduction to Presentation of Data and Missing Data

12.1 Presentation of Data

In pharmaceuticals, a research may be relating to clinical or non-clinical. During the process of research several data are collected relating to various attributes. The data is collected either one to one interaction, based on experimental observations, telephonic interviews, questionnaires, scheduled interactions, data retrieved etc. Such data is crude and the output for an attribute may be same but might have been presented in the crude data as two different notations, but both are same. Hence, crude data has to be fine tuned for making the output uniform. This process is not considered as manipulation but as data cleaning, data uniforming or data cleansing. In a research report, as a proof the entire data collected (crude data), is compiled and may be included in the rare side of the book as annexure/appendix. Such data cannot draw any conclusions as it is huge. To draw conclusions, it is necessary to bring down the entire data to chronological or logical order. Especially, a research is initiated with an objective and several times the research lands up to a different result. This is very commonly observed in research and this is leading to new research questions and their solving. With respect to the current context, the researcher based on his experience with the research, he/she should be in a position to present the data not only for his understanding and drawing conclusions, but also to a third person who reads the research for immediate understanding and draw conclusions. It is necessary to realize at this juncture, a research proposal is drafted in future tense, where as a research report, research paper are usually drafted in simple past tense.

Data can be presented in Tables and Figures. Such Tables and Figures again should not be confusing in drawing conclusions. Hence, where ever necessary an attribute should be placed in a Table, Figure or both formats. In the current day scenario, Microsoft Excel is making all the processes easier where as earlier it was manual as hand drawings, calculations using calculators which were tedious. The objective of planning is that making huge data represent in minimum number of Tables and Figures. For instance, in the past year several patients visited the hospital and the data is available in a crude manner. From this data, it is difficult to identify the number of patients with respect to gender wise, age wise, type of disease, inpatient or out-patient etc. This can be compiled into the following one Table 12.1, which gives information in one stretch.

TABLE 12.1 Demography of Patients

S. No	Age	Gender	No. of In-patients	No. of Out-patients
1	20-40 years	Male		
		Female		
2	40-60 years	Male		
		Female		
3	60-80 years	Male		
		Female		

Hence, Tables are necessary to have detailed values but Figures have limitations with representing end results only in several circumstances.

With respect to Figures 12.1 to 12.13, illustrates several types such as histograms, line graphs, trend graphs, bar graphs, scatter plots, bubble plots, filter plots, contour plots, surface plots, stock/outlier plots, radar/spider/web plots, pie plots etc.

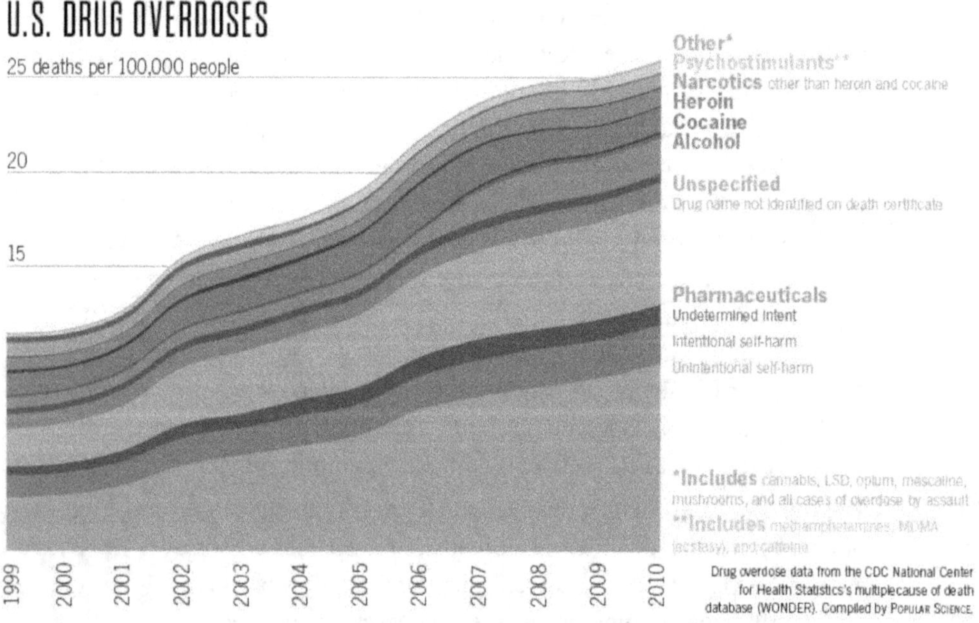

FIGURE 12.1 Area Plot

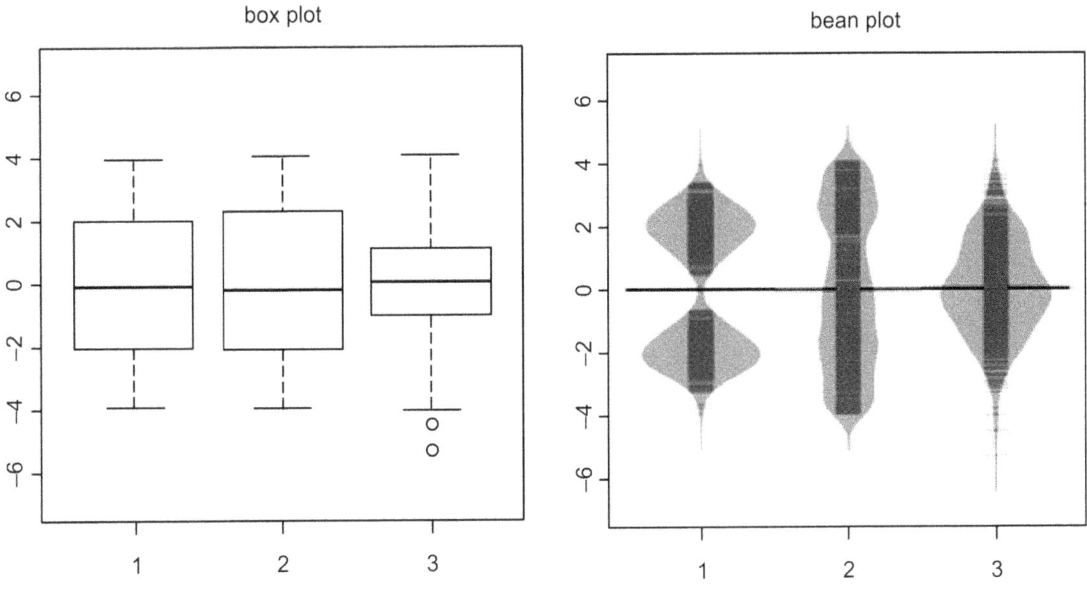

FIGURE 12.2 Box and Bean Plot

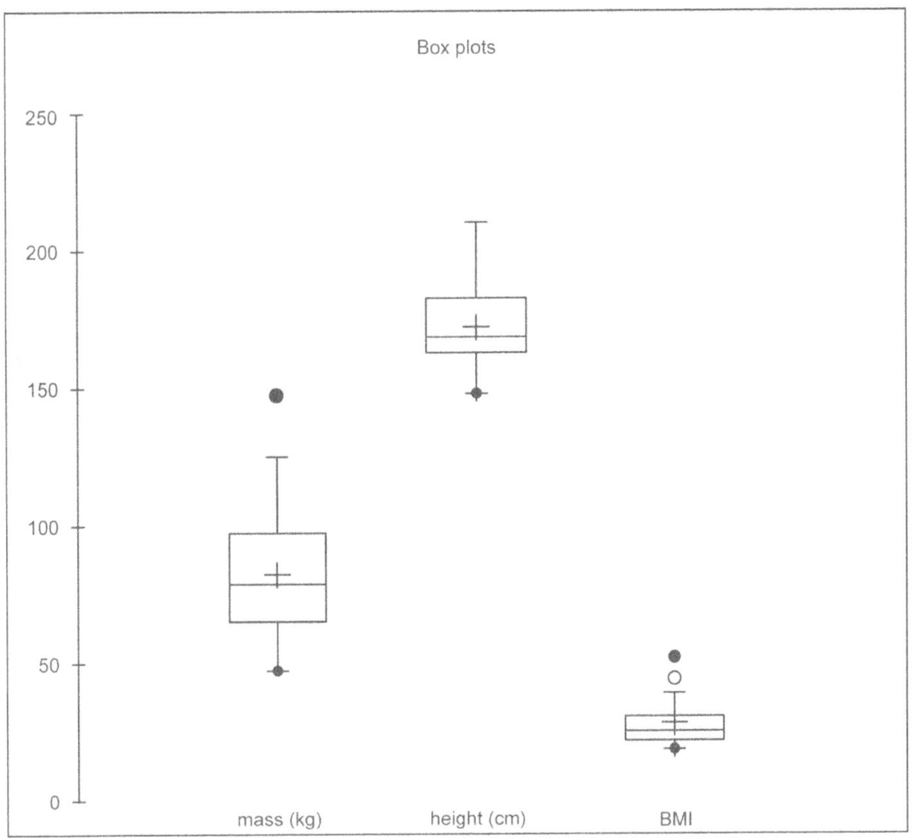

FIGURE 12.3 Box or Outlier Plot

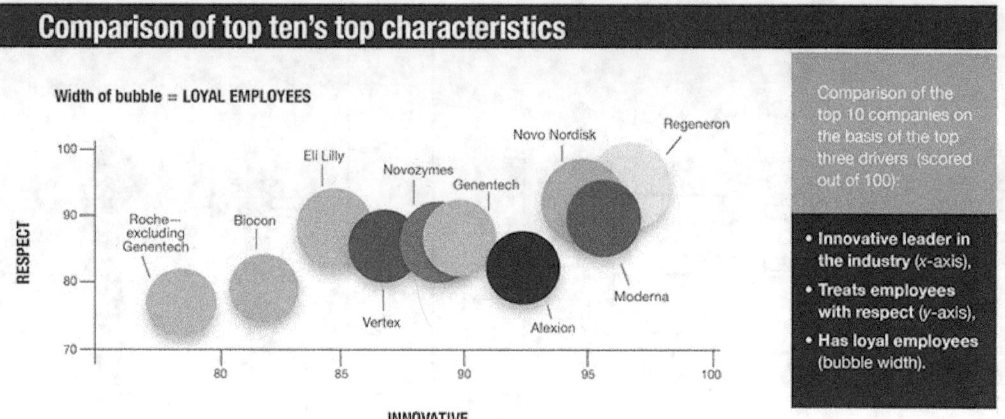

FIGURE 12.4 Bubble Plot

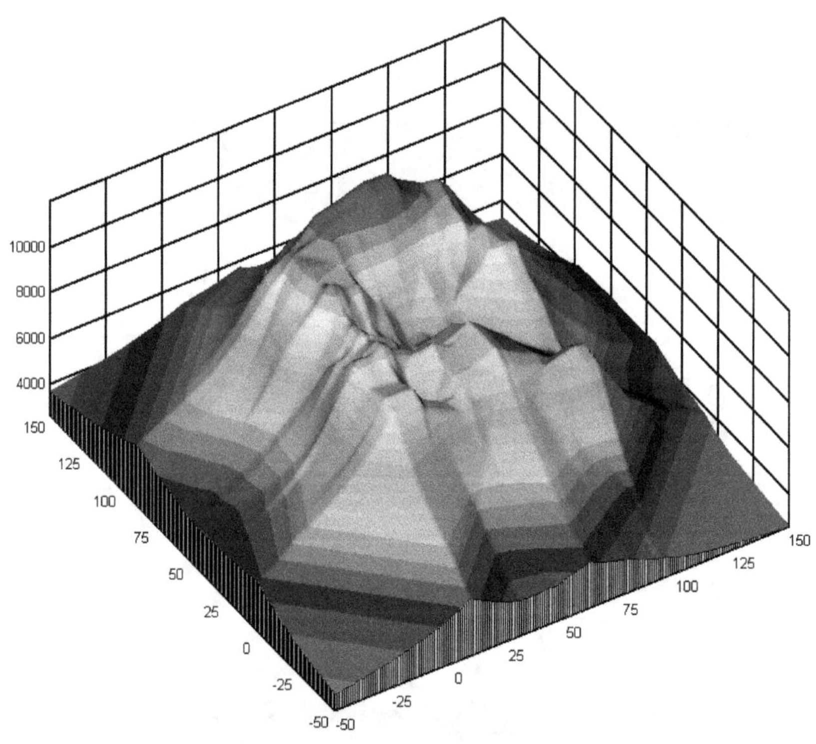

FIGURE 12.5 Contour Plot 3D

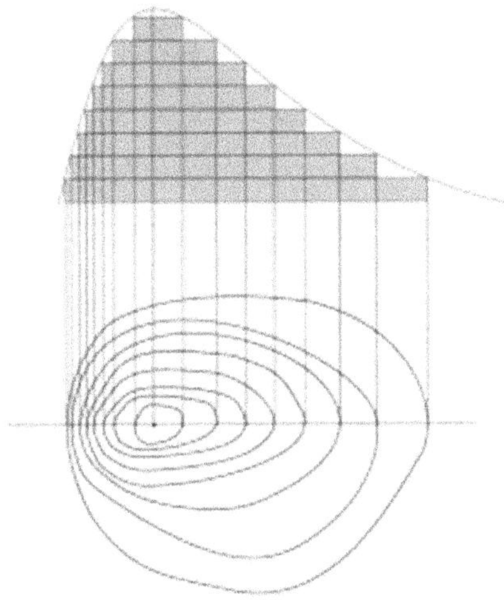

FIGURE 12.6 Contour Plot

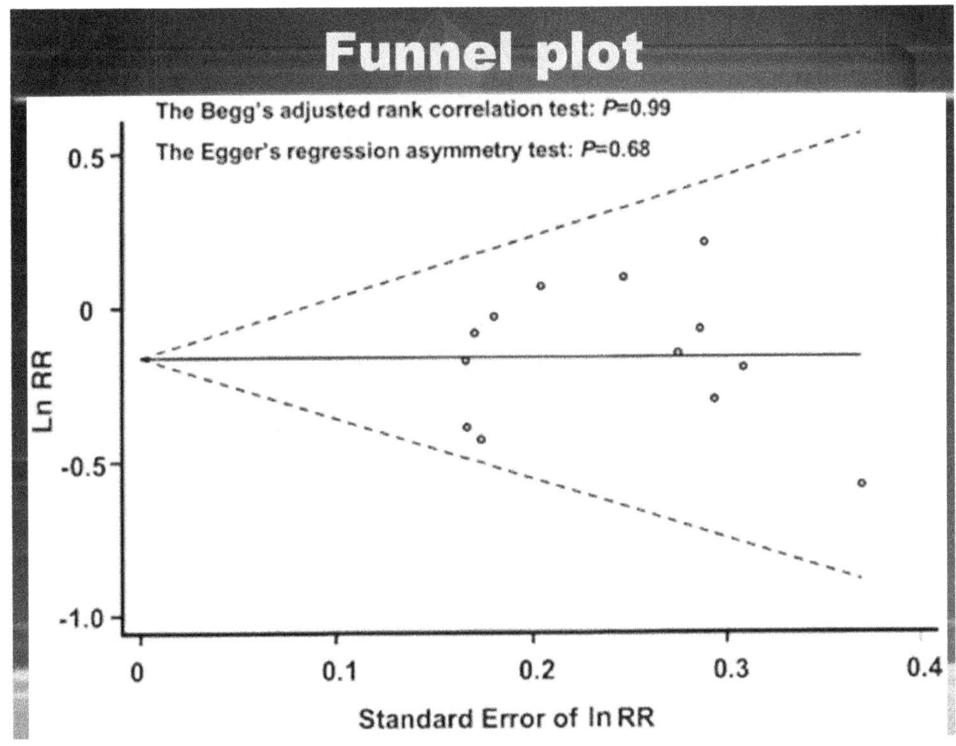

FIGURE 12.7 Funnel Plot

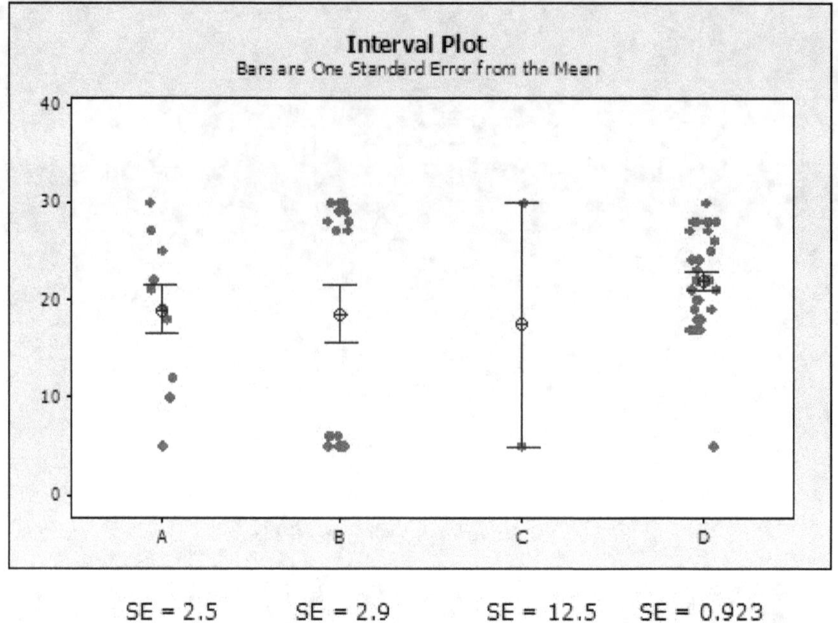

FIGURE 12.8 Interval Plot

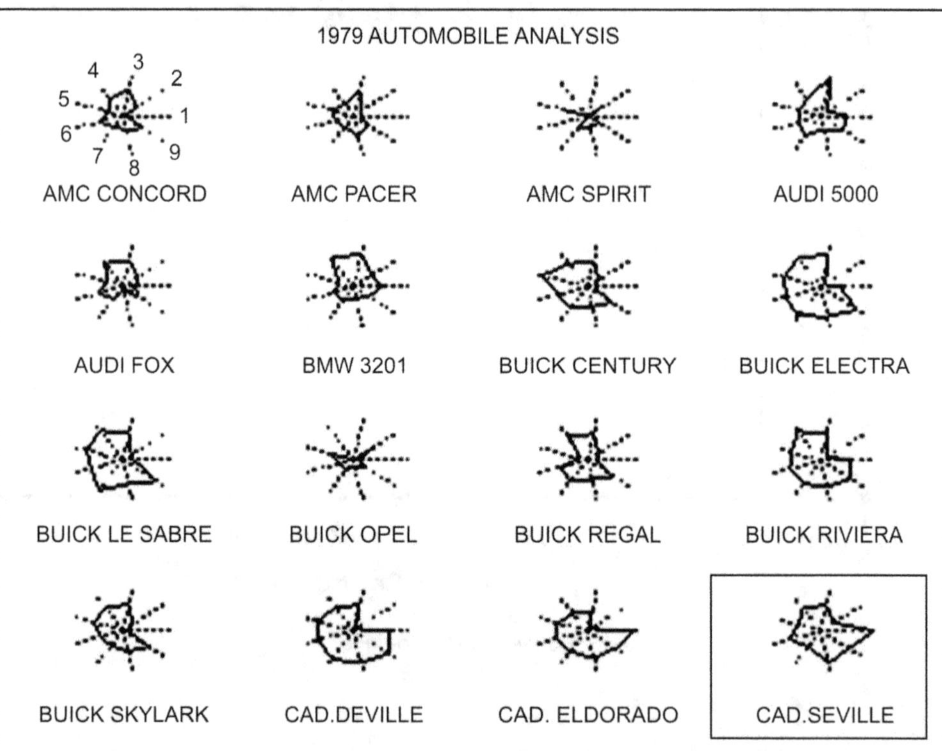

FIGURE 12.9 Radar Plot

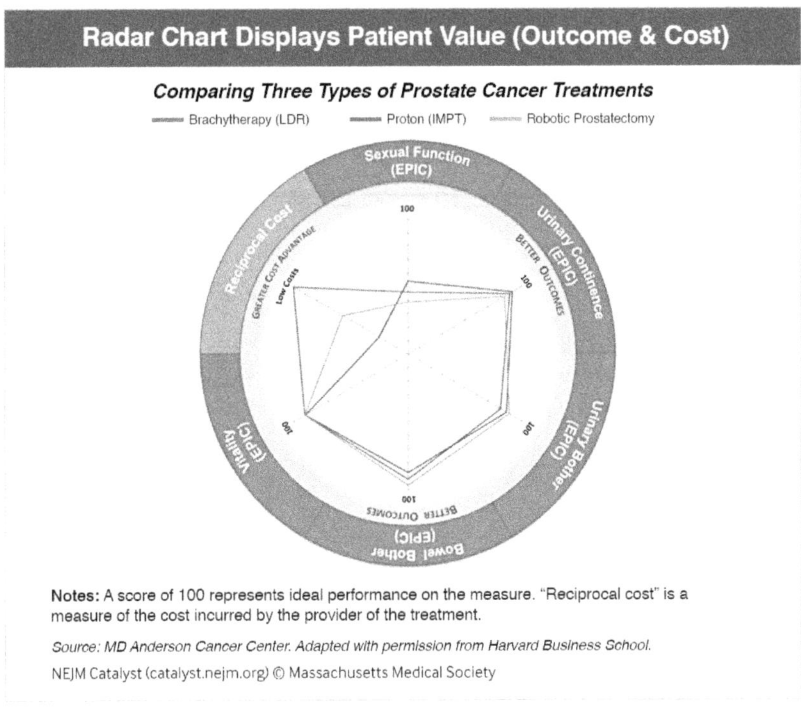

Notes: A score of 100 represents ideal performance on the measure. "Reciprocal cost" is a measure of the cost incurred by the provider of the treatment.

Source: MD Anderson Cancer Center. Adapted with permission from Harvard Business School.

NEJM Catalyst (catalyst.nejm.org) © Massachusetts Medical Society

FIGURE 12.10 Radar Plot relating to Prostrate Cancer Treatment

SCATTER PLOT

What is the relationship between the X and Y Plot?

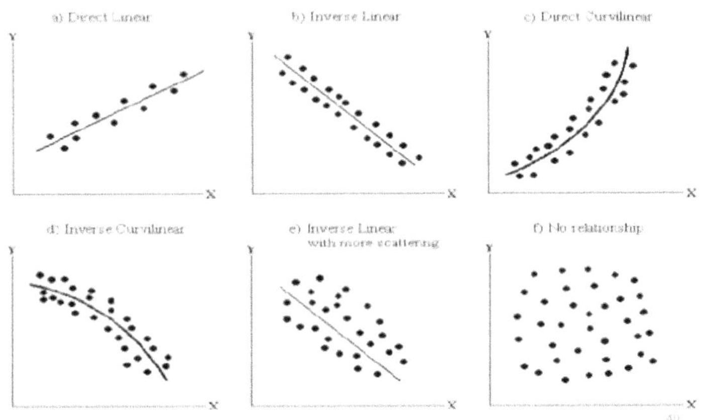

FIGURE 12.11 Scatter Plot

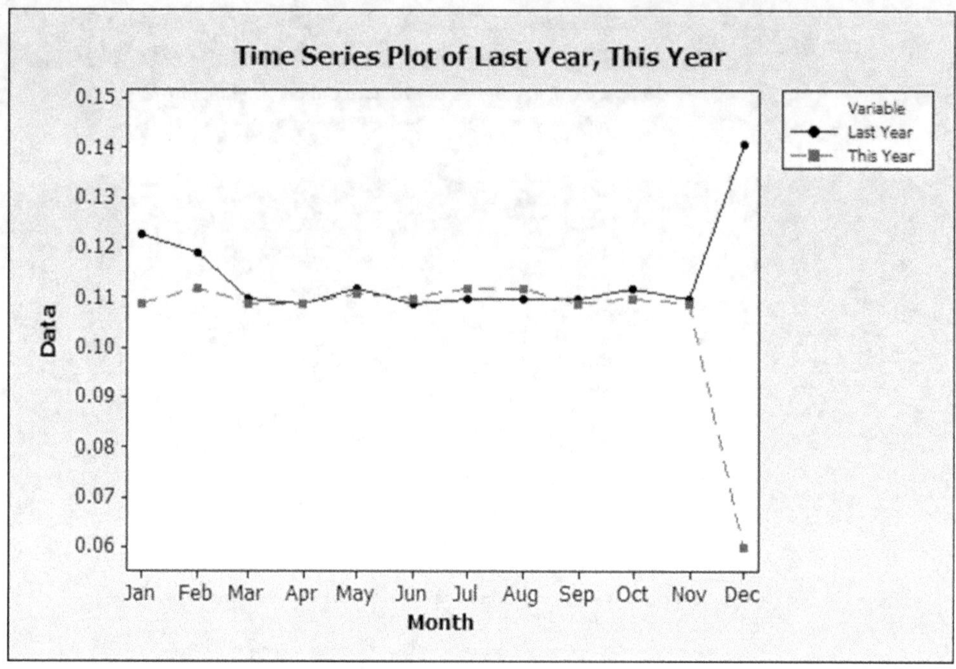

FIGURE 12.12 Time Series Plot

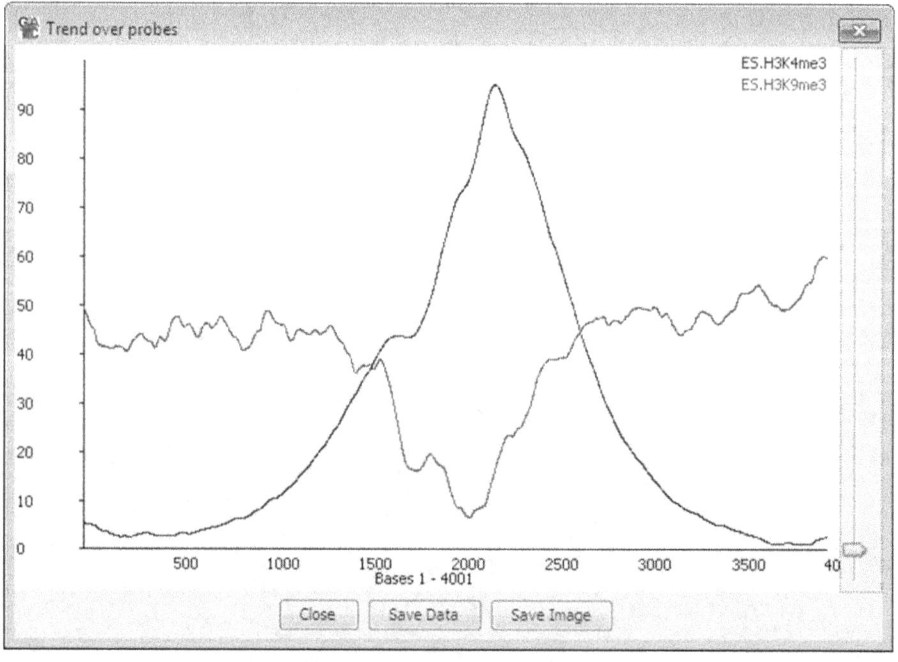

FIGURE 12.13 Trend Plot

At this level of study, readers can be expected in pharmaceuticals being applying various Tables and plots/Figures. The role of web plot/radar plot/spider plot is rarely seen and the plot is helpful in comparison of products within a company or among companies. For instance, let us assume a buyer wants to buy Maruti car. The company has several Maruti cars and among the one which one has to be selected. After judgment, the buyer has selected Maruti 800 without A/c. This can be illustrated with a table and the plot as mentioned below:

TABLE 12.2 Assessment of Various Models of Maruti Car

Car Model/Attribute	Size	Weight	Seating Comfort	Air Conditioned	Speed	Mileage
			Rating (1 to 7)			
Maruti 800	6	6	5	0	4	5
Maruti 800 A/c	6	6	5	6	4	4
Maruti X	6	5	5	6	4	4
Maruti Y	6	5	5	6	5	4

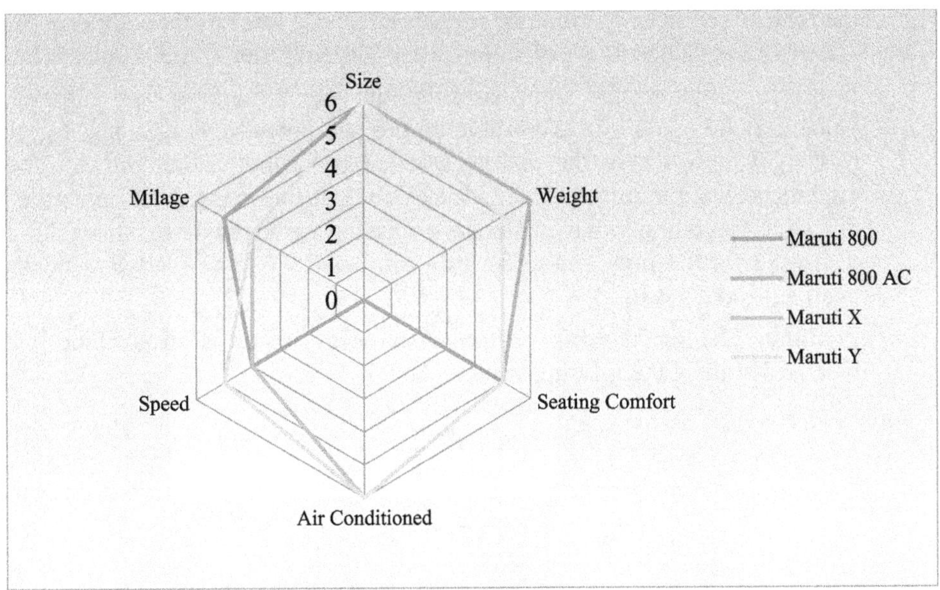

FIGURE 12.14 Comparison of Various Models of Maruti Car w.r.t Various Attributes

From the above Table 12.2 and Figure 12.14, the buyer has selected Maruti 800 even though he/she rated zero for the attribute air conditioning. As a whole, the ideal car is one which has for all the attributes uniform rating or even higher than uniform w.r.t some of the attributes.

12.2 Missing Data

During a research process, a series of data is collected from patients, product attributes or from animals. During the time period, a situation may arise; a patient did not turn up his visit to the hospital so as to provide the data. Such data is called as missing data. Especially, in case of pre-clinical studies, an animal from the group may die.

Under certain circumstances, the missing data becomes crucial and several times based on statistical significance, the missing data may be omitted for conducting the statistical test for the entire leftover data.

Alternatively, in certain circumstances, especially in two-way cross over designs, missing data is prominently seen in the table where data is compiled. A missing data can be estimated and used based on the rest of the data that is available. Such missing data in cell "Y_{ij}" can be calculated with the following equation

$$Y_{ij} = \frac{rY_i + cY_j - y}{(r-1)(c-1)}$$

Where, Y_{ij} = observation missing in the ith row and jth column, r = number of rows in the table, c=number of columns in the table, Y_i = total of the values in the ith row, Y_j = total of the values in the jth column and y=grand total of all the observations

In certain circumstance, upon consultation with the appropriate authority, a missing value may be taken into consideration the last preceding value and for all the further missing values where the patient stopped reporting or withdrawn. Yet in certain circumstances, the missing value may be taken into consideration as the mean of the available preceding values. Hence, a missing value may be statistically concluded as discarded for the final end tests or an estimated value derived statistically among the available values is used.

Problem 12.1 on Missing Value: A table of values of an attribute is as illustrated below. Estimate the missing value.

Estimation of a Single Missing Data Point				
	Columns			
	1	*2*	*3*	*Total*
Rows				
1	*3*	*5*	*6*	*14*
2	*7*	*4*	*9*	*20*
3	*4*	*---*	*6*	*10*
Total	*14*	*9*	*21*	*44*

Solution:

$$Y_{ij} = \frac{rY_i + cY_j - y}{(r-1)(c-1)} = \frac{3(10)+3(9)-44}{(3-1)(3-1)} = 3.25$$

Hence, the missing value of 3.25, which is an estimate based on the rest of the values and can be used for analysis of the entire table data.

13 Probability, Permutations and Combinations

13.0 Introduction

In pharmaceuticals probability plays a critical role in understanding the occurrence of an event. This can be interpreted in several ways i.e., what is the probability of selecting a patient from a population into the group, what is the probability of occurrence of an error by the researcher in collecting the data, what is the probability until which variations in the attributes of a product can be permitted and are of quality. In case of permutations and combinations, out of a population of patients (say 1, 00, 000) how many ways we can pick 10 patients (say).

13.1 Probability

In general terms probability is defined as the chance of occurrence of an event or not an event. For instance, when we toss a coin once, the chance of occurrence of head or tail has equal role among the total two possibilities. Hence the probability of occurrence of head is given by occurrence of head/total possible events i.e., ½ = 0.5. Similarly, the probability of occurrence of tails is also ½ = 0.5.

Hence probability when tossing a coin =

$$\left[\left[\frac{\text{occurrence of event}}{2}\right] + \left[\frac{\text{occurrence of non-event}}{2}\right]\right] = 1$$

Hence, the range of probability values lies between 0 and 1 or in the percentage of 0 to 100.

Now let us imagine an experiment, where a coin in tossed twice and what is the probability of getting a head. When a coin is tossed twice, the various possibilities are head, head; head, tail; tail, head; tail, tail. Theoretically, there are three possibilities of getting head out of the four. Hence, the probability of getting heads when a coin is tossed twice is ¾.

Problem 13.1 on tossing two coins

Two coins were tossed 500 times simultaneously, it was observed that the number of two coins showing two heads is 115, one head is 300 and no heads is 85 times. Calculate the probability of occurrence of each event.

Solution:

$$\text{Probability of event two head} = \frac{\text{No. of events with two heads}}{\text{Total number of trials}} = \frac{115}{500} = 0.23$$

$$\text{Probability of event one head} = \frac{\text{No. of events with one heads}}{\text{Total number of trials}} = \frac{300}{500} = 0.6$$

$$\text{Probability of event one heads} = \frac{\text{No. of events with no heads}}{\text{Total number of trials}} = \frac{85}{500} = 0.17$$

To recollect back the probability concept further, let us take the playing dies. Each die contains six faces and every face has one of, one to six numbers. If you observe, the chance of getting 1, 2, 3, 4, 5, 6 for a throw of the die is 1/6.

Problem 13.2 on playing dies:

A die is thrown 100 times and the frequency of outcome of 1, 2, 3, 4, 5 and 6 are 10, 23, 17, 4, 11 and 35 respectively. What is the probability of corresponding outcome?

Solution:

$$\text{Probability of event 1} = \frac{\text{No. of events with 1}}{\text{Total number of trials}} = \frac{10}{100} = 0.1$$

$$\text{Probability of event 2} = \frac{\text{No. of events with 2}}{\text{Total number of trials}} = \frac{23}{100} = 0.23$$

$$\text{Probability of event 3} = \frac{\text{No. of events with 3}}{\text{Total number of trials}} = \frac{17}{100} = 0.17$$

$$\text{Probability of event 4} = \frac{\text{No. of events with 4}}{\text{Total number of trials}} = \frac{4}{100} = 0.04$$

$$\text{Probability of event 5} = \frac{\text{No. of events with 5}}{\text{Total number of trials}} = \frac{11}{100} = 0.11$$

$$\text{Probability of event 6} = \frac{\text{No. of events with 6}}{\text{Total number of trials}} = \frac{35}{100} = 0.35$$

Now let us consider pack of playing cards. One has to understand first of all playing cards, since most are not aware of. A park of cards contains hearts (♥)-red, diamond (♦)-red, spade (♠)-black and clubs (♣)-black. Each symbol has A, 2, 3, 4, 5, 6, 7, 8, 9, 10, J (Jockey), Q (Queen), K (King) cards. In addition to this the pack contains one jocker to play. If, one plays a pack of cards, you will come across with a total of 52 cards (excluding jocker card). The chance of getting any one card is given by 1/52 since the total probability is a maximum of 1 (or 100 percent). Now, what is the chance of getting a red card, it is 26/52=1/2=0.5 (or 50 percent).

In pharmaceutical or medical research, the data collected when graphically represented, the probability representation will be either discrete or continuous distribution. Examples for the former are binomial, poisson where as for the latter are exponential, normal, t-distribution.

13.2 Permutations and Combinations

In an easy way to understand, let us imagine playing cards. Out of 52 playing cards, if you want to select any three cards, in how many ways you get the three cards. In case of permutation, it speaks about picking three cards as well as their arrangement. In case of combinations it speaks only about selection of three cards. To understand about the permutations and combinations, we should have an understanding about factorial. At this point of time n factorial (n!) is represented by n * (n-1)!. For instance, $5! = 5 * 4 * 3 * 2 * 1 = 120$. By convention $0! = 1$.

Among the two types of permutations i.e., linear and circular, not to make things very complicated, the current topic is discussed with linear permutation. The number of 'n' dissimilar things taken 'r' at a time is given by '$^{n}P_r$'. If, $n \geq 1$ and $0 \leq r \leq n$, then $^{n}P_r = n!/(n-r)!$.

As a fundamental, $^{n}P_n = n!$ and $^{n}P_0 = 1$.

Problem 13.3 on Permutations:

Out of pack of 52 playing cards, in how many permutations three cards can be picked.

Solution:

$$^{56}P_3 = 52! / (52-3)! = 1.326 * 10^5 = 1, 32, 600 \text{ ways.}$$

Now let us see about combinations. If 'n' dissimilar items when taken 'r' at a time, then the number of combinations is given by $^{n}C_r = {}^{n}P_r/r! = n! / (n-r)!r!$.

Problem 13.4 on Combinations:

Out of pack of 52 playing cards, in how many combinations three cards can be picked.

Solution:

$$^{52}C_3 = {}^{52}P_3/3! = 52! / (52-3)!3! = 2.210 * 10^4 = 22, 100.$$

The same can be applied in pharmaceuticals, when selecting patients etc., depending on the objective and plan of study.

14 Statistics, Bio-statistics and their Relation to Distribution Trends

14.0 Introduction

Statistics are a collection of numerical data, analysing and interpreting. Statistics are playing a critical role in regular day to day life right from the basic amenities to the high end medical devices. For instance, every individual is unique and in a cloth show room only selected sizes of apparels are available. This can be considered that the size design of the clothing was made limited a few number of sizes and made available in the market. Whereas, in case of the personal clothing stitched at a tailor, the clothing measurements are taken with respect to individual's body size. Hence, statistics are making available large volumes of the product in the market where as individual is limited to compromise to select a product that is best fit among the available. Hence, statistics are making the economy of the country to flourish with prior estimations and making available in the market the products. Then how the selected sizes are made available in the market? This is purely on statistical studies. This can be interpreted that scientifically several individual's body size for a shirt were measured and compiled, a statistical analysis is made and based on this, selected sizes are made available in the market as readymade apparel.

Likewise in pharmaceuticals, right from etiology of the disease to post-marketing surveillance of a drug product, statistics are playing a critical role. Hence, statistics originate from collection of data from a population and since collection of data from population is cumbersome, time consuming and expensive, statistics are drawn from a sample of a population and projected to the population.

Hence, measurement of parameters (attributes) in question should be as precise as possible. Collection of parameters may lead to errors and these errors may be considered as systematic and non-systematic (random) errors. In case of systematic, the occurrence of error is either too high or too low and lack in accuracy, and such errors are not suitable for statistical analysis. Where as in random errors, the error occurs by chance (sometimes high and sometimes low) and such errors lack in precision, and can be statistically analysed for possibility of occurrence. For instance, during the tablet punching process, the machine is set for required tablet thickness, hardness, disintegration time, drug content etc., but errors in tablets occur on random. Such random error occurs due to long run of the tablet machine for a batch in the day. Even though, the tablet machine operator monitors periodically the various attributes of the tablet during the punching process, the operator rectifies immediately the machine to meet the standards set forth for the tablet. The entire batch of the tablets punched is ensured for quality parameters and for statistical significance so that only approved tablets are packed and released into the market.

Hence, in a pharmaceutical industry, it is necessary not only establishing the equipment, operating the equipment, producing the product and making it available in the market, but also necessary to ensure that quality, reproducible product is made available in the market. For instance, to ensure available tablet in the market is of desired hardness, the pharmaceutical industry initially manufacture a population of tablets, select an empirical sample and hardness of each tablet is measured. The trend (distribution) in the hardness of the tablets is determined by a graph and from this a statistical significance, confidential interval, probability of occurrence is predicted or established. Later, the probability of a tablet deviating from the set standard is estimated. As the statistical parameters are established in the pharmaceutical industry, later on batches are easy to ensure for quality of the tablets in terms of how many tablets have to be collected from the batch, how many have to be tested for a tablet parameter, later measure the tablet parameter in the current batch and see whether fall in the acceptable limit or not. If in limits, the batch passes and if not in limits, the batch fails and the entire may be directed by the authority for re-processing or discarding the batch. The rationale behind pharmacopoeial monographs with respect to standard limits of various attributes of Active Pharmaceutical Ingredients (APIs) and dosage forms can be considered of statistical back ground. For instance, for an assay, the procedure says (assumption), take 20 tablets, weigh the entire twenty tablets and powder them in a mortar and pestle. From the resulting powder mixture, weigh an equivalent powder equivalent to labeled content of one tablet. Perform the assay experimentally and based upon calculation, it is observed for the value within the limits i.e., not less than 90 percent and not more than 110 percent. If the assay value is within the limits, the batch of tablets passes else fails.

At this juncture, a demarcation between mathematical statistics and bio-statistics should be clarified. For instance, in a sample of healthy individuals, the height, weights are measured. No two individuals have the same height and weight. Does it mean this is an error? This is not to be so because all the individuals are healthy. This can be interpreted that all the individuals heights and weights may be mathematical statistically insignificant, but are bio-statistically significant because all the individuals are healthy and the variation is due to idiosyncrasy. Likewise, if a blood pressure is measured in healthy volunteers, all the healthy individuals does not have exactly 120/80, but have minor variations from the normal value. This can be considered that mathematically the values may be significantly different, but bio-statistically the values are possessing in-significant difference, since the volunteers are healthy.

Mathematics and its principles, theroms and derivations are not only helping in biological system, but also in every segment of science. To justify this statement, lines, ellipse, parabolic shapes or curves have been derived with mathematical equations and based on these equations technologies (manmade satellites) have reached Mars and Jupiter. The equations are helping in knowing how much fuel is required, what angle the rocket has to be directed to reach its destination. With the same principles, India achieved in launching a satellite and sent it to the moon. In the same way curves/trends/distributions such as binomial, Gaussian (or normal), poisson, student 't', χ^2 (Chi-square), F (or variance ratio) are helping to theoretically predict the chance of occurrence or non-occurrence and based on practical available sample, upon testing, the chance of occurrence or non-occurrence in the population is judged.

14.1   Bernoulli Distribution

The distribution is a discrete probability distribution and was established by Swiss mathematician Jacob Bernoulli. Here the random variable takes the value of one of the two outcomes i.e., success, yes, true or one for probability of occurrence (say 'p') and a value of failure, no, false or zero for probability of non-occurrence (say 'q=1-p'). It is just similar to tossing a coin, and the probability of either head or tails is equal to ½. Bernoulli distribution is a special case of binomial distribution; where in a single trial is conducted. For the performance of a fixed number of trials, the fixed probability of success on each trial is called as Bernoulli trial. Hence, the distribution of heads and tails during a coin tossing is one example of Bernoulli distribution. When a compare and contrast is made among distributions, a binomial distribution is the number of successes in n trials, a geometric distribution is the number of failures before the first success and a negative binomial distribution is represented by the number of failures before the xth success. The relationship between Bernoulli and Binomial distribution is a sum of independent Bernoulli random variable is a Binomial random variable. The expected value of Bernoulli random variable x is probability 'p' and for variance is p(1-p) i.e., pq. The various values of Bernoulli distribution are as follows:

Probability mass function	$f(x) = p^x\,(1-p)^{1-x}$
Cumulative distribution function	$F(0) = 1 - p,\ F(1) = 1$
Parameter restriction	$0 \le p \le 1$
Domain	$x = \{0, 1\}$
Mean	p
Mode	[2p]
Variance	p (1-p)
Skewness	$\dfrac{1 - 2p}{\sqrt{p\,(1-p)}}$
Kurtosis	$\dfrac{6p^2 - 6p + 1}{p\,(1-p)}$

14.2   Chebyshev's Theorem

Irrespective of the type of distribution the data belongs, if we have the mean and standard deviation of a data, we can predict the percentage occurrence of a value within the said interval. In this case, there is a necessity to know how many standard deviations from the mean, the value is away. Hence, if 'k' is the number of standard deviations away the value is from the mean, then the percentage of occurrence of the value within the said interval is given by

$$\text{Percentage of occurrence} = \left[1 - \frac{1}{k^2}\right] \times 100, \text{ where } k > 1$$

and $\qquad k = \dfrac{\text{the within number}}{\text{standard deviation}}$

Problem 14.1 relating to Chebyshev's Theorem

Using Chebyshev's theorem, find the percentage of the values that will fall between 123 and 179 for a data set with mean of 151 and standard deviation of 14.

Solution:

Step 1: Calculation of k-value:

$$k = \frac{\text{the within number}}{\text{standard deviation}} = \frac{x - \mu}{\sigma} = \frac{123 - 151}{14} = \frac{-28}{14} = 2$$

Step 2: Using Chebyshev's value:

$$\textbf{Percentage occurance} = \left[1 - \frac{1}{2^2}\right] \times 100 = \left[1 - \frac{1}{4}\right] \times 100 = \frac{3}{4} \times 100 = 0.75 \times 100 = 75\%$$

Step 3: Hence, a value falling under the said interval is at least 75 percent.

Problem 14.2 relating to Chebyshev's Theorem

Suppose that average score of a maths test is 84 with a standard deviation of four points. According to Chebyshev's theorem, at least what percent of the tests have a grade of at least of 72 and at most of 96.

Solution:

Step 1: Calculation of k-value:

$$k = \frac{\text{the within number}}{\text{standard deviation}} = \frac{x - \mu}{\sigma} = \frac{96 - 84}{4} = 3$$

Step 2: Using Chebyshev's value:

$$\textbf{Percentage occurance} = \left[1 - \frac{1}{3^2}\right] \times 100 = \left[1 - \frac{1}{9}\right] \times 100 = \frac{8}{9} \times 100 = 0.88 \times 100 = 88\%$$

Step 3: Hence, it indicates that 88 percent of the class scores within the said interval of 72 to 96 marks (interval)

14.3 Binomial Distribution

In pharmaceutical research several dichotomous data are obtained such as LD_{50} determination (animal live *or* die after dosing), ED_{50} determination (drug effective *or* not), sample defects (acceptable *or* not), clinical trials (successful *or* not), formulation modification (old *or* new preferred), coin tossing (head *or* tail) and such data falls under binomial distribution, where probability is 0.5.

Let us consider a New Chemical Entity (NCE) for which LD_{50} has to be determined. For this, a group of six animals are selected (or in multiple groups consisting of 6 animals in each). The chance of all the six animals, five animals, four animals, three animals, two animals, one animal or zero animal dying is found to have a trend of binomial distribution. Hence theoretically, if we consider chance of occurrence of death of animals as 'p' and chance of non-occurrence of death of animals (i.e., animals alive) as 'q', then the total value of "p + q = 1". Therefore, "q = 1 − p". Hence, if a maximum value of p=1, the least value of q=0 and vice-versa. Hence, the probability of occurrence of an incident is 1 or less. In terms of percentage, p value takes the maximum of 100. If Number of animals (N) = 6, p = probability of occurrence of death = total number of animals dead/total no. of animals and q = probability of non-occurrence of death i.e., animals living = no. of animals living/total number of animals, then

The probability of occurrence by binomial distribution $= \dfrac{N!}{k!(N-k)!}p^k q^{n-k}$

$$= p^0 q^N + \frac{N!}{1!(N-1)!}p^1 q^{N-1} + \frac{N!}{2!(N-2)!}p^2 q^{N-2} + \frac{N!}{3!(N-3)!}p^3 q^{N-3} + ... + p^N q^0$$

where, k is number of animals death

i.e., $6!/0!(6-0)!\ p^0 q^6 + 6!/1!(6-1)!\ p^1 q^{6-1} + 6!/2!(6-2)!\ p^2 q^{6-2} + 6!/3!(6-3)!\ p^3 q^{6-3} + ... + 6!/6!(6-6)!\ p^6 q^0$

i.e., $6!/0!(6-0)!\ p^0 6/6^6 + 6!/1!(6-1)!\ 1/6^1 5/6^{6-1} + 6!/2!(6-2)!\ 2/6^2 4/6^{6-2} + 6!/3!(6-3)!\ 3/6^3 3/6^{6-3} + ... + 6!/6!(6-6)!\ 6/6^6 q^0$

i.e., $6!/0!(6-0)!\ p^0 1^6 + 6!/1!(6-1)!\ 0.16^1 0.83^{6-1} + 6!/2!(6-2)!\ 0.33^2 0.66^{6-2} + 6!/3!(6-3)!\ 0.5^3 0.5^{6-3} + ... + 6!/6!(6-6)!\ 6/6^6 q^0$

i.e., $6!/0!(6-0)!\ p^0 * 1^6 + 6!/1!(6-1)!\ 0.16^1 0.83^5 + 6!/2!(6-2)!\ 0.33^2 0.66^4 + 6!/3!(6-3)!\ 0.5^3 0.5^3 + ... + 6!/6!(6-6)!\ 6/6^6 q^0$

i.e., $6!/0!(6-0)!* p^0 * 1 + 6!/1!(6-1)!\ 0.16 * 0.39 + 6!/2!(6-2)!\ 0.10 * 0.18 + 6!/3!(6-3)!\ 0.12 * 0.12 + 6!/4!(6-4)!\ 0.003 * 0.33 + 6!/5!(6-5)!\ 0.83 * 0.16 + 6!/6!(6-6)!*1^6 q^0$

i.e., $1 + 6!/1!(6-1)!\ 0.62 + 6!/2!(6-2)!\ 0.018 + 6!/3!(6-3)!\ 0.014 + 6!/4!(6-4)!\ 0.00099 + 6!/5!(6-5)!\ 0.132 + 1$

i.e., $1 + 6 * 0.62 + 15 * 0.018 + 20 * 0.014 + 15 * 0.00099 + 6 * 0.132 + 1$

i.e., $1 + 3.72 + 0.27 + 0.28 + 0.014 + 0.792 + 1$

Hence, from the above equation calculations, the following, Table 14.1, Figure 14.1 illustrates the various factors:

TABLE 14.1 Establishing Theoretical Equation and Calculation for Binomial Distribution

Death of Animals (out of 6)	Factor of Binomial Equation	Coefficient of Binomial	Probability (factor times coefficient)	Probability as percentage (p %)
6	p^0q^6	1	1/64=0.015625	1.56
5	p^1q^5	6	6/64=0.09375	9.38
4	p^2q^4	15	15/64=0.234375	23.44
3	p^3q^3	20	20/64=0.3125	31.25
2	p^4q^2	15	15/64=0.234375	23.43
1	p^5q^1	6	6/64=0.09375	9.38
0	p^6q^0	1	1/64=0.015625	1.56
Total		**64**	**1.0**	**100**

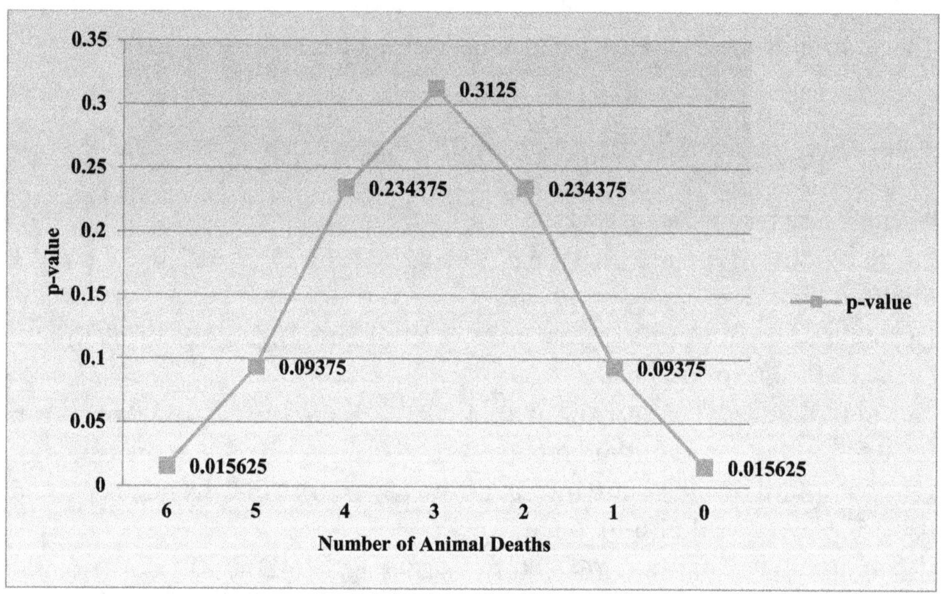

FIGURE 14.1 Binomial Distribution of No. of Death with respect to Probability of Occurance (Based on Theoretical Calculations)

All the above calculations were made based on theoretical binomial equation and estimating the probability of an incidence of 1, 2, 3, 4, 5, 6, 0 animals living (or dying) after administering drug.

Problem 14.3 on Binomial Distribution: If an antibiotic is administered to four patients and if 'p' is considered as cure and 'q' is considered as not-cured, what is the probability of three patients getting cured when probability of success to antibiotic is 0.75 (i.e., p =0.75).

Solution:

$$P = \begin{bmatrix} N \\ X \end{bmatrix} p^x q^{N-X}$$

Where,
$$\begin{bmatrix} N \\ X \end{bmatrix} = \frac{N!}{X!(N-X)!}$$

$$P = \frac{4!}{3!(4-3)!}(0.75)^3 (0.25)^{4-3}$$

$$= \frac{4 \times 3 \times 2 \times 1}{3 \times 2 \times 1 \times 1} \times (0.42188) \times (0.25) = 0.42188$$

Problem 14.4 on Normal Approximation to Binomial Distribution: Sixty subjects were asked to use two variations of a formula, A and B. Preference was indicated based on the formula's "feel" in mouth, and the results are as follows:

Prefer Formula A	Prefer Formula B	No Preference
32	16	12

Conduct a suitable statistical test and come to conclusions.

Solution:

Let H_0: p = 0.5 and H_A: p ≠ 0.5

Percentage preferring = 32/48 = 66.7 %

$$Z = \frac{\left[[p_A - 0.5] - \frac{1}{2N}\right]}{\sqrt{\frac{pq}{N}}} = \frac{\left[|0.667 - 0.5| - \frac{1}{98}\right]}{\sqrt{\frac{0.5 \times 0.5}{48}}} = 2.17$$

There is a significant preference at p < 0.05 for formula A among those who express a preference. The conclusion is that 48 subjects who expressed a preference, 2/3 preferred formula A (p, 0.05), and there were 12 subjects who had no preference.

Note: The problem may also be analyzed by chi-square test or by non-parametric techniques.

Now, let us take a practical example. Let us select 100 tablets of 500 mg drug containing tablets from market. If the technologies are uniform, the weight of the tablets should be uniform among the companies. But, it varies between companies. At the same time, within a company itself, when weight of 100 tablets are measured at the fourth decimal level, every tablet weight is unique and when a plot of individual weight of the tablet and the count of the number of tablets with respect to weight is made, the trend is as shown in the following Table 14.2 and the Figure 14.2.

TABLE 14.2 Weight of 100 Tablets for a 500 mg Drug Containing Tablet

Weight of Tablet	Count of Tablet	Weight of Tablet	Count of Tablet	Weight of Tablet	Count of Tablet	Weight of Tablet	Count of Tablet	Weight of Tablet	Count of Tablet
0.4355	1	0.5782	1	0.6013	1	0.6621	1	0.78	1
0.4359	1	0.5784	1	0.6019	1	0.6652	1	0.7806	1
0.5115	1	0.5791	1	0.6022	2	0.6874	1	0.7833	1
0.5194	1	0.5809	1	0.6035	1	0.6942	1	0.7878	1
0.5224	1	0.5828	1	0.6036	1	0.6961	2	0.7896	1
0.5229	1	0.5869	1	0.6041	1	0.6977	1	0.7914	1
0.5291	1	0.5875	1	0.6047	1	0.7137	1	0.7916	1
0.53	1	0.5884	1	0.6099	1	0.7172	1	0.7965	1
0.5394	1	0.5895	1	0.6102	1	0.718	1	0.7966	1
0.5427	1	0.5901	1	0.6113	1	0.7284	1	0.7968	1
0.5453	1	0.5905	1	0.6199	1	0.7433	1	0.8023	1
0.5598	1	0.5919	1	0.6239	1	0.7448	1	0.8058	1
0.5637	1	0.5933	1	0.6256	1	0.7574	1	0.8118	1
0.5645	1	0.5945	1	0.6265	1	0.7637	1	0.8335	1
0.5711	1	0.5956	1	0.6278	1	0.7643	1	0.8378	1
0.5723	1	0.5958	1	0.638	1	0.7659	1	0.8539	1
0.5734	1	0.5965	1	0.6436	1	0.7719	1	0.9727	1
0.575	1	0.5973	1	0.6492	1	0.774	1	0.9765	1
0.5757	1	0.598	1	0.6493	1	0.778	1	Grand Total	100
0.5777	1	0.5981	1	0.6521	1	0.7793	1		

Note: All the tablets in the table mentioned does not reflect from one company and hence the disparity in weight is observed due to varying excipient compositions and manufacturing technologies.

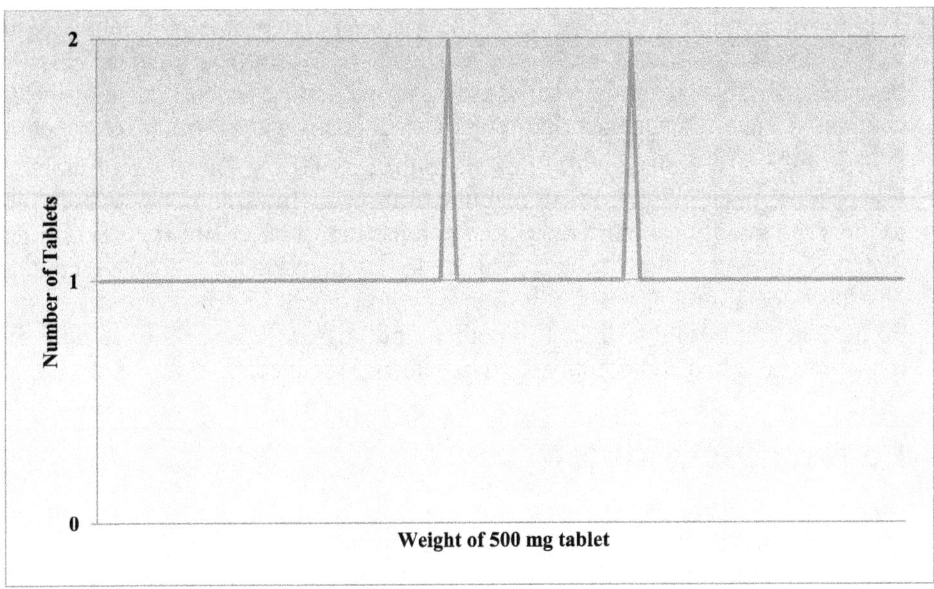

FIGURE 14.2 Plot of Number of Tablets vs. Actual Weight of 500 mg Tablet
(Plot of 100 tablets with their weights)

The above graph indicates, all the hundred tablets have unique weight values (until fourth decimal) and a few have same values. In this case, out of 100 tablets, two tablets have same value and one another two tablets have the same value and the remaining 96 tablets have unique values.

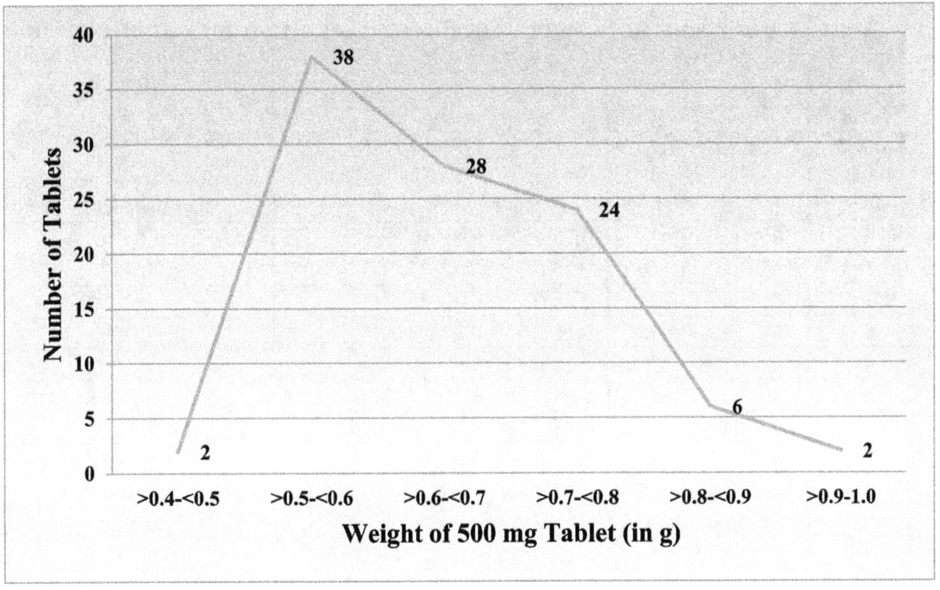

FIGURE 14.3 Trend of Number of Tablets vs. Weight of Tablets (500 mg one hundred tablets)

The above mentioned graph, Figure 14.3, is a similar plot of 100 tablets with respect to weight and as the x-axis scale was changed, a distribution trend is observed. This is because, the tablet weights were rounded up to first or second decimal instead of fourth decimal. Hence, a frequency distribution of tablets is observed, unlike the earlier graph.

It is necessary to understand at this stage that, a 500 mg paracetamol tablet may contain less or more than 500 mg due to manufacturing variations and/or with additional overages to meet the quality standards until the completion of shelf life (i.e., expiry date-indicates that the contents of the tablet reduced to 90 percent from labeled content). Hence, pharmacopoeial tests are not only framed with respect to drug content i.e., not more than 90 percent and not more than 110 percent, but also with respect to sample size of tablets that are to be tested and comply to statistical significance.

14.4 Poisson Distribution

When the 'p' value is changed in a binomial equation, for various values of 'N', the frequency distribution is observed asymmetrical, unlike when p=0.5 (in symmetric conditions). Such distributions are skewed and when p-value is very less, the distribution converts into Poisson distribution (Fig.14.4). Here, a binomial distribution has converted to Poisson distribution to the circumstances. This can be illustrated with determination of LD_{25} wherein, 25 percent of the animals die from a total number of 10 animals and the values can be predicted using generalized notation of binomial equation i.e., $\dfrac{N!}{k!(N-k)!}p^k q^{N-k}$ and this can be further illustrated with the following Table 14.3 (where p=0.25, q=0.75)

TABLE 14.3 Establishing Theoretical Equation and Calculation for Poisson Distribution

No. of Animals Dead	N!/k!(N-k)!	$p^k q^{N-k}$	$\dfrac{N!}{k!(N-k)!}p^k q^{N-k}$ (probability of occurrence of the incident)
0	10!/0!(10-0)!=1	$0.25^0 0.75^{10}=0.056$	0.056
1	10!/1!(10-1)!=10	$0.25^1 0.75^9=0.01877$	0.1877
2	10!/2!(10-2)!=45	$0.25^2 0.75^8=0.00625$	0.2816
3	10!/3!(10-3)!=120	$0.25^3 0.75^7=0.002085685$	0.2503
4	10!/4!(10-4)!=210	$0.25^4 0.75^6=0.000695228$	0.1460
5	10!/5!(10-5)!=252	$0.25^5 0.75^5=0.000231742$	0.0584
6	10!/6!(10-6)!=210	$0.25^6 0.75^4=0.0000772476$	0.0162
7	10!/7!(10-7)!=120	$0.25^7 0.75^3=0.0000257492$	0.0031
8	10!/8!(10-8)!=45	$0.25^8 0.75^2=0.00000858306$	0.0004
9	10!/9!(10-9)!=10	$0.25^9 0.75^1=0.00000286102$	0.00002861
10	10!/10!(10-10)!=1	$0.25^{10} 0.75^0=0.000000953674$	0.000000953
		Total	**0.9997 (=1)**

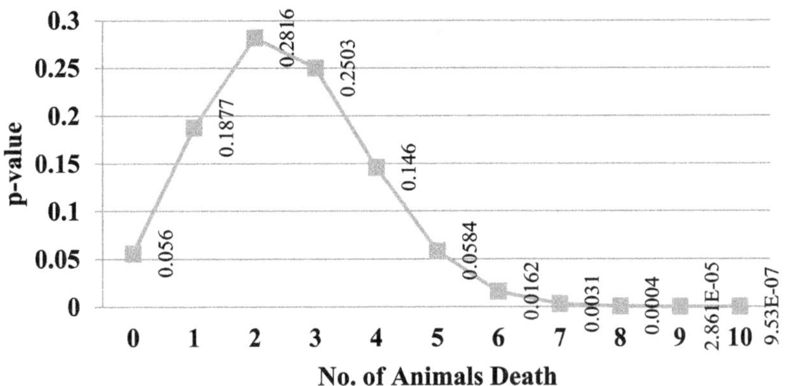

Figure 14.4 Theoretical Poisson Distribution

From the above experiment, it can be interpreted that the probability of 9 out of 10 or 10 out of 10 deaths is less than 0.0001 or one death in 10000. For the probability of 2 or 3 deaths it is 0.2816 + 0.2503=0.5319, which is 53%. To achieve less than 5 deaths, the probability is 0.1877 +0.2816 + 0.2503 + 0.1460 = 0.8656 (i.e., 86.5 %). The chance of 6 or more deaths is less than 2%.

A Poisson distribution can be described when an average frequency of an event occurrence is known. A Poisson distribution is defined as

$$P = \frac{\lambda^x e^{-\lambda}}{x!}$$

Where

    λ = Poisson factor or average frequency

    x = Observed number of events per sample

    P = Poisson distribution

The relation with asymmetrical distribution and Poisson distribution is given by

$$\lambda = Np$$

Where,

    λ = Poisson factor

    p = probability and is much less than (1-p) and (1-p) tending towards one [(1-p) → 1]

    N=Number of observations

A Poisson distribution study can be conducted from studies conducted during a specified time period (say, past 10 years etc.,) or within a certain area or volume. A Poisson distribution can be illustrated with distribution and chance of occurrence of a red blood/white blood cell in a haemocytometer individual cell.

When a Poisson distribution study is being conducted on several studies conducted, it is necessary that the Poisson factor (or average frequency) should be constant from one study with the other.

As an example, the average death rate for a disease is found to be 15%, the chance of occurrence in 10 disease patients can be interpreted by Poisson factor. The Poisson factor $(\lambda) = Np = 10 \times 15/100 = 10 \times 0.15 = 1.5$. When the values of '$x$' are represented by 0, 1, 2, 3, 4, 5, ..., 10. The probabilities can be given by

$$P = 1.5^0 \ e^{-1.5}/0!, \ 1.5^1 \ e^{-1.5}/1!, \ 1.5^2 \ e^{-1.5}/2!, \ 1.5^3 \ e^{-1.5}/3!, \ 1.5^4 \ e^{-1.5}/4!, \ 1.5^5 \ e^{-1.5}/5!,$$
$$1.5^6 \ e^{-1.5}/6!, \ 1.5^7 \ e^{-1.5}/7!, \ 1.5^8 \ e^{-1.5}/8!, \ 1.5^9 \ e^{-1.5}/9!, \ 1.5^{10} \ e^{-1.5}/10!$$

and the individual probabilities can be illustrated in the following table 14.4.

TABLE 14.4 Cumulative Probability for a Poisson Distribution

x	P	Cumulative sum of P %
0	0.223	22.3
1	0.335	55.8
2	0.251	80.9
3	0.126	93.5
4	0.047	98.2
5	0.014	99.6
6	0.004	100
7	0.000756	100.0756
8	0.001418	100.2174
9	0.000023638	100.2197
10	0.0000035457	100.2201

From the above table, it illustrates that 100 percent probability of occurrence is fulfilled by x=6, which indicated death cases up to six patients.

As a second example, a study was conducted over a period of 1960-1973 for the occurrence of human rabies. During the period, it has been observed the sequence of occurrences as 1, 3, 2, 1, 1, 1, 1, 0, 1, 1, 3, 1, 1, 1.

So, during the 14 years span, it has been observed that a total of 18 occurrences. Hence, mean annual frequency of occurrence=18/14=1.29 (= λ). Basically, λ=Np and here N=1 (one year of observation) and p=18/14=1.29

If the above occurrences are the actual practical reality values, then the theoretical values are as mentioned in the following Table 14.5:

TABLE 14.5 Probability of Occurance of Human Rabies for a Poisson Distribution

Cases per year (x)	Number of years in which incidence occurred	Number of cases observed	Poisson Distribution $P = \lambda^x \ e^{-\lambda}/x! = 1.29^x \ e^{-1.29}/x!$	Number of Cases Expected (18 P)
0	1	0	0.276	18 * 0.276 = 4.96 (~5)
1	10	10	0.355	18 * 0.355 = 6.39 (~6)
2	1	2	0.229	18 * 0.229 = 4.122 (~4)
3	2	6	0.098	18 * 0.098 = 1.76 (~2)
4	0	0	0.031	18 * 0.031 = 0.558 (~1)
Total	14	18	0.989 (~1)	18

14.5   Gaussian or Normal Distribution

The distribution is also called as normal error curve. When the 'N' value of a binomial distribution is increased and when probability 'p' is equal to 0.5, the distribution tends towards a normal distribution instead of binomial or poisson.

A normal distribution is given by

$$(\textit{Phi})\ \Phi(x) = \frac{e^{\frac{-[(x-\mu)\sigma]^2}{2}}}{\sigma\sqrt{2\pi}}$$

Where,

   μ = population mean

   σ = population standard deviation

   x = deviate from mean

A standardised normal distribution equation can be obtained when, $\mu = 0$ and $\sigma = 1$, then

$$(\textit{Phi})\ \Phi(x) = \frac{e^{\frac{-x^2}{2}}}{\sqrt{2\pi}}$$

To understand the features of normal distribution curve, let us consider the equation when $x = 0$, then

$$(\textit{Phi})\ \Phi(x) = \frac{e^{-0}}{\sqrt{2\pi}} = \frac{1}{\sqrt{2\pi}} = 0.40$$

and Phi (Φ) takes as the maximum value.

This indicates the distribution is symmetrical i.e., $\Phi(x) = \Phi(-x)$, which means the distribution has two opposite side curves and as a whole the entire curve has a central dome-like portion with either sides as two tails. The two tails have inflection at $x=1$ and $x=-1$. Then, $\Phi(1) = \Phi(-1) = 0.24$. In several cases, the tails tend towards to infinity (i.e., $x \to \infty$, $x \to -\infty$) and $\Phi(x) \to 0$.

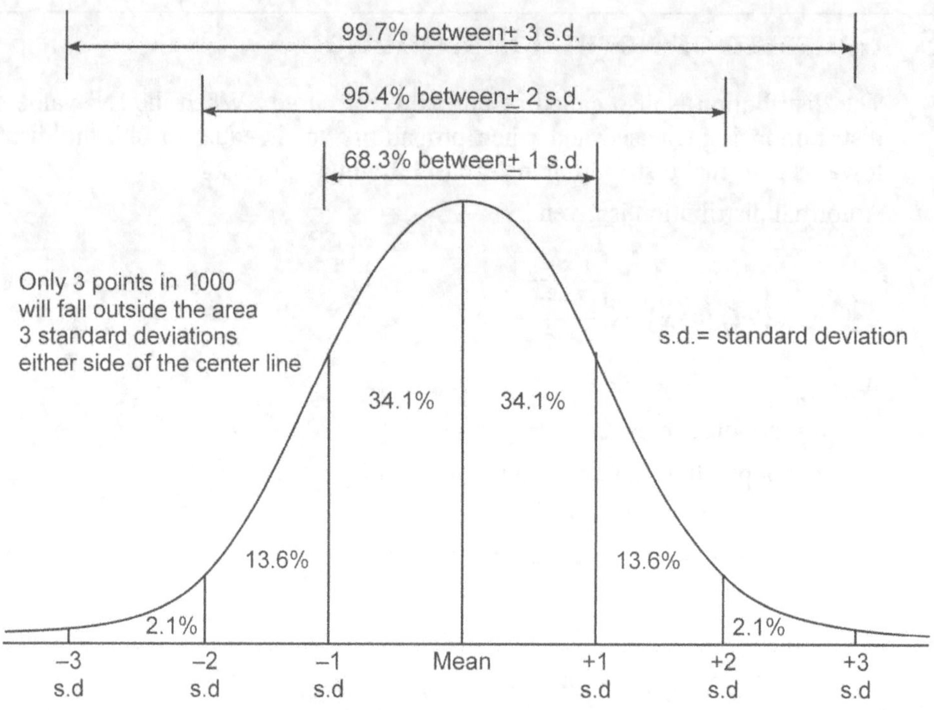

FIGURE 14.5 Normal Distribution

In the above normal distribution, Figure 14.5, when a vertical line is drawn exactly at the peak and parallel to y-axis, the line coincides on x-axis at the mean value of the attribute measured. The deviations from the mean are responsible for symmetrical curves. The entire area under the curve can be considered as probability and has the maximum value as 1 or 100 percent.

It is believed that 50 % of the population fall under +/- 0.675 standard deviation of mean, 68.3 % of the population fall under +/- 1 standard deviation of mean, 95 % of the population fall under +/- 1.96 standard deviation of mean, 99 % of the population fall under +/- 2.576 standard deviation of mean, 99.9 % of the population fall under 3.291 standard deviation of the mean.

As the curve is symmetrical, 50 % of the population have values below the mean, 25 % have values less than 0.675 standard deviation units below the mean and conversely, 25 % have values more than 0.675 units above the mean, 2.5 % (1 in 40) of the population have values less than 1.96 standard deviations below the mean, 0.5% (1 in 200) have values less than 2.576 units below the mean and 0.05 % (1 in 2000) have values less than 3.291 units below the mean.

At the extremes of the tails, the p values are extremely low and the occurrences are 1 in 10, 000; 1 in 1, 00, 000 where the standard deviations are 3.891 and more.

The area under the Gaussian or normal distribution can be given by

$$\text{Area} = P = \int \Phi (x) \, dx$$

A Gaussian or normal distribution curve becomes a sigmoid or quantal curve when the probability or area under the curve is considered as a cumulative value. Such curve may not be of use while deciding the statistical significance (single or two tailed) but such curves are helpful as quantal drug response curves. The probability values of sigmoid can be obtained for a sigmoid curve by drawing a straight line between two end points of the sigmoid curve and the line passing through the center of the sigmoid curve and finally interpolating the probability values from x-axis to the straight line (diagonal line) to the a scale (probability scale) parallel to y-axis. The following Figure 14.6 is an illustration of conversion of normal curve to quantal (sigmoid) and projection of probability from x-axis to probability scale (axis parallel to y-axis).

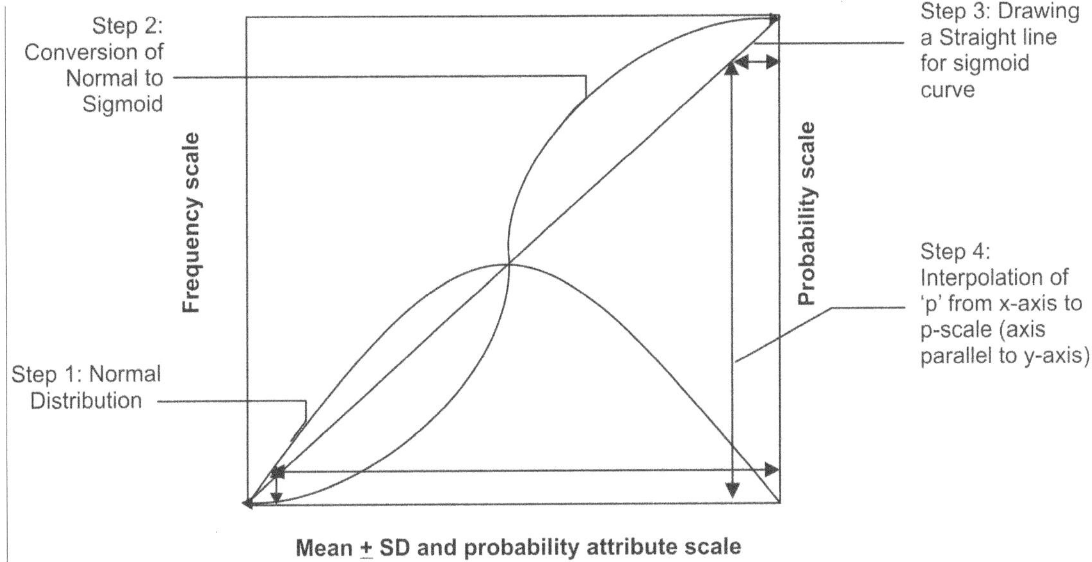

FIGURE 14.6 Conversion of Normal Distribution to Sigmoid Distribution (Cumulative Gaussian distribution)

The application of normal distribution is widely observed when attributes from a population or a sample were compiled. When a test of statistical significance is observed for a sample in the population, any other sample drawn from the same population should also fulfill statistical significance. Hence, sample selected should be heterogeneous and the attributes should represent the population side. A homogenous sampling may lead to deviation from normal distribution significance. In other words, a sample should be homogeneous but cover all the heterogeneous factors of the population so that the sample can be judged that it is representing the population.

It has been observed in several circumstances, sample representing the normal distribution, but analysis of an attribute in the sample not to be a normal distribution. Such variations led to several non-parametric tests. In addition to this, several statistical tests were developed based on normal distribution and are currently in use.

15 Measures of Central Tendency and Variability

15.0 Introduction

Let us imagine, a sample of one thousand one hundred and three tablets were drawn from a batch manufactured. If the thickness of the entire sample of tablets drawn were measured by Vernier Calipers, then Table 15.1, illustrates the entire tablets thicknesses. If it is very difficult to draw a conclusion for a sample drawn then, how can we draw a conclusion for the entire batch (say 10 million tablets). The thickness statistic of 1103 tablets were huge and to draw a conclusion, a one value is calculated, which is called as central tendency.

Central tendency is an approach to draw a conclusion by representation of one value for a group of values for a sample drawn or for an entire population. The three different types of measures of central tendency are mean, median and mode.

15.1 Measures of Central Tendency

15.1.1 Un-grouped

A. Mean:

The three different types of mean are arithmetic mean (average value), geometric mean, and harmonic mean.

Arithmetic mean is also called as average value. It is the most commonly used measurement. It is defined as the ratio of sum of measurement to the number of measurements. Arithmetic mean is given by

$$\textit{Arithmetic mean} \ = \ \bar{Y} = \frac{\Sigma Y}{N}$$

Where, $\bar{Y}$ = Arithmetic mean, Y = individual measurement, ΣY = sum of all individual measurements, N = Number of measurements.

Geometric mean is an appropriate measure of central tendency when the attribute being measured is of exponential type. In pharmaceuticals such type of data are derived when measuring radioactive emission, plasma concentration of certain drugs.

Geometric mean is the appropriate measure of central tendency when compared with arithmetic mean under such circumstances. Geometric mean is given by

$$Geometic\ Mean = \overline{G_y} = (Y_1\ X\ Y_2\ X\ Y_3\ X \dots\dots\dots)^{1/N}$$

$$\log G = \frac{\sum \log Y}{N}$$

Harmonic mean is a measure of central tendency for attributes that are reciprocal such as relating to titers in serological work, intervals between events such as pulse intervals, volumes of distribution in pharmacokinetics. Harmonic mean is a measure of reciprocal of the arithmetic mean of the reciprocals of the original measurements. Harmonic mean is given by

$$Harmonic\ mean = \overline{H} = \frac{1}{\left[\frac{\sum 1/Y}{N}\right]} = \frac{N}{\sum 1/Y}$$

B. Median:

Median is a type of measure of central tendency where in the entire data under test gets divided into two equally sized groups after arranging the data in a rank order. For an odd-number rank the median is given by $(N + 1)/2$ and for an even-numbered rank the median is between $N/2$ and $(N + 2)/2$.

C. Mode:

Mode is the third type of measure of central tendency, where in the value which is occurring most commonly within the group.

Hence, it is necessary to understand that arithmetic mean and geometric mean are obtained with calculation whereas, median and mode are obtained by inspection.

15.1.2 Grouped

A. Mean:

Step 1: For each class interval, calculate the mid class value.

Step 2: Multiply the mid class value with frequency of class interval.

Step 3: **Finally Mean = Total of (mid class * frequency)/Total frequency**

B. Median:

Step 1: For each class interval, calculate the mid class value.

Step 2: Calculate mid value of the frequency and the obtained value falls in the corresponding class interval (group).

Step 3: For a precise calculation of median, the formula is

$$Estimated\ Median = L + \frac{\frac{n}{2} - B}{G} \times w$$

Where, L = lower class boundary of the group containing the median, n = total number of values, B = cumulative frequency of groups before the median group, G = frequency of median group, w=group width

C. Mode:

Step 1: Identify the highest frequency and the corresponding group is called modal group.

Step 2: For a precise calculation of mode, the formula is

$$\textit{Estimated Mode} = L + f_\infty - f_{m-1}\,(f_m - f_{m-1}) - (f_m + f_{m+1}) \times w$$

Where, L = lower class boundary of the group containing the mode (modal group), f_∞ = frequency of modal group, f_{m-1} = frequency of the group before the modal group, f_m = frequency of modal group, f_{m+1} = frequency of the group after the modal group, w = width of the group.

15.2   Measures of Variability

In a pharmaceutical industry, while manufacturing a tablet dosage form, theoretically all the attributes are fixed to a rounded figure. For instance, 500 mg (or 0.5000g) of paracetamol in the tablet. During the manufacturing process several errors such as human, machine occurs leading to deviation from the fixed value of the attribute. Hence, when a batch of 10 million tablets were manufactured, the drug content in each tablet varies and deviates either on the lower or upper side of 500 mg. This spread in variation in values from the theoretically expected is the measure of variability.

The different measures of variability are range, deviation from mean, sum of squared deviations and mean square deviation, variance, standard deviation and coefficient of variation.

A. Range:

Range is the simplest measurement of variability. It contains two values that is, the lowest and the highest and all the values of the sample or the population falls between the two values.

B. Deviation from the Mean:

Let us image 100 tablets were punched and should weigh theoretically 500 mg (0.5000 g). After punching, the entire tablets were weighed individually. Some possess with weight lower than 500 mg and some with higher than 500 mg. The sum of deviation i.e., negative differences and positive differences from theoretical value of 500 mg, when measured and found that the value is zero indicating that the number of tablets with negative differences and number of tablets with positive differences in weight may be equal or may not be equal but the sum is making the value zero.

If all the 100 tablets punched each exactly weigh 500 mg (0.5000g), then the arithmetic mean weight of 100 tablets will be 500 mg (0.5000g). As practically it is not reached, the arithmetic mean of the 100 tablets varies from the theoretical value, which is called as deviation from the mean.   Hence, theoretical mean value is different from practical mean value and hence it can be considered as practical mean as a deviate from the theoretical mean.

It is necessary to understand that population mean value differs from sample mean and this is due to errors in sampling from the population. As the sample size increases, the sample mean tend towards population mean. Hence, sample collected should exactly represent the population characteristics. If the sample size is very large and contains all the representations of the population characteristics, the sample mean and population mean becomes equal.

Now let us imagine, the practical mean value is considered as the reference mean for the batch. Several individual tablet weights represent deviating from the practical mean and the corresponding tablet weight is a deviate from the mean. The relation between theoretical mean, practical mean (also called as provisional estimate), and the individual tablet weight is given by

$$\textbf{\textit{Arithmetic mean}} = \bar{Y} = Y' + \frac{\Sigma(Y - Y')}{N}$$

Where, $\bar{Y}$ = arithmetic mean (theoretical mean), Y' = practical mean (or provisional estimate), Y = individual tablet weight, N = Number of tablets considered for the test (or sample size)

The above equation is helpful to determine the arithmetic mean when other values are known.

C. Sum of Squared Deviations and Mean Square Deviation:

The sum of squared deviations and mean square deviation are factors of standard deviation or the variance.

$$\textit{Sum of Squared deviation} = SY = \sum (Y - \bar{Y}\bar{Y})^2$$

$$\textit{Mean Square deviation} = \frac{SY}{N} = \frac{\Sigma(Y - \bar{Y}\bar{Y})^2}{N}$$

The other notation of sum of squared deviation can be derived as follows:

$$\textit{Sum of Squared deviation} = SY = \sum (Y - \bar{Y}\bar{Y})^2$$

$$SY = \sum (Y^2 - 2Y.\bar{Y}\bar{Y} + \bar{Y}^2)$$

As mean ($\bar{Y}$) is a constant, the above equation can be re-arranged as follows:

$$SY = \sum Y^2 - 2\bar{Y}.\sum Y + \sum \bar{Y}^2$$

As, $\Sigma Y/N = \bar{Y}$, and $\Sigma(\bar{Y})^2 = N(\bar{Y})^2$, then substituting the value in the above equation

$$SY = \sum Y^2 - 2\frac{\Sigma Y}{N}.\sum Y + \frac{N\,(\Sigma Y)^2}{N^2}$$

$$SY = \sum Y^2 - \frac{(\sum Y)^2}{N}$$

D. Variance:

Variance is defined as the ratio of sum of squared deviations divided by the number of degrees of freedom. The equation is given by

$$s_Y^2 = \frac{Sum\ of\ squared\ deviation}{Degree\ of\ freedom} = \frac{(Y - \bar{Y})^2}{N - 1}$$

E. Standard Deviation:

Square root of variance is called as the standard deviation. Standard deviation is given by

$$s_Y = \sqrt{s_y^2} = \sqrt{\frac{Sum\ of\ squared\ deviation}{Degree\ of\ freedom}} = \sqrt{\frac{\Sigma(Y - \bar{Y})^2}{N - 1}}$$

or

$$s_Y = \sqrt{\frac{\sum Y^2 - \frac{(\sum Y)^2}{N}}{N - 1}}$$

F. Coefficient of Variation:

Coefficient of variation is defined as the ratio of standard deviation to mean. Coefficient of variation is given by

$$Coefficient\ of\ variation = C.V = \frac{standard\ deviation}{mean}\ x\ 100 = \frac{s_y}{\bar{Y}}\ x\ 100$$

or

Coefficient of variation is defined as the ratio of standard deviation to mean multiplied by 100.

$$CV = \frac{SD}{\bar{Y}}\ x\ 100$$

Note: The second equation is more reliable as it is applicable to different units used (i.e., kg or lb)

Problem 15.1 on Standard deviation:

The distribution of the number of previous pregnancies of a group of women attending an antenatal clinic is as follows:

No. of Pregnancies	0	1	2	3	4
No. of Women	18	27	31	19	5

Calculate the mean and standard deviation from the frequency distribution.

Solution:

$$S.D = \sqrt{\dfrac{\Sigma y^2 - \dfrac{(\Sigma y)^2}{N}}{N-1}}$$

The total number of previous pregnancies is

$\Sigma y = (0 \times 18) + (1 \times 27) + (2 \times 31) + (3 \times 19) + (4 \times 5) = 0 + 27 + 62 + 57 + 20 = 166$

$\Sigma y^2 = (0^2 \times 18) + (1^2 \times 27) + (2^2 \times 31) + (3^2 \times 19) + (4^2 \times 5) = 0 + 27 + 124 + 171 + 80 = 402$

The average no. of previous pregnancies is

$$\bar{y} = 166/100 = 1.66$$

The standard deviation is

$$S.D = \sqrt{\dfrac{402 - \left(\dfrac{27556}{100}\right)}{100-1}}$$

$$S.D = \sqrt{\dfrac{402 - 27556}{99}}$$

$$S.D = \sqrt{\dfrac{126.44}{99}} = \sqrt{1.277} = 1.13$$

TABLE 15.1 Thickness of 1103 Paracetamol Tablets using Vernier Calipers (in cm)

Tablet No	Thickness Main Scale Reading (MSR)	Vernier Coincidence (VC)	Least Count (LC)	Thickness of Tablet=[MSR +(VC * LC)] (in cm)	Tablet No	Thickness Main Scale Reading (MSR)	Vernier Coincidence (VC)	Least Count (LC)	Thickness of Tablet=[MSR +(VC * LC)] (in cm)	Tablet No	Thickness Main Scale Reading (MSR)	Vernier Coincidence (VC)	Least Count (LC)	Thickness of Tablet=[MSR +(VC * LC)] (in cm)	Tablet No	Thickness Main Scale Reading (MSR)	Vernier Coincidence (VC)	Least Count (LC)	Thickness of Tablet=[MSR +(VC * LC)] (in cm)
1	0.4	5	0.01	0.45	276	0.4	5	0.01	0.45	551	0.4	5	0.01	0.45	826	0.4	5	0.01	0.45
2	0.4	5	0.01	0.45	277	0.4	5	0.01	0.45	552	0.4	6	0.01	0.46	827	0.4	6	0.01	0.46
3	0.4	5	0.01	0.45	278	0.4	6	0.01	0.46	553	0.4	5	0.01	0.45	828	0.4	5	0.01	0.45
4	0.4	5	0.01	0.45	279	0.4	5	0.01	0.45	554	0.4	5	0.01	0.45	829	0.4	5	0.01	0.45
5	0.4	5	0.01	0.45	280	0.4	5	0.01	0.45	555	0.4	5	0.01	0.45	830	0.4	6	0.01	0.46
6	0.4	5	0.01	0.45	281	0.4	5	0.01	0.45	556	0.4	6	0.01	0.46	831	0.4	6	0.01	0.46
7	0.4	5	0.01	0.45	282	0.4	5	0.01	0.45	557	0.4	5	0.01	0.45	832	0.4	5	0.01	0.45
8	0.4	5	0.01	0.45	283	0.4	5	0.01	0.45	558	0.4	5	0.01	0.45	833	0.4	5	0.01	0.45
9	0.4	5	0.01	0.45	284	0.4	5	0.01	0.45	559	0.4	5	0.01	0.45	834	0.4	6	0.01	0.46
10	0.4	5	0.01	0.45	285	0.4	6	0.01	0.46	560	0.4	6	0.01	0.46	835	0.4	6	0.01	0.46
11	0.4	5	0.01	0.45	286	0.4	5	0.01	0.45	561	0.4	5	0.01	0.45	836	0.4	5	0.01	0.45
12	0.4	5	0.01	0.45	287	0.4	5	0.01	0.45	562	0.4	6	0.01	0.46	837	0.4	6	0.01	0.46
13	0.4	5	0.01	0.45	288	0.4	6	0.01	0.46	563	0.4	5	0.01	0.45	838	0.4	6	0.01	0.46
14	0.4	5	0.01	0.45	289	0.4	5	0.01	0.45	564	0.4	5	0.01	0.45	839	0.4	6	0.01	0.46
15	0.4	5	0.01	0.45	290	0.4	5	0.01	0.45	565	0.4	5	0.01	0.45	840	0.4	6	0.01	0.46
16	0.4	5	0.01	0.45	291	0.4	6	0.01	0.46	566	0.4	5	0.01	0.45	841	0.4	6	0.01	0.46
17	0.4	5	0.01	0.45	292	0.4	6	0.01	0.46	567	0.4	5	0.01	0.45	842	0.4	6	0.01	0.46
18	0.4	5	0.01	0.45	293	0.4	5	0.01	0.45	568	0.4	6	0.01	0.46	843	0.4	6	0.01	0.46
19	0.4	5	0.01	0.45	294	0.4	5	0.01	0.45	569	0.4	5	0.01	0.45	844	0.4	6	0.01	0.46
20	0.4	5	0.01	0.45	295	0.4	6	0.01	0.46	570	0.4	6	0.01	0.46	845	0.4	6	0.01	0.46
21	0.4	5	0.01	0.45	296	0.4	6	0.01	0.46	571	0.4	5	0.01	0.45	846	0.4	6	0.01	0.46
22	0.4	5	0.01	0.45	297	0.4	6	0.01	0.46	572	0.4	5	0.01	0.45	847	0.4	5	0.01	0.45
23	0.4	5	0.01	0.45	298	0.4	5	0.01	0.45	573	0.4	5	0.01	0.45	848	0.4	5	0.01	0.45
24	0.5	7	0.01	0.57	299	0.4	6	0.01	0.46	574	0.4	5	0.01	0.45	849	0.4	5	0.01	0.45
25	0.4	5	0.01	0.45	300	0.4	6	0.01	0.46	575	0.4	6	0.01	0.46	850	0.4	6	0.01	0.46
26	0.4	5	0.01	0.45	301	0.4	6	0.01	0.46	576	0.4	5	0.01	0.45	851	0.4	5	0.01	0.45
27	0.4	5	0.01	0.45	302	0.4	6	0.01	0.46	577	0.4	5	0.01	0.45	852	0.4	5	0.01	0.45
28	0.4	5	0.01	0.45	303	0.4	5	0.01	0.45	578	0.4	5	0.01	0.45	853	0.4	6	0.01	0.46
29	0.4	5	0.01	0.45	304	0.4	5	0.01	0.45	579	0.4	6	0.01	0.46	854	0.4	6	0.01	0.46
30	0.4	5	0.01	0.45	305	0.4	6	0.01	0.46	580	0.4	5	0.01	0.45	855	0.4	6	0.01	0.46
31	0.4	5	0.01	0.45	306	0.4	6	0.01	0.46	581	0.4	6	0.01	0.46	856	0.4	6	0.01	0.46
32	0.4	5	0.01	0.45	307	0.4	5	0.01	0.45	582	0.4	6	0.01	0.46	857	0.4	6	0.01	0.46
33	0.4	6	0.01	0.46	308	0.4	6	0.01	0.46	583	0.4	5	0.01	0.45	858	0.4	5	0.01	0.45
34	0.4	6	0.01	0.46	309	0.4	6	0.01	0.46	584	0.4	5	0.01	0.45	859	0.4	5	0.01	0.45

TABLE 15.1 *Contd...*

Tablet No	Thickness Main Scale Reading (MSR)	Vernier Coincidence (VC)	Least Count (LC)	Thickness of Tablet=[MSR +(VC * LC)] (in cm)	Tablet No	Thickness Main Scale Reading (MSR)	Vernier Coincidence (VC)	Least Count (LC)	Thickness of Tablet=[MSR +(VC * LC)] (in cm)	Tablet No	Thickness Main Scale Reading (MSR)	Vernier Coincidence (VC)	Least Count (LC)	Thickness of Tablet=[MSR +(VC * LC)] (in cm)	Tablet No	Thickness Main Scale Reading (MSR)	Vernier Coincidence (VC)	Least Count (LC)	Thickness of Tablet=[MSR +(VC * LC)] (in cm)
35	0.4	5	0.01	0.45	310	0.4	6	0.01	0.46	585	0.4	5	0.01	0.45	860	0.4	6	0.01	0.46
36	0.4	6	0.01	0.46	311	0.4	6	0.01	0.46	586	0.4	5	0.01	0.45	861	0.4	6	0.01	0.46
37	0.4	6	0.01	0.46	312	0.4	6	0.01	0.46	587	0.4	5	0.01	0.45	862	0.4	5	0.01	0.45
38	0.4	6	0.01	0.46	313	0.4	6	0.01	0.46	588	0.4	5	0.01	0.45	863	0.4	5	0.01	0.45
39	0.4	5	0.01	0.45	314	0.4	6	0.01	0.46	589	0.4	6	0.01	0.46	864	0.4	6	0.01	0.46
40	0.4	5	0.01	0.45	315	0.4	5	0.01	0.45	590	0.4	6	0.01	0.46	865	0.4	6	0.01	0.46
41	0.4	5	0.01	0.45	316	0.4	5	0.01	0.45	591	0.4	6	0.01	0.46	866	0.4	5	0.01	0.45
42	0.4	5	0.01	0.45	317	0.4	6	0.01	0.46	592	0.4	5	0.01	0.45	867	0.4	6	0.01	0.46
43	0.4	5	0.01	0.45	318	0.4	6	0.01	0.46	593	0.4	5	0.01	0.45	868	0.4	6	0.01	0.46
44	0.4	5	0.01	0.45	319	0.4	6	0.01	0.46	594	0.4	5	0.01	0.45	869	0.4	6	0.01	0.46
45	0.4	5	0.01	0.45	320	0.4	6	0.01	0.46	595	0.4	5	0.01	0.45	870	0.4	5	0.01	0.45
46	0.4	5	0.01	0.45	321	0.4	6	0.01	0.46	596	0.4	6	0.01	0.46	871	0.4	6	0.01	0.46
47	0.4	6	0.01	0.46	322	0.4	5	0.01	0.45	597	0.4	6	0.01	0.46	872	0.4	6	0.01	0.46
48	0.5	7	0.01	0.57	323	0.4	5	0.01	0.45	598	0.4	4	0.01	0.44	873	0.4	6	0.01	0.46
49	0.4	5	0.01	0.45	324	0.4	5	0.01	0.45	599	0.4	6	0.01	0.46	874	0.4	6	0.01	0.46
50	0.4	6	0.01	0.46	325	0.4	6	0.01	0.46	600	0.4	5	0.01	0.45	875	0.4	6	0.01	0.46
51	0.4	6	0.01	0.46	326	0.4	6	0.01	0.46	601	0.4	6	0.01	0.46	876	0.4	5	0.01	0.45
52	0.4	5	0.01	0.45	327	0.4	6	0.01	0.46	602	0.4	6	0.01	0.46	877	0.4	6	0.01	0.46
53	0.4	6	0.01	0.46	328	0.4	5	0.01	0.45	603	0.4	6	0.01	0.46	878	0.4	5	0.01	0.45
54	0.4	5	0.01	0.45	329	0.4	6	0.01	0.46	604	0.4	6	0.01	0.46	879	0.4	6	0.01	0.46
55	0.4	6	0.01	0.46	330	0.4	6	0.01	0.46	605	0.4	6	0.01	0.46	880	0.4	5	0.01	0.45
56	0.4	5	0.01	0.45	331	0.4	5	0.01	0.45	606	0.4	6	0.01	0.46	881	0.4	5	0.01	0.45
57	0.4	6	0.01	0.46	332	0.4	6	0.01	0.46	607	0.4	6	0.01	0.46	882	0.4	6	0.01	0.46
58	0.4	5	0.01	0.45	333	0.4	6	0.01	0.46	608	0.4	6	0.01	0.46	883	0.4	6	0.01	0.46
59	0.4	4	0.01	0.44	334	0.4	6	0.01	0.46	609	0.4	6	0.01	0.46	884	0.4	5	0.01	0.45
60	0.4	5	0.01	0.45	335	0.4	6	0.01	0.46	610	0.4	6	0.01	0.46	885	0.4	5	0.01	0.45
61	0.4	6	0.01	0.46	336	0.4	6	0.01	0.46	611	0.4	6	0.01	0.46	886	0.4	5	0.01	0.45
62	0.4	5	0.01	0.45	337	0.4	6	0.01	0.46	612	0.4	6	0.01	0.46	887	0.4	6	0.01	0.46
63	0.4	6	0.01	0.46	338	0.4	6	0.01	0.46	613	0.4	6	0.01	0.46	888	0.4	6	0.01	0.46
64	0.4	6	0.01	0.46	339	0.4	6	0.01	0.46	614	0.4	6	0.01	0.46	889	0.4	6	0.01	0.46
65	0.4	6	0.01	0.46	340	0.4	6	0.01	0.46	615	0.4	6	0.01	0.46	890	0.4	6	0.01	0.46
66	0.4	6	0.01	0.46	341	0.4	5	0.01	0.45	616	0.4	6	0.01	0.46	891	0.4	6	0.01	0.46
67	0.4	6	0.01	0.46	342	0.4	6	0.01	0.46	617	0.4	5	0.01	0.45	892	0.4	6	0.01	0.46
68	0.4	6	0.01	0.46	343	0.4	5	0.01	0.45	618	0.4	6	0.01	0.46	893	0.4	6	0.01	0.46
69	0.4	6	0.01	0.46	344	0.4	6	0.01	0.46	619	0.4	5	0.01	0.45	894	0.4	5	0.01	0.45

TABLE 15.1 Contd...

Tablet No	Thickness Main Scale Reading (MSR)	Vernier Coincidence (VC)	Least Count (LC)	Thickness of Tablet=[MSR +(VC * LC)] (in cm)	Tablet No	Thickness Main Scale Reading (MSR)	Vernier Coincidence (VC)	Least Count (LC)	Thickness of Tablet=[MSR +(VC * LC)] (in cm)	Tablet No	Thickness Main Scale Reading (MSR)	Vernier Coincidence (VC)	Least Count (LC)	Thickness of Tablet=[MSR +(VC * LC)] (in cm)	Tablet No	Thickness Main Scale Reading (MSR)	Vernier Coincidence (VC)	Least Count (LC)	Thickness of Tablet=[MSR +(VC * LC)] (in cm)
70	0.4	6	0.01	0.46	345	0.4	6	0.01	0.46	620	0.4	6	0.01	0.46	895	0.4	5	0.01	0.45
71	0.4	6	0.01	0.46	346	0.4	6	0.01	0.46	621	0.4	6	0.01	0.46	896	0.4	5	0.01	0.45
72	0.4	6	0.01	0.46	347	0.4	6	0.01	0.46	622	0.4	6	0.01	0.46	897	0.4	6	0.01	0.46
73	0.4	6	0.01	0.46	348	0.4	5	0.01	0.45	623	0.4	6	0.01	0.46	898	0.4	6	0.01	0.46
74	0.4	6	0.01	0.46	349	0.4	6	0.01	0.46	624	0.4	6	0.01	0.46	899	0.4	6	0.01	0.46
75	0.4	6	0.01	0.46	350	0.4	5	0.01	0.45	625	0.4	6	0.01	0.46	900	0.4	6	0.01	0.46
76	0.4	6	0.01	0.46	351	0.4	6	0.01	0.46	626	0.4	6	0.01	0.46	901	0.4	6	0.01	0.46
77	0.4	6	0.01	0.46	352	0.4	5	0.01	0.45	627	0.4	5	0.01	0.45	902	0.4	6	0.01	0.46
78	0.4	6	0.01	0.46	353	0.4	6	0.01	0.46	628	0.4	6	0.01	0.46	903	0.4	6	0.01	0.46
79	0.4	6	0.01	0.46	354	0.4	6	0.01	0.46	629	0.4	5	0.01	0.45	904	0.4	5	0.01	0.45
80	0.4	6	0.01	0.46	355	0.4	5	0.01	0.45	630	0.4	5	0.01	0.45	905	0.4	6	0.01	0.46
81	0.4	6	0.01	0.46	356	0.4	6	0.01	0.46	631	0.4	6	0.01	0.46	906	0.4	6	0.01	0.46
82	0.4	6	0.01	0.46	357	0.4	6	0.01	0.46	632	0.4	6	0.01	0.46	907	0.4	6	0.01	0.46
83	0.4	6	0.01	0.46	358	0.4	5	0.01	0.45	633	0.4	6	0.01	0.46	908	0.4	5	0.01	0.45
84	0.4	6	0.01	0.46	359	0.4	5	0.01	0.45	634	0.4	6	0.01	0.46	909	0.4	6	0.01	0.46
85	0.4	5	0.01	0.45	360	0.4	5	0.01	0.45	635	0.4	6	0.01	0.46	910	0.4	6	0.01	0.46
86	0.4	6	0.01	0.46	361	0.4	5	0.01	0.45	636	0.4	6	0.01	0.46	911	0.4	6	0.01	0.46
87	0.4	6	0.01	0.46	362	0.4	6	0.01	0.46	637	0.4	6	0.01	0.46	912	0.4	6	0.01	0.46
88	0.4	5	0.01	0.45	363	0.4	5	0.01	0.45	638	0.4	6	0.01	0.46	913	0.4	6	0.01	0.46
89	0.4	6	0.01	0.46	364	0.4	6	0.01	0.46	639	0.4	6	0.01	0.46	914	0.4	6	0.01	0.46
90	0.4	6	0.01	0.46	365	0.4	6	0.01	0.46	640	0.4	6	0.01	0.46	915	0.4	5	0.01	0.45
91	0.4	6	0.01	0.46	366	0.4	6	0.01	0.46	641	0.4	6	0.01	0.46	916	0.4	6	0.01	0.46
92	0.4	6	0.01	0.46	367	0.4	5	0.01	0.45	642	0.4	6	0.01	0.46	917	0.4	5	0.01	0.45
93	0.4	6	0.01	0.46	368	0.4	5	0.01	0.45	643	0.4	6	0.01	0.46	918	0.4	5	0.01	0.45
94	0.4	2	0.01	0.42	369	0.4	6	0.01	0.46	644	0.4	5	0.01	0.45	919	0.4	5	0.01	0.45
95	0.4	6	0.01	0.46	370	0.4	5	0.01	0.45	645	0.4	5	0.01	0.45	920	0.4	5	0.01	0.45
96	0.4	6	0.01	0.46	371	0.4	5	0.01	0.45	646	0.4	5	0.01	0.45	921	0.4	5	0.01	0.45
97	0.4	6	0.01	0.46	372	0.4	5	0.01	0.45	647	0.4	6	0.01	0.46	922	0.4	6	0.01	0.46
98	0.4	6	0.01	0.46	373	0.4	5	0.01	0.45	648	0.4	6	0.01	0.46	923	0.4	5	0.01	0.45
99	0.4	6	0.01	0.46	374	0.4	6	0.01	0.46	649	0.4	6	0.01	0.46	924	0.4	6	0.01	0.46
100	0.4	6	0.01	0.46	375	0.4	6	0.01	0.46	650	0.4	6	0.01	0.46	925	0.4	6	0.01	0.46
101	0.4	6	0.01	0.46	376	0.4	5	0.01	0.45	651	0.4	5	0.01	0.45	926	0.4	6	0.01	0.46
102	0.4	6	0.01	0.46	377	0.4	5	0.01	0.45	652	0.4	5	0.01	0.45	927	0.4	6	0.01	0.46
103	0.4	6	0.01	0.46	378	0.4	5	0.01	0.45	653	0.4	6	0.01	0.46	928	0.4	6	0.01	0.46

TABLE 15.1 *Contd...*

Tablet No	Thickness Main Scale Reading (MSR)	Vernier Coincidence (VC)	Least Count (LC)	Thickness of Tablet=[MSR +(VC * LC)] (in cm)	Tablet No	Thickness Main Scale Reading (MSR)	Vernier Coincidence (VC)	Least Count (LC)	Thickness of Tablet=[MSR +(VC * LC)] (in cm)	Tablet No	Thickness Main Scale Reading (MSR)	Vernier Coincidence (VC)	Least Count (LC)	Thickness of Tablet=[MSR +(VC * LC)] (in cm)	Tablet No	Thickness Main Scale Reading (MSR)	Vernier Coincidence (VC)	Least Count (LC)	Thickness of Tablet=[MSR +(VC * LC)] (in cm)
104	0.4	6	0.01	0.46	379	0.4	5	0.01	0.45	654	0.4	5	0.01	0.45	929	0.4	6	0.01	0.46
105	0.4	6	0.01	0.46	380	0.4	5	0.01	0.45	655	0.4	6	0.01	0.46	930	0.4	5	0.01	0.45
106	0.4	6	0.01	0.46	381	0.4	5	0.01	0.45	656	0.4	5	0.01	0.45	931	0.4	5	0.01	0.45
107	0.4	6	0.01	0.46	382	0.4	6	0.01	0.46	657	0.4	6	0.01	0.46	932	0.4	6	0.01	0.46
108	0.4	6	0.01	0.46	383	0.4	6	0.01	0.46	658	0.4	6	0.01	0.46	933	0.4	5	0.01	0.45
109	0.4	6	0.01	0.46	384	0.4	5	0.01	0.45	659	0.4	5	0.01	0.45	934	0.4	5	0.01	0.45
110	0.4	5	0.01	0.45	385	0.4	5	0.01	0.45	660	0.4	6	0.01	0.46	935	0.4	5	0.01	0.45
111	0.4	6	0.01	0.46	386	0.4	6	0.01	0.46	661	0.4	6	0.01	0.46	936	0.4	6	0.01	0.46
112	0.4	5	0.01	0.45	387	0.4	5	0.01	0.45	662	0.4	6	0.01	0.46	937	0.4	6	0.01	0.46
113	0.4	6	0.01	0.46	388	0.4	6	0.01	0.46	663	0.4	6	0.01	0.46	938	0.4	6	0.01	0.46
114	0.4	6	0.01	0.46	389	0.4	6	0.01	0.46	664	0.4	6	0.01	0.46	939	0.4	6	0.01	0.46
115	0.4	6	0.01	0.46	390	0.4	6	0.01	0.46	665	0.4	6	0.01	0.46	940	0.4	6	0.01	0.46
116	0.4	5	0.01	0.45	391	0.4	5	0.01	0.45	666	0.4	5	0.01	0.45	941	0.4	5	0.01	0.45
117	0.4	5	0.01	0.45	392	0.4	6	0.01	0.46	667	0.4	6	0.01	0.46	942	0.4	6	0.01	0.46
118	0.4	6	0.01	0.46	393	0.4	6	0.01	0.46	668	0.4	6	0.01	0.46	943	0.4	6	0.01	0.46
119	0.4	6	0.01	0.46	394	0.4	5	0.01	0.45	669	0.4	6	0.01	0.46	944	0.4	6	0.01	0.46
120	0.4	5	0.01	0.45	395	0.4	5	0.01	0.45	670	0.4	6	0.01	0.46	945	0.4	5	0.01	0.45
121	0.4	6	0.01	0.46	396	0.4	6	0.01	0.46	671	0.4	6	0.01	0.46	946	0.4	6	0.01	0.46
122	0.4	6	0.01	0.46	397	0.4	6	0.01	0.46	672	0.4	5	0.01	0.45	947	0.4	6	0.01	0.46
123	0.4	6	0.01	0.46	398	0.4	6	0.01	0.46	673	0.4	6	0.01	0.46	948	0.4	6	0.01	0.46
124	0.4	6	0.01	0.46	399	0.4	6	0.01	0.46	674	0.4	6	0.01	0.46	949	0.4	6	0.01	0.46
125	0.4	5	0.01	0.45	400	0.4	5	0.01	0.45	675	0.4	5	0.01	0.45	950	0.4	5	0.01	0.45
126	0.4	5	0.01	0.45	401	0.4	5	0.01	0.45	676	0.4	5	0.01	0.45	951	0.4	6	0.01	0.46
127	0.4	6	0.01	0.46	402	0.4	6	0.01	0.46	677	0.4	6	0.01	0.46	952	0.4	5	0.01	0.45
128	0.4	5	0.01	0.45	403	0.4	5	0.01	0.45	678	0.4	5	0.01	0.45	953	0.4	6	0.01	0.46
129	0.4	6	0.01	0.46	404	0.4	5	0.01	0.45	679	0.4	5	0.01	0.45	954	0.4	6	0.01	0.46
130	0.4	6	0.01	0.46	405	0.4	6	0.01	0.46	680	0.4	6	0.01	0.46	955	0.4	5	0.01	0.45
131	0.4	5	0.01	0.45	406	0.4	5	0.01	0.45	681	0.4	6	0.01	0.46	956	0.4	6	0.01	0.46
132	0.4	6	0.01	0.46	407	0.4	5	0.01	0.45	682	0.4	6	0.01	0.46	957	0.4	6	0.01	0.46
133	0.4	5	0.01	0.45	408	0.4	5	0.01	0.45	683	0.4	6	0.01	0.46	958	0.4	6	0.01	0.46
134	0.4	5	0.01	0.45	409	0.4	5	0.01	0.45	684	0.4	6	0.01	0.46	959	0.4	6	0.01	0.46
135	0.4	5	0.01	0.45	410	0.4	6	0.01	0.46	685	0.4	6	0.01	0.46	960	0.4	6	0.01	0.46
136	0.4	6	0.01	0.46	411	0.4	5	0.01	0.45	686	0.4	6	0.01	0.46	961	0.4	6	0.01	0.46
137	0.4	5	0.01	0.45	412	0.4	5	0.01	0.45	687	0.4	6	0.01	0.46	962	0.4	6	0.01	0.46
138	0.4	5	0.01	0.45	413	0.4	6	0.01	0.46	688	0.4	4	0.01	0.44	963	0.4	5	0.01	0.45

TABLE 15.1 *Contd...*

Tablet No	Thickness Main Scale Reading (MSR)	Vernier Coincidence (VC)	Least Count (LC)	Thickness of Tablet=[MSR+(VC * LC)] (in cm)	Tablet No	Thickness Main Scale Reading (MSR)	Vernier Coincidence (VC)	Least Count (LC)	Thickness of Tablet=[MSR+(VC * LC)] (in cm)	Tablet No	Thickness Main Scale Reading (MSR)	Vernier Coincidence (VC)	Least Count (LC)	Thickness of Tablet=[MSR+(VC * LC)] (in cm)	Tablet No	Thickness Main Scale Reading (MSR)	Vernier Coincidence (VC)	Least Count (LC)	Thickness of Tablet=[MSR+(VC * LC)] (in cm)
139	0.4	5	0.01	0.45	414	0.4	5	0.01	0.45	689	0.4	5	0.01	0.45	964	0.4	5	0.01	0.45
140	0.4	5	0.01	0.45	415	0.4	5	0.01	0.45	690	0.4	5	0.01	0.45	965	0.4	6	0.01	0.46
141	0.4	5	0.01	0.45	416	0.4	6	0.01	0.46	691	0.4	6	0.01	0.46	966	0.4	5	0.01	0.45
142	0.4	5	0.01	0.45	417	0.4	6	0.01	0.46	692	0.4	6	0.01	0.46	967	0.4	6	0.01	0.46
143	0.4	5	0.01	0.45	418	0.4	5	0.01	0.45	693	0.4	6	0.01	0.46	968	0.4	5	0.01	0.45
144	0.4	5	0.01	0.45	419	0.4	5	0.01	0.45	694	0.4	5	0.01	0.45	969	0.4	6	0.01	0.46
145	0.4	5	0.01	0.45	420	0.4	6	0.01	0.46	695	0.4	6	0.01	0.46	970	0.4	6	0.01	0.46
146	0.4	6	0.01	0.46	421	0.4	5	0.01	0.45	696	0.4	5	0.01	0.45	971	0.4	6	0.01	0.46
147	0.4	6	0.01	0.46	422	0.4	5	0.01	0.45	697	0.4	5	0.01	0.45	972	0.4	5	0.01	0.45
148	0.4	6	0.01	0.46	423	0.4	5	0.01	0.45	698	0.4	5	0.01	0.45	973	0.4	5	0.01	0.45
149	0.4	5	0.01	0.45	424	0.4	5	0.01	0.46	699	0.4	6	0.01	0.46	974	0.4	5	0.01	0.45
150	0.4	5	0.01	0.45	425	0.4	5	0.01	0.45	700	0.4	6	0.01	0.46	975	0.4	5	0.01	0.45
151	0.4	6	0.01	0.46	426	0.4	5	0.01	0.45	701	0.4	5	0.01	0.45	976	0.4	5	0.01	0.45
152	0.4	7	0.01	0.47	427	0.4	5	0.01	0.45	702	0.4	6	0.01	0.46	977	0.4	6	0.01	0.46
153	0.4	6	0.01	0.46	428	0.4	6	0.01	0.46	703	0.4	6	0.01	0.46	978	0.4	5	0.01	0.45
154	0.4	6	0.01	0.46	429	0.4	6	0.01	0.46	704	0.4	5	0.01	0.45	979	0.4	6	0.01	0.46
155	0.4	6	0.01	0.46	430	0.4	5	0.01	0.45	705	0.4	6	0.01	0.46	980	0.4	5	0.01	0.45
156	0.4	6	0.01	0.46	431	0.4	5	0.01	0.45	706	0.4	5	0.01	0.45	981	0.4	6	0.01	0.46
157	0.4	5	0.01	0.45	432	0.4	6	0.01	0.46	707	0.4	5	0.01	0.45	982	0.4	5	0.01	0.45
158	0.4	5	0.01	0.45	433	0.4	5	0.01	0.45	708	0.4	5	0.01	0.45	983	0.4	5	0.01	0.45
159	0.4	5	0.01	0.45	434	0.4	5	0.01	0.45	709	0.4	6	0.01	0.46	984	0.4	6	0.01	0.46
160	0.4	5	0.01	0.45	435	0.4	6	0.01	0.46	710	0.4	6	0.01	0.46	985	0.4	6	0.01	0.46
161	0.4	5	0.01	0.45	436	0.4	5	0.01	0.45	711	0.4	6	0.01	0.46	986	0.4	6	0.01	0.46
162	0.4	6	0.01	0.46	437	0.4	6	0.01	0.46	712	0.4	6	0.01	0.46	987	0.4	6	0.01	0.46
163	0.4	6	0.01	0.46	438	0.4	5	0.01	0.45	713	0.4	6	0.01	0.46	988	0.4	6	0.01	0.46
164	0.4	6	0.01	0.46	439	0.4	5	0.01	0.45	714	0.4	6	0.01	0.46	989	0.4	5	0.01	0.45
165	0.4	5	0.01	0.45	440	0.4	5	0.01	0.45	715	0.4	5	0.01	0.45	990	0.4	6	0.01	0.46
166	0.4	6	0.01	0.46	441	0.4	6	0.01	0.46	716	0.4	6	0.01	0.46	991	0.4	5	0.01	0.45
167	0.4	6	0.01	0.46	442	0.4	6	0.01	0.46	717	0.4	6	0.01	0.46	992	0.4	6	0.01	0.46
168	0.4	6	0.01	0.46	443	0.4	6	0.01	0.46	718	0.4	5	0.01	0.45	993	0.4	5	0.01	0.45
169	0.4	5	0.01	0.45	444	0.4	5	0.01	0.45	719	0.4	6	0.01	0.46	994	0.4	6	0.01	0.46
170	0.4	5	0.01	0.45	445	0.4	5	0.01	0.45	720	0.4	5	0.01	0.45	995	0.4	6	0.01	0.46
171	0.4	5	0.01	0.45	446	0.4	5	0.01	0.45	721	0.4	5	0.01	0.45	996	0.4	6	0.01	0.46
172	0.4	5	0.01	0.45	447	0.4	6	0.01	0.46	722	0.4	6	0.01	0.46	997	0.4	6	0.01	0.46

TABLE **15.1** Contd...

Tablet No	Thickness Main Scale Reading (MSR)	Vernier Coincidence (VC)	Least Count (LC)	Thickness of Tablet=[MSR +(VC * LC)] (in cm)	Tablet No	Thickness Main Scale Reading (MSR)	Vernier Coincidence (VC)	Least Count (LC)	Thickness of Tablet=[MSR +(VC * LC)] (in cm)	Tablet No	Thickness Main Scale Reading (MSR)	Vernier Coincidence (VC)	Least Count (LC)	Thickness of Tablet=[MSR +(VC * LC)] (in cm)	Tablet No	Thickness Main Scale Reading (MSR)	Vernier Coincidence (VC)	Least Count (LC)	Thickness of Tablet=[MSR +(VC * LC)] (in cm)
173	0.4	6	0.01	0.46	448	0.4	5	0.01	0.45	723	0.4	5	0.01	0.45	998	0.4	4	0.01	0.44
174	0.4	5	0.01	0.45	449	0.4	5	0.01	0.45	724	0.4	6	0.01	0.46	999	0.4	6	0.01	0.46
175	0.4	5	0.01	0.45	450	0.4	5	0.01	0.45	725	0.4	5	0.01	0.45	1000	0.4	5	0.01	0.45
176	0.4	5	0.01	0.45	451	0.4	6	0.01	0.46	726	0.4	5	0.01	0.45	1001	0.4	6	0.01	0.46
177	0.4	6	0.01	0.46	452	0.4	6	0.01	0.46	727	0.4	6	0.01	0.46	1002	0.4	6	0.01	0.46
178	0.4	5	0.01	0.45	453	0.4	6	0.01	0.46	728	0.4	6	0.01	0.46	1003	0.4	5	0.01	0.45
179	0.4	5	0.01	0.45	454	0.4	5	0.01	0.45	729	0.4	5	0.01	0.45	1004	0.4	6	0.01	0.46
180	0.4	5	0.01	0.45	455	0.4	6	0.01	0.46	730	0.4	6	0.01	0.46	1005	0.4	5	0.01	0.45
181	0.4	5	0.01	0.45	456	0.4	4	0.01	0.44	731	0.4	6	0.01	0.46	1006	0.4	5	0.01	0.45
182	0.4	5	0.01	0.45	457	0.4	5	0.01	0.45	732	0.4	5	0.01	0.45	1007	0.4	5	0.01	0.45
183	0.4	5	0.01	0.45	458	0.4	5	0.01	0.45	733	0.4	6	0.01	0.46	1008	0.4	6	0.01	0.46
184	0.4	6	0.01	0.46	459	0.4	6	0.01	0.46	734	0.4	6	0.01	0.46	1009	0.4	6	0.01	0.46
185	0.4	5	0.01	0.45	460	0.4	6	0.01	0.46	735	0.4	5	0.01	0.45	1010	0.4	5	0.01	0.45
186	0.4	6	0.01	0.46	461	0.4	6	0.01	0.46	736	0.4	6	0.01	0.46	1011	0.4	5	0.01	0.45
187	0.4	5	0.01	0.45	462	0.4	6	0.01	0.46	737	0.4	5	0.01	0.45	1012	0.4	5	0.01	0.45
188	0.4	5	0.01	0.45	463	0.4	5	0.01	0.45	738	0.4	6	0.01	0.46	1013	0.4	6	0.01	0.46
189	0.4	6	0.01	0.46	464	0.4	6	0.01	0.46	739	0.4	6	0.01	0.46	1014	0.4	6	0.01	0.46
190	0.4	5	0.01	0.45	465	0.4	6	0.01	0.46	740	0.4	6	0.01	0.46	1015	0.4	5	0.01	0.45
191	0.4	5	0.01	0.45	466	0.4	5	0.01	0.45	741	0.4	6	0.01	0.46	1016	0.4	6	0.01	0.46
192	0.4	5	0.01	0.45	467	0.4	5	0.01	0.45	742	0.4	6	0.01	0.46	1017	0.4	6	0.01	0.46
193	0.4	5	0.01	0.45	468	0.4	6	0.01	0.46	743	0.4	5	0.01	0.45	1018	0.4	6	0.01	0.46
194	0.4	6	0.01	0.46	469	0.4	5	0.01	0.45	744	0.4	5	0.01	0.45	1019	0.4	5	0.01	0.45
195	0.4	6	0.01	0.46	470	0.4	6	0.01	0.46	745	0.4	6	0.01	0.46	1020	0.4	5	0.01	0.45
196	0.4	6	0.01	0.46	471	0.4	5	0.01	0.45	746	0.4	5	0.01	0.45	1021	0.4	5	0.01	0.45
197	0.4	5	0.01	0.45	472	0.4	6	0.01	0.46	747	0.4	5	0.01	0.45	1022	0.4	5	0.01	0.45
198	0.4	5	0.01	0.45	473	0.4	6	0.01	0.46	748	0.4	6	0.01	0.46	1023	0.4	5	0.01	0.45
199	0.4	5	0.01	0.45	474	0.4	5	0.01	0.45	749	0.4	6	0.01	0.46	1024	0.4	6	0.01	0.46
200	0.4	6	0.01	0.46	475	0.4	6	0.01	0.46	750	0.4	6	0.01	0.46	1025	0.4	6	0.01	0.46
201	0.4	6	0.01	0.46	476	0.4	6	0.01	0.46	751	0.4	6	0.01	0.46	1026	0.4	5	0.01	0.45
202	0.4	5	0.01	0.45	477	0.4	6	0.01	0.46	752	0.4	6	0.01	0.46	1027	0.4	5	0.01	0.45
203	0.4	5	0.01	0.45	478	0.4	6	0.01	0.46	753	0.4	6	0.01	0.46	1028	0.4	5	0.01	0.45
204	0.4	6	0.01	0.46	479	0.4	5	0.01	0.45	754	0.4	6	0.01	0.46	1029	0.4	5	0.01	0.45
205	0.4	5	0.01	0.45	480	0.4	6	0.01	0.46	755	0.4	6	0.01	0.46	1030	0.4	6	0.01	0.46
206	0.4	6	0.01	0.46	481	0.4	6	0.01	0.46	756	0.4	6	0.01	0.46	1031	0.4	5	0.01	0.45
207	0.4	5	0.01	0.45	482	0.4	6	0.01	0.46	757	0.4	6	0.01	0.46	1032	0.4	5	0.01	0.45

TABLE 15.1 Contd...

Tablet No	Thickness Main Scale Reading (MSR)	Vernier Coincidence (VC)	Least Count (LC)	Thickness of Tablet=[MSR +(VC * LC)] (in cm)	Tablet No	Thickness Main Scale Reading (MSR)	Vernier Coincidence (VC)	Least Count (LC)	Thickness of Tablet=[MSR +(VC * LC)] (in cm)	Tablet No	Thickness Main Scale Reading (MSR)	Vernier Coincidence (VC)	Least Count (LC)	Thickness of Tablet=[MSR +(VC * LC)] (in cm)	Tablet No	Thickness Main Scale Reading (MSR)	Vernier Coincidence (VC)	Least Count (LC)	Thickness of Tablet=[MSR +(VC * LC)] (in cm)
208	0.4	6	0.01	0.46	483	0.4	5	0.01	0.45	758	0.4	6	0.01	0.46	1033	0.4	5	0.01	0.45
209	0.4	5	0.01	0.45	484	0.4	6	0.01	0.46	759	0.4	6	0.01	0.46	1034	0.4	6	0.01	0.46
210	0.4	5	0.01	0.45	485	0.4	6	0.01	0.46	760	0.4	6	0.01	0.46	1035	0.4	5	0.01	0.45
211	0.4	5	0.01	0.45	486	0.4	6	0.01	0.46	761	0.4	6	0.01	0.46	1036	0.4	6	0.01	0.46
212	0.4	5	0.01	0.45	487	0.4	5	0.01	0.45	762	0.4	6	0.01	0.46	1037	0.4	5	0.01	0.45
213	0.4	6	0.01	0.46	488	0.4	4	0.01	0.44	763	0.4	6	0.01	0.46	1038	0.4	6	0.01	0.46
214	0.4	6	0.01	0.46	489	0.4	6	0.01	0.46	764	0.4	6	0.01	0.46	1039	0.4	5	0.01	0.45
215	0.4	5	0.01	0.45	490	0.4	6	0.01	0.46	765	0.4	6	0.01	0.46	1040	0.4	6	0.01	0.46
216	0.4	6	0.01	0.46	491	0.4	5	0.01	0.45	766	0.4	6	0.01	0.46	1041	0.4	5	0.01	0.45
217	0.4	5	0.01	0.45	492	0.4	5	0.01	0.45	767	0.4	5	0.01	0.45	1042	0.4	6	0.01	0.46
218	0.4	5	0.01	0.45	493	0.4	5	0.01	0.45	768	0.4	5	0.01	0.45	1043	0.4	5	0.01	0.45
219	0.4	6	0.01	0.46	494	0.4	5	0.01	0.45	769	0.4	6	0.01	0.46	1044	0.4	6	0.01	0.46
220	0.4	5	0.01	0.45	495	0.4	5	0.01	0.45	770	0.4	5	0.01	0.45	1045	0.4	6	0.01	0.46
221	0.4	6	0.01	0.46	496	0.4	5	0.01	0.45	771	0.4	5	0.01	0.45	1046	0.4	5	0.01	0.45
222	0.4	5	0.01	0.45	497	0.4	5	0.01	0.45	772	0.4	5	0.01	0.45	1047	0.4	5	0.01	0.45
223	0.4	5	0.01	0.45	498	0.4	5	0.01	0.45	773	0.4	6	0.01	0.46	1048	0.4	5	0.01	0.45
224	0.4	5	0.01	0.45	499	0.4	5	0.01	0.45	774	0.4	5	0.01	0.45	1049	0.4	5	0.01	0.45
225	0.4	6	0.01	0.46	500	0.4	6	0.01	0.46	775	0.4	6	0.01	0.46	1050	0.4	5	0.01	0.45
226	0.4	6	0.01	0.46	501	0.4	5	0.01	0.45	776	0.4	6	0.01	0.46	1051	0.4	6	0.01	0.46
227	0.4	5	0.01	0.45	502	0.4	5	0.01	0.45	777	0.4	6	0.01	0.46	1052	0.4	6	0.01	0.46
228	0.4	6	0.01	0.46	503	0.4	6	0.01	0.46	778	0.4	6	0.01	0.46	1053	0.4	6	0.01	0.46
229	0.4	6	0.01	0.46	504	0.4	6	0.01	0.46	779	0.4	6	0.01	0.46	1054	0.4	6	0.01	0.46
230	0.4	6	0.01	0.46	505	0.4	6	0.01	0.46	780	0.4	6	0.01	0.46	1055	0.4	6	0.01	0.46
231	0.4	6	0.01	0.46	506	0.4	6	0.01	0.46	781	0.4	4	0.01	0.44	1056	0.4	6	0.01	0.46
232	0.4	6	0.01	0.46	507	0.4	6	0.01	0.46	782	0.4	5	0.01	0.45	1057	0.4	6	0.01	0.46
233	0.4	6	0.01	0.46	508	0.4	6	0.01	0.46	783	0.4	6	0.01	0.46	1058	0.4	6	0.01	0.46
234	0.4	6	0.01	0.46	509	0.4	6	0.01	0.46	784	0.4	6	0.01	0.46	1059	0.4	6	0.01	0.46
235	0.4	6	0.01	0.46	510	0.4	6	0.01	0.46	785	0.4	5	0.01	0.45	1060	0.4	6	0.01	0.46
236	0.4	5	0.01	0.45	511	0.4	6	0.01	0.46	786	0.4	6	0.01	0.46	1061	0.4	6	0.01	0.46
237	0.4	5	0.01	0.45	512	0.4	6	0.01	0.46	787	0.4	6	0.01	0.46	1062	0.4	6	0.01	0.46
238	0.4	6	0.01	0.46	513	0.4	5	0.01	0.45	788	0.4	6	0.01	0.46	1063	0.4	6	0.01	0.46
239	0.4	5	0.01	0.45	514	0.4	6	0.01	0.46	789	0.4	6	0.01	0.46	1064	0.4	6	0.01	0.46
240	0.4	6	0.01	0.46	515	0.4	5	0.01	0.45	790	0.4	6	0.01	0.46	1065	0.4	6	0.01	0.46
241	0.4	6	0.01	0.46	516	0.4	6	0.01	0.46	791	0.4	6	0.01	0.46	1066	0.4	6	0.01	0.46

TABLE 15.1 *Contd...*

Tablet No	Thickness Main Scale Reading (MSR)	Vernier Coincidence (VC)	Least Count (LC)	Thickness of Tablet=[MSR +(VC * LC)] (in cm)	Tablet No	Thickness Main Scale Reading (MSR)	Vernier Coincidence (VC)	Least Count (LC)	Thickness of Tablet=[MSR +(VC * LC)] (in cm)	Tablet No	Thickness Main Scale Reading (MSR)	Vernier Coincidence (VC)	Least Count (LC)	Thickness of Tablet=[MSR +(VC * LC)] (in cm)	Tablet No	Thickness Main Scale Reading (MSR)	Vernier Coincidence (VC)	Least Count (LC)	Thickness of Tablet=[MSR +(VC * LC)] (in cm)
242	0.4	6	0.01	0.46	517	0.4	5	0.01	0.45	792	0.4	6	0.01	0.46	1067	0.4	6	0.01	0.46
243	0.4	6	0.01	0.46	518	0.4	5	0.01	0.45	793	0.4	6	0.01	0.46	1068	0.4	5	0.01	0.45
244	0.4	6	0.01	0.46	519	0.4	5	0.01	0.45	794	0.4	6	0.01	0.46	1069	0.4	6	0.01	0.46
245	0.4	5	0.01	0.45	520	0.4	7	0.01	0.47	795	0.4	5	0.01	0.45	1070	0.4	6	0.01	0.46
246	0.4	6	0.01	0.46	521	0.4	5	0.01	0.45	796	0.4	6	0.01	0.46	1071	0.4	6	0.01	0.46
247	0.4	6	0.01	0.46	522	0.4	5	0.01	0.45	797	0.4	5	0.01	0.45	1072	0.4	6	0.01	0.46
248	0.4	6	0.01	0.46	523	0.4	5	0.01	0.45	798	0.4	6	0.01	0.46	1073	0.4	6	0.01	0.46
249	0.4	5	0.01	0.45	524	0.4	6	0.01	0.46	799	0.4	6	0.01	0.46	1074	0.4	5	0.01	0.45
250	0.4	5	0.01	0.45	525	0.4	5	0.01	0.45	800	0.4	6	0.01	0.46	1075	0.4	6	0.01	0.46
251	0.4	6	0.01	0.46	526	0.4	6	0.01	0.46	801	0.4	6	0.01	0.46	1076	0.4	5	0.01	0.45
252	0.4	6	0.01	0.46	527	0.4	5	0.01	0.45	802	0.4	5	0.01	0.45	1077	0.4	6	0.01	0.46
253	0.4	5	0.01	0.45	528	0.4	6	0.01	0.46	803	0.4	6	0.01	0.46	1078	0.4	5	0.01	0.45
254	0.4	5	0.01	0.45	529	0.4	5	0.01	0.45	804	0.4	6	0.01	0.46	1079	0.4	5	0.01	0.45
255	0.4	5	0.01	0.45	530	0.4	6	0.01	0.46	805	0.4	6	0.01	0.46	1080	0.4	5	0.01	0.45
256	0.4	4	0.01	0.44	531	0.4	6	0.01	0.46	806	0.4	5	0.01	0.45	1081	0.4	5	0.01	0.45
257	0.4	5	0.01	0.45	532	0.4	5	0.01	0.45	807	0.4	6	0.01	0.46	1082	0.4	5	0.01	0.45
258	0.4	6	0.01	0.46	533	0.4	6	0.01	0.46	808	0.4	5	0.01	0.45	1083	0.4	5	0.01	0.45
259	0.4	5	0.01	0.45	534	0.4	5	0.01	0.45	809	0.4	6	0.01	0.46	1084	0.4	5	0.01	0.45
260	0.4	5	0.01	0.45	535	0.4	5	0.01	0.45	810	0.4	5	0.01	0.45	1085	0.4	5	0.01	0.45
261	0.4	5	0.01	0.45	536	0.4	6	0.01	0.46	811	0.4	6	0.01	0.46	1086	0.4	6	0.01	0.46
262	0.4	5	0.01	0.45	537	0.4	5	0.01	0.45	812	0.4	5	0.01	0.45	1087	0.4	6	0.01	0.46
263	0.4	6	0.01	0.46	538	0.4	6	0.01	0.46	813	0.4	6	0.01	0.46	1088	0.4	6	0.01	0.46
264	0.4	6	0.01	0.46	539	0.4	6	0.01	0.46	814	0.4	5	0.01	0.45	1089	0.4	6	0.01	0.46
265	0.4	6	0.01	0.46	540	0.4	6	0.01	0.46	815	0.4	6	0.01	0.46	1090	0.4	5	0.01	0.45
266	0.4	6	0.01	0.46	541	0.4	5	0.01	0.45	816	0.4	5	0.01	0.45	1091	0.4	6	0.01	0.46
267	0.4	6	0.01	0.46	542	0.4	6	0.01	0.46	817	0.4	6	0.01	0.46	1092	0.4	5	0.01	0.45
268	0.4	5	0.01	0.45	543	0.4	6	0.01	0.46	818	0.4	6	0.01	0.46	1093	0.4	6	0.01	0.46
269	0.4	6	0.01	0.46	544	0.4	6	0.01	0.46	819	0.4	6	0.01	0.46	1094	0.4	5	0.01	0.45
270	0.4	6	0.01	0.46	545	0.4	6	0.01	0.46	820	0.4	6	0.01	0.46	1095	0.4	5	0.01	0.45
271	0.4	6	0.01	0.46	546	0.4	6	0.01	0.46	821	0.4	6	0.01	0.46	1096	0.4	5	0.01	0.45
272	0.4	6	0.01	0.46	547	0.4	5	0.01	0.45	822	0.4	6	0.01	0.46	1097	0.4	5	0.01	0.45
273	0.4	6	0.01	0.46	548	0.4	5	0.01	0.45	823	0.4	6	0.01	0.46	1098	0.4	5	0.01	0.45
274	0.4	5	0.01	0.45	549	0.4	5	0.01	0.45	824	0.4	5	0.01	0.45	1099	0.4	6	0.01	0.46
275	0.4	6	0.01	0.46	550	0.4	6	0.01	0.46	825	0.4	6	0.01	0.46	1100	0.4	6	0.01	0.46
															1101	0.4	5	0.01	0.45
															1102	0.4	5	0.01	0.45
															1103	0.4	6	0.01	0.46

16 Standard Error, Confidence Level/Confidence Interval/ Confidence Limits, Statistical Errors, Hypothesis

16.1 Standard Error

Let us imagine a population of 100 tablets whose thickness has to be determined. As the numbers of tablets are less in number, a researcher measures the thickness of every individual tablet by Vernier calipers. He records all the values and plots a graph No. of tablets (y-axis) vs. thickness of tablet (x-axis). It is expected for a normal (or student 't') distribution curve.

Let us imagine, the entire 100 tablets mean thickness is "$\bar{x}$". Now, let us divide the entire 100 tablets into five groups as g1, g2, g3, g4, g5 with number of tablets in each group as n1, n2, n3, n4, n5 and their corresponding group mean thickness as $\bar{x}_1, \bar{x}_2, \bar{x}_3, \bar{x}_4, \bar{x}_5$ respectively.

Does, a plot of No. of tablets (y-axis) vs. thickness of tablet (x-axis) with respect to groups means and the population mean have a normal distribution? The answer is yes.

When the numbers of tablets in each group are not equal, then

The total population mean is given by, $\bar{x} = \dfrac{\Sigma\left(n_g a_g\right)}{\Sigma\left(n_g\right)}$

Where

    n_g = No. of tablets in each group

    a_g = Average thickness of tablets within the group

If the number of tablets in each group is equal, then the equation is given by

The total population mean $\bar{x} = \Sigma\,(a_g) \,/\, G_n$, where G_n is the total number of groups.

Now let us switch to a new concept, that is, if a sample of ten tablets from the population was drawn separately and sample mean ($\bar{x}_s$) and sample standard deviation (σ_s) are calculated. Based on these values, we can estimate the possible standard deviation of the mean with respect to total population being studied. This estimate is called standard error of mean and it is represented by

$$\text{Standard Error (S.E)} = \sqrt{\left(\text{standard deviation}\right)^2 / \text{sample size}} = \sqrt{\left(\sigma\right)^2 / N} = \sigma / \sqrt{N}$$

Where,

$$\sigma = \sqrt{\frac{\Sigma\left(x_i - \bar{x}\right)^2}{N-1}}$$

Then the final equation of **Standard Error** $= \sqrt{\dfrac{\Sigma\left(x_i - \bar{x}\right)^2}{N(N-1)}}$

Where (N-1) is called the degrees of freedom (df), Where N is equal to number of independent variable minus 1 is the number of parameters used in the test for intermittent calculation to achieve final calculation of standard error. Here, one parameter that is mean ($\bar{x}$) is used for intermittent calculation.

Note: Degrees of freedom (df) can be better illustrated of selecting one hat per day among 7 hats on every day of the week without selecting the same hat again. Hence degree of freedom is (N-1)≡(7-1)≡6. This means that the individual has six freedoms to select for six days of his choice and on last day he does not have any freedom (choice) but by force has to select the final left over hat.

Problem 16.1 on Standard Error:

The mean of eight plasma volumes is 3.001 and the standard deviation is 0.311. Calculate the standard error of mean.

Solution:

Standard Error = s/√n = 0.311/√8 = 0.111

Problem 16.2 on Standard Error:

If mean pulse rate of population was 70 per minute and standard deviation was 8 beats, calculate the minimum size of sample to verify the earlier findings.

[Hint: Standard error of mean does not exceed or is not larger than the 1/50th of the population mean.]

Solution:

$$SE = \frac{SD}{\sqrt{n}} = \frac{1}{50} \times \text{Mean}$$

$$SE = \frac{8}{\sqrt{n}} = \frac{1}{50} \times 70$$

at 95% confidence limits,

$$n = \left(\frac{50}{70} \times 8 \times 2\right)^2 = \frac{6400}{49} = 130.6$$

16.2 Estimation of Confidence Level/ Confidence Interval/Confidence Limits

Confidence Limit is the deviate from the mean value until which the individual independent variable is available in the acceptable region of a normal distribution curve. A confidence Limit is the one the researcher is in confident level in saying the statistical test conducted is significant to his comfort. In other words, the level is expected to increase the comfort in judging the statistical test. To determine the confidence level, it is necessary to fix the probability at which the statistical study is tested and in several circumstances, it is considered as 5 % (0.05) probability. The equation for calculating the confidence limit for the study conducted is given by

Confidence Limit (C. L or $\bar{Y}$ or deviate) (probability) = [μ ± (σ * t∞(probability)/√N)]

Where μ = mean; σ = standard deviation; $t_{\infty(probability)}$ = standard deviate value from the mean with reference to the normal distribution curve at the defined probability; N = sample size

For instance, if μ = 2.25; σ = 0.3986; $t_{\infty(95\%)}$ = 1.96; N=100 for one hundred patients with respect to their plasma cholesterol concentrations, then C. L (95%) = 2.25 ± 0.0781 ≈ 2.17 to 2.33

The difference between confidence level, confidence interval and confidence limits are confidence level is an attribute with respect to researcher, confidence interval is the standard deviation range from the mean in the distribution curve and confidence limits are the extreme values of the standard deviation from the mean.

16.3 Application of Confidence Level/Confidence Interval/Confidence Limits in Pharmaceuticals

In pharmaceuticals, samples are drawn and analyzed for pharmacopoeial compliance. It is observed that pharmacopoeial parameters are statistical conclusions, but all pharmaceutical industries does not establish distribution curves for products and this can be further strengthened by drawing sample by statistical calculation and analyzing various pharmacopoeial parameters by statistical methods and drawing conclusion statistically. It is assumed that high end industries follow statistics and the current example narrates who wish to initiate.

A question arises, whether is it possible to initiate? The answer is yes. This is because industries maintain quality data of past batches or an industry can freshly start with the current batch that is being manufactured. In case data is collected from past records, the data is called as retrospective data where as if the data is collected from current batch, the data becomes prospective data.

The immediate question is that what are the various attributes (parameters) and statistical methods. For this, all the pharmacopoeial tests are the attributes and methods are what is the sample size, how to judge a parameter of the sample is significant with the population. For instance, a pharmaceutical industry wishes for tablets and various attributes are tablet weight, thickness, hardness, friability, assay, disintegration time, dissolution time, uniformity of drug content etc.

Steps and procedure to be followed:

Step 1: Draw a sample of 1000 tablets from the current batch. Measure the various parameters (i.e., thickness, hardness, weight, dissolution time, disintegration time etc.). Ensure drawing sample both heterogeneous (different lots) and homogenous (same lot) so that possible variations in the manufacture process are also included.

Step 2: Plot a graph of attribute (say weight of tablet) on x-axis (abscissa) and No. of tablets with same weight on y-axis (ordinate). After plotting the graph, a normal (or 't') distribution curve is expected. Figure 16.1, illustrates a plot of 1000 tablets with respect to weight and corresponding numbers. It gives a clear indication of normal distribution.

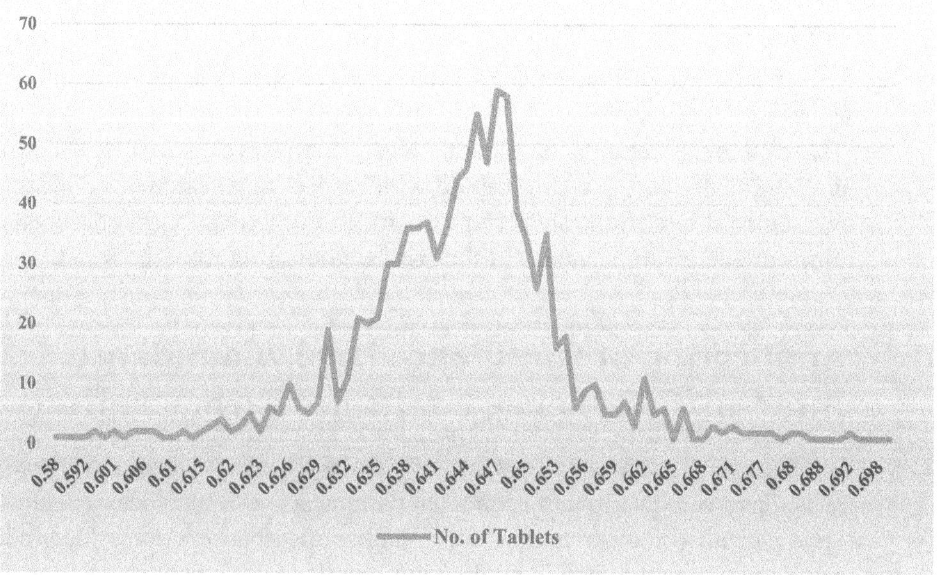

FIGURE 16.1 Weight of 1000 tablets with Corresponding Frequency in Numbers

Step 3: Calculate the average weight of the entire 1000 tablets. This can be considered as average (mu-μ). Similarly a standard deviation (σ) can be calculated. It has been observed that $\mu = 0.643709$ g and $\sigma = 0.012585$ g.

Step 4: Calculation of Confidence Limit, which is usually at 5% probability and 95 % confidence level.

$$\textbf{Confidence limit (C. L or } \boldsymbol{Y} \textbf{ or deviate)}_{\text{(probability)}} = [\mu \pm (\sigma * t_{\infty\,\text{(probability)}} / \sqrt{N})]$$

Where μ = mean; σ = standard deviation; $t_{\infty\,\text{(probability)}}$ (or z value) = standard deviate value from the mean with reference to the normal distribution standard curve at the defined probability for two tailed; N=Population size

Since, μ = 0.643709 g; σ = 0.012585; t_∞ (or z) = 1.96; N=1000 for one thousand tablets with respect to weight, then C. L (95%) = $[\mu \pm (\sigma * t_{\infty\,\text{(probability)}} / \sqrt{N})]$ = $[0.643709 \pm (0.012585 * 1.96 / \sqrt{1000})]$ = $[0.643709 \pm (0.012585 * 0.06198064214)]$ = $[0.643709 \pm (7.800263813 \times 10^{-4})]$ = $[0.643709 \pm 0.0007800263813]$. Hence, tablets in between the range of 0.6444 g to 0.642929 g can be accepted. If a sample of tablets from a new batch and their average weight is not within the range set, the sample/batch fails the weight which is also called as deviate from the z-value.

For a disintegration test (for tablets), Indian Pharmacopoeia 1996 indicates to test on 6 tablets and if 1(17 % fail) or 2 (33 % fail) tablets fail, a repetition of test on additional 12 tablets is suggested. It is indicated that the batch passes when not less than 16 tablets (89 % pass) of the total 18 tablets disintegrate.

Figures 16.2, 16.3 illustrates the trend of diameter and thickness of Paracetamol Tablets indicating a right tailed and two-tailed respectively.

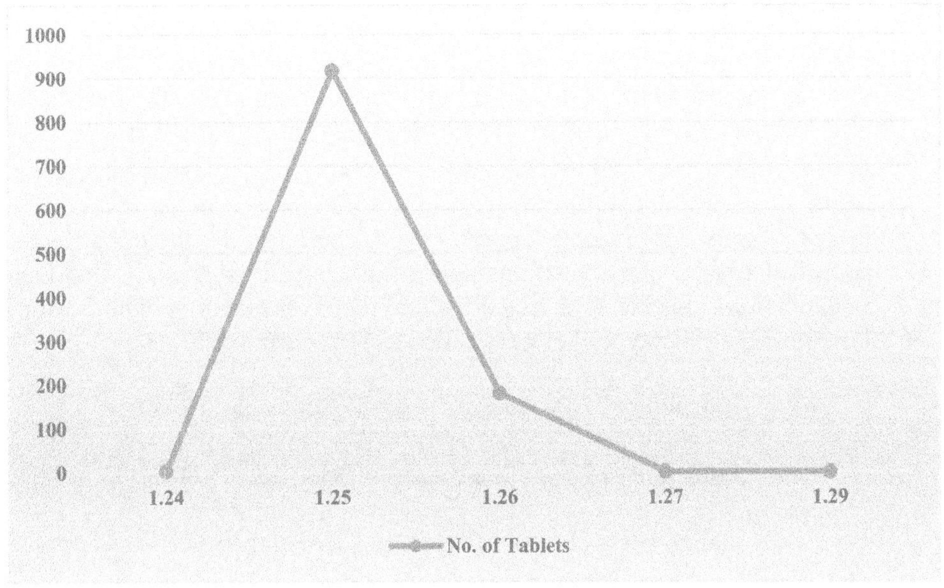

FIGURE 16.2 Trend of Diameter of 1103 Paracetamol Tablets (in cm)

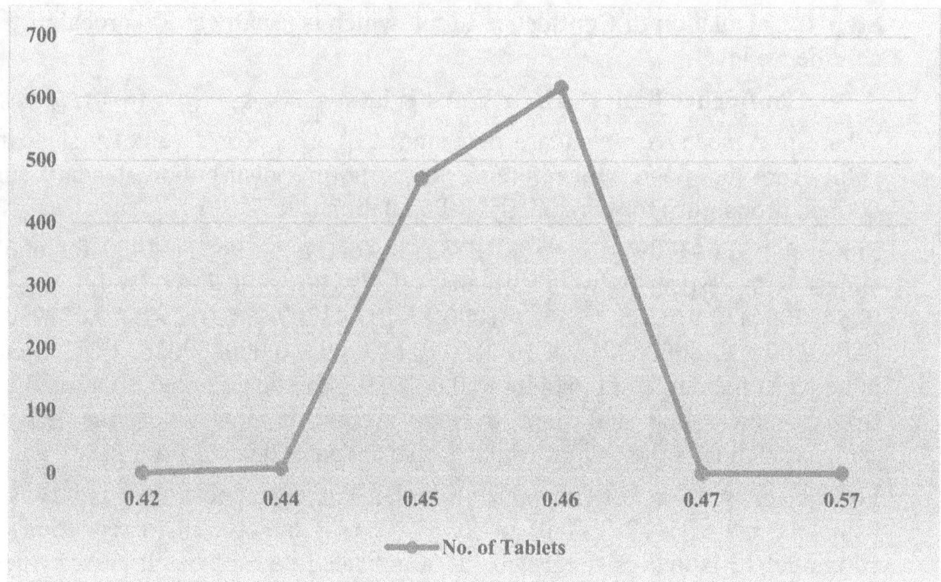

FIGURE 16.3 Trend of Thickness of 1103 Paracetamol Tablets (in cm)

16.4 Statistical Errors

When a sample attribute is analyzed by statistics, there is a chance of occurrence of error in the statistical test conducted. Such errors are called as statistical errors. Statistical errors are classified into "Type I error" and "Type II error".

In case of a "Type I error", the error has occurred in a statistical test by incorrectly rejecting a true null hypothesis. This means that the researcher has identified an effect that is actually not present. In case of a "Type II error", the error has occurred in a statistical test by incorrectly retaining a false null hypothesis. This means that the researcher was unable to detect the effect that is present. A type I error is called as false positive and a type II error is called as false negative.

$$\text{Probability of Type I error} = \alpha = P(\text{Reject } H_0 \mid H_0 \text{ is true})$$

$$\text{Probability of Type II error} = \beta = P(\text{Do not reject } H_0 \mid H_0 \text{ is false})$$

$$\text{and Power} = (1 - \beta) = (\text{Reject } H_0 \mid H_0 \text{ is false})$$

This can be explained with an example:

Let us imagine a hypothesis (proposal) is made saying "Rinsing tooth paste with water prevents against cavities". For this, the researcher develops a null hypothesis saying "Rinsing tooth paste with water has no effect against cavities" with a desperate intention of nullifying the null hypothesis. Simultaneously, the researcher also proposes an alternate hypothesis saying "Rinsing tooth paste with water prevents against cavities". To study the hypothesis made, the researcher has to select some volunteers (say sample size of 50 patients) and divides them into two groups i.e., control group and test group using random technique. Initially, every individual volunteer was selected after fulfilling inclusion and exclusion criteria made before conducting the study. This means that the volunteer status of tooth condition were scored with respect to number present, scoring of teeth (if necessary every individual teeth) with respect to decay, any cavity already present, level of tooth cavity etc. Both the groups are provided with the tooth paste and the control group does not rinse the tooth paste with water whereas the test group rinse the tooth paste with water. The test was conducted for a period of 1 year with the researcher taking the scores of every individual every month. After 12 months, the researcher has the data of all the volunteers for statistical analysis. The researcher during the process of scoring may lead to errors that are considered as "Type I error" and "Type II error" and at this stage needs imagination of possible errors.

It is necessary to understand that if we reject null hypothesis there is a risk of committing type I error and if we accept null hypothesis there is a risk of committing type II error. Controlling both the errors is not possible. If we reduced type I error, this may lead to increase in type II error. Hence, an optimum type I error probability of occurrence (say 5%) and type II error probability of occurrence (say 10%) are fixed. It is also necessary to understand that when a study is conducted on a large population, the errors are minimized. As it is not possible with large population and as we are using very small samples of a population, we try to fix the optimum levels of type I and type II errors and calculate a statistically significant number of sample sizes for the study.

Let us imagine another example, in a class of 10 students, let the null hypothesis is framed as all the students are regular to classes and the alternate hypothesis is all the students are not regular. Here, the researcher developed the null hypothesis to nullify it and accept the alternate hypothesis. An error occur when the teacher gives absent when student was present or the vice-versa of when the students present giving absent. A type I error of incorrectly rejecting the true null hypothesis occurs when all the students were present for class but wrongly rejected the null hypothesis and the probability of rejecting the null hypothesis is given by 'α' usually accepted value is 5%. In case of type II error, in-correctly retaining a false null-hypothesis that is, null-hypothesis is wrong but was accepted. The probability of occurrence of type II error is given by 'β', which usually takes a value of 10%. This implies that scientists accept errors to a permissible limit. If the type I error is up to 5% and type II error is up to 10%. It is in the acceptable limit.

In terms of probability, "α-alpha" denotes probability of occurrence of type I error and "β-beta" denotes probability of occurrence of type II error. For a statistical significant test, the test should have optimum "α-alpha" and as low as possible "β-beta".

A statistical test is said to be working well provided the "Power" of the statistical test is high. A "Power" of a statistical test is represented by "1-β". In order to achieve good Power for a statistical test, the Power depends on

i.   The statistical significance criterion selected for the test i.e., p=5% usually in pharmaceuticals

ii.   The magnitude of the effect of interest in the population

iii. The sample size used to detect the effect

This can be interpreted better with the normal distribution curve.

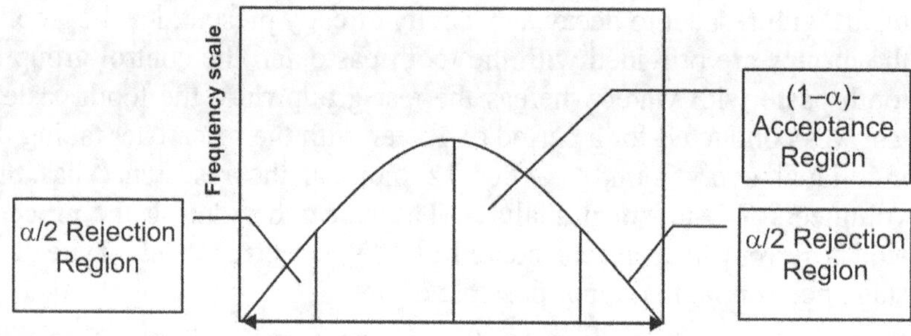

FIGURE 16.4 Normal Distribution with Type I Error

If the total probability, Figure 16.4, under the normal distribution is considered as 1 or 100 % (maximum value) and the probability of type I error (α-alpha) for a two tailed test is α/2 + (1-α) + α/2. If a value falls in α/2 region i.e., a value in the lower region (for left tailed) and a value in the higher region (for right tailed), the null hypothesis is rejected. This implies, the alternate hypothesis which is accepted, falls in the acceptance region of (1-α). The total probability under the curve is given by $\alpha + (1 - \alpha)$.

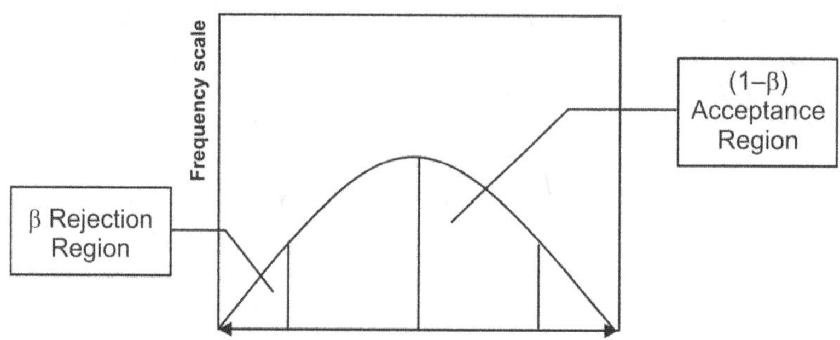

FIGURE 16.5 Normal Distribution with Type II Error

Likewise, when type II error and its probability (β) are considered, Figure 16.5, the value of 'β' should be low so as the power (1-β) is high enough tending towards unity indicating the statistical test is working well. If a plot for type II error for a normal curve is made, 'β' must be expected in the 'α/2' rejection region and '1- β' in the acceptable region.

Hence, it is necessary to keep in mind, a distribution curve with respect to an attribute in question, probability curves with respect to type 1 and type II errors while understanding the concepts, for instance Figure 16.6 for hypothesis.

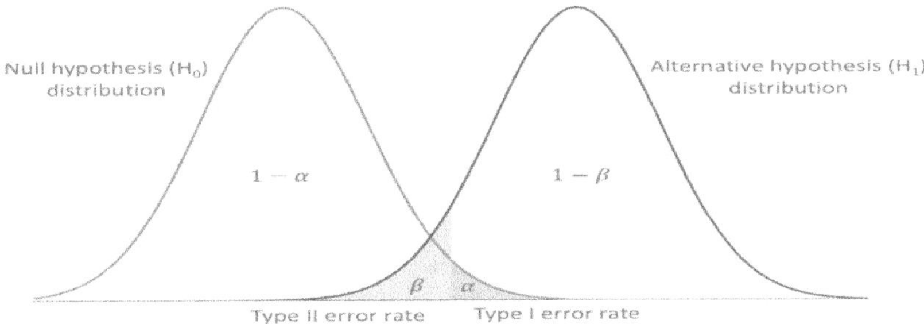

Figure 16.6 Hypothesis, Type I and Type II errors

Hence a final decision can be taken as mentioned in Table 16.1.

TABLE 16.1 Types of Error in Significance Testing

Conclusion of Significance Test	Reality	
	Null Hypothesis is true	**Null Hypothesis is false**
Reject Null hypothesis	Type I Error (probability = significance) i.e. (p = α)	Correct Conclusion (p = Power) i.e., (p = 1-β)
Accept Null hypothesis (or do not reject null hypothesis)	Correct Conclusion (probability = 1 – significance) i.e., (p=1-α)	Type II Error (probability = 1- Power) i.e., (p = β)

Problem 16.3 on Normal distribution:

Calculate the probability of a value falling between -1.96 and +1.28 for the standard normal curve.

Solution:

The area corresponding to Z = -1.96 is 0.025. The area corresponding to +1.28 is 0.9. The difference is 0.875.

Thus the probability of observing a value between -1.96 and +1.28 is 0.875.

Problem 16.4 on Normal distribution: What is the probability that a tablet will weigh between 185 mg and 210 mg if tablet weights have an approximately normal distribution with mean 200 mg and a standard deviation of 10? Hint: Use Z transformation (normal distribution)

Solution: For a normal distribution curve, the value for z is given by the formulation

$$x = \mu \pm \frac{\sigma z}{\sqrt{N}}$$

Where, x = tablet weight, μ = mean, σ = standard deviation, z= standard value of deviation from standard normal distribution curve, N=Population size

As, N=1, then the equation is

$$x = \mu \pm \sigma z$$

After re-arranging the equation, $z = \dfrac{x-\mu}{\sigma} = \dfrac{185-200}{10} = -1.5$

$$z = \frac{x - \mu}{\sigma} = \frac{210 - 200}{10} = 1$$

The cumulative area, in a standard normal distribution curve, corresponding to $z = -1.5$ and $z = +1$ are 0.0668 and 0.8413 respectively.

Therefore, the probability of finding a tablet weighing between 185 and 210 mg is 0.84-0.07=0.77

Problem 16.5 on Normal distribution:

When inspecting 100 tablets for quality, what is the probability of observing a proportion of defective tablets equal to or greater than 0.10, if the true proportion defective is 0.07?

Solution: The equation of normal approximation to the binomial distribution is

$$z = \frac{|p - p_0| - \dfrac{1}{2n}}{\sqrt{\dfrac{p_o q_o}{n}}}$$

Where, p = observed proportion, p_0 = true probability of success (= 0.5), n = number of binomial trials, the sample size, 1/2n is Yates continuity correction for improvement of approximation.

Therefore,

$$z = \frac{|0.1 - 0.07| - \dfrac{1}{200}}{\sqrt{\dfrac{0.07 \times 0.93}{100}}} = 0.98$$

From cumulative normal distribution area chart, the probability of a value less than Z = 0.98 is approximately 0.84. The probability of a value greater than Z = 0.98 is $1 - 0.84 = 0.16$. Therefore, the probability of observing a proportion greater than 0.1 when inspecting 100 tablets from this batch is approximately 0.16.

Problem 16.6 on Binomial Data:

Suppose that of 1000 tablets inspected, 25 were found to be defective. Find the confidence limits in this binomial case at 99 % confidence interval.

Solution:

The equation for confidence limits for a binomial data is as follows:

$$\text{Confidence Limits} = p \pm Z \sqrt{\frac{pq}{N}}$$

Here the proportion of good tablets = 975/1000 = 0.975

At 99 % confidence interval,

$$\text{Confidence Limits} = 0.975 \pm 2.58\sqrt{\frac{(0.025)(0.975)}{1000}} = 0.975 \pm 0.013$$

Problem 16.7 on Binomial Data

Quality control data gathered from many batches showed that 4% of tablets manufactured with a target weight o f200 mg weighed more than 220 mg or less than 180 mg, the upper and lower QC limits. Examination of a new batch shows that 32 of 500 tablets (6.4%) are out of specifications. Is this result unexpected based on the previous history of the batch (4%, or 20 tablets, are expected to be out of limits).

[**Hint:** Comparison of proportions].

Solution:

Let, H_0: $p_0 = 0.04$ and H_A: $p_0 \neq 0.04$

$$Z = \frac{[p - p_0] - \dfrac{1}{2N}}{\sqrt{\dfrac{p_0 q_0}{N}}} = \frac{\left[|0.064 - 0.040| - \frac{1}{1000}\right]}{\sqrt{\dfrac{(0.04)(0.96)}{500}}} = 2.62$$

The new batch has significantly more tablets out of limits than are normally observed. A 95% confidence interval on the true proportion of out-of-limit tablets in this batch is

$$\text{Confidence Limits} = p \pm Z\sqrt{\frac{pq}{N}} = 0.064 \pm 1.96\sqrt{\frac{(0.064)(0.936)}{500}}$$

$$= 0.064 \pm 0.021$$

Problem 16.8 on Binomial Data:

Diseased animals were treated with either placebo (control) or drug. Sixty on of 75 of the control animals survived, whereas 69 of 75 animals given the drug survived. Is the drug more effective than the control in preventing death? The data is as follows:

Fourfold Table Showing Number of Animals Alive and Dead After Three Months			
	Alive	Dead	Total
Control	61	14	75
Drug	69	6	75
Total	130	20	150

Solution:

Let the H_0: $P_{drug} = P_{placebo}$ and H_A: $P_{drug} \neq P_{placebo}$, where P_{drug} is the probability that an animal will survive the drug treatment and $P_{placebo}$ is the probability that an animal will survive placebo treatment.

This is the binomial analog of the independent groups two sample 't' test. In the 't' test, the variances were pooled under the assumption of equal variability in the two groups. Here, all the data are pooled to estimate a common p, the best estimate of the true probability under the null hypothesis, which states that the two populations have the same proportion of survivors. The pooled $p = p_0 = 130/150 = 0.867$ (overall proportion of survivors)

Then,

$$Z = \frac{\left[\left|p_1 - p_2\right| - \frac{1}{N}\right]}{\sqrt{(p_0)(q_0)\left(\frac{1}{N_1} + \frac{1}{N_2}\right)}} = \frac{\left[\left|0.92 - 0.813\right| - \frac{1}{75}\right]}{\sqrt{(0.867)(0.133)\left(\frac{1}{75} + \frac{1}{75}\right)}} = 1.68$$

In this case, the difference is significant at the 10 % level, not significant at the usual 5% level.

16. 5 Hypothesis and Steps involved in Statistical Analysis

Hypothesis is an assumption made for a problem before solving it. A statistician develops a null hypothesis as well as alternate hypothesis and tries to solve the problem. Before conducting the statistical test, the researcher defines the level of significance. After conducting the statistical test, based on the result the statistician either rejects or accepts a null hypothesis. In other words, if null hypothesis is rejected, the statistician accepts the alternate hypothesis or the vice-versa. As the word indicates, a null-hypothesis is developed with an intension to nullify the hypothesis. For instance, two samples each of twenty tablets are available. The two samples are collected with an objective to determine the drug content (assay value) and say whether they are from same batch or two different batches manufactured. Here, initially, the statistician defines the null-hypothesis (H_0) in such a way that, the two samples of tablets are from the same batch. As an alternate hypothesis (H_A) the statistician defines the two samples of tablets are from different batches. The two hypotheses are only assumptions. After conducting the appropriate statistical test, based on the results obtained, the statistician compares with theoretical deviate value and finally gives a decision whether to accept the null hypothesis or not. After making the decision on the hypothesis, the statistician comes to a conclusion with respect to the two samples of tablets.

The steps involved in statistical analysis are as follows:

Step 1: Defining a null hypothesis

Step 2: Defining an alternative hypothesis

Step 3: Defining the probability limits and to be considered two tailed or single tailed (right or left tail)

Step 4: Identifying the appropriate statistical test and explaining the reason behind why the test is appropriate.

Step 5: Calculating the provided data with respect to the statistical test equation.

Step 6: Mentioning a statement saying the calculated statistical test value is greater than the standard statistical test value (from standard charts) or the vice versa.

Step 7: Using the calculated and standard values, after deciding the hypothesis, concluding with respect to the given problem.

17 Student "t" Distribution and its Applications

17.0 Introduction

Gossett has developed a distribution derived from normal distribution and it was named as student 't' distribution. Several sample means drawn from several large samples of the same population have a normal distribution where as in case of student 't' distribution, as the sample sizes are smaller than normal, the distribution is slightly different from normal and it is called as student 't' distribution. In other words, means of large samples have Gaussian distribution whereas means of small samples have student 't' distribution. The characteristic features of student 't' distribution are that the bell shaped curve is slightly flattened at the top and has two elongated tails at either ends of the curve.

Student 't' curve can be illustrated, Figure 17.1, as follows:

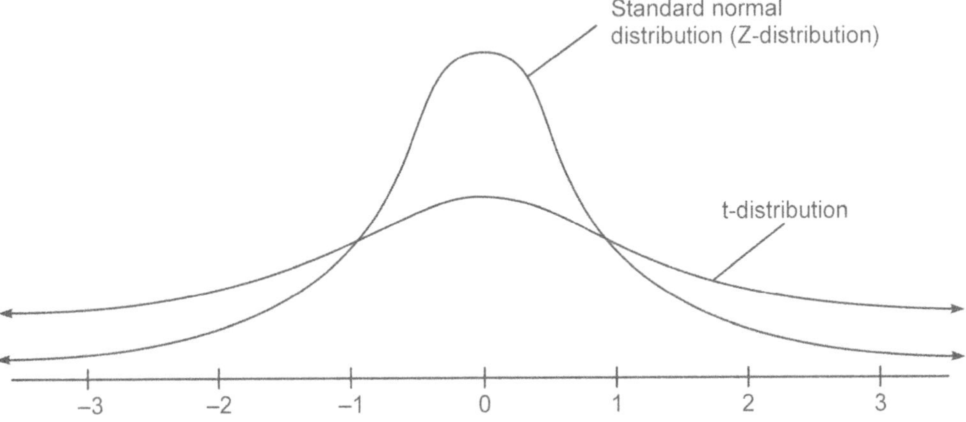

FIGURE 17.1 Student 't' Distribution with Comparison with Normal Distribution

For a student 't' distribution, the confidence limit is given by

$$\textbf{Confidence Limit (C. L or } \bar{Y} \textbf{ or deviate)}_{\text{(probability)}} = [\bar{x} \pm (s * t_{\text{(probability)}}/\sqrt{N})]$$

Where $\bar{x}$ = mean; s = standard deviation; "$t_{(probability)}$=" = standard deviate value with reference to the student 't' distribution curve at the defined probability; N=sample size

As other applications, Student 't' test is used to find out whether there is significant difference between means of two treatment groups/drugs effect/drug quality parameters etc. The principal features for student 't' test are

i. The two treatment groups should fulfill individually a normal distribution.

ii. The variance between the groups should be almost the same and the current distribution test helps for groups having variance up to 4 factor variation, else a different Behrens-Fisher test is used.

iii. The two groups should be independent. This means that influence of treatment of one group does not influence on the other group. For instance, in a study of two group of patients with a placebo and drug treatment groups, if a placebo treatment group patient given with white colour tablet discloses to drug treatment group patient that he has been given with placebo (white colour tablet), then the result would not be independent. Likewise, two groups of animals are planned for two treatments and during the process, if all the animals are put in one cage with food. Competition for food and other interactions favour the stronger animal and influence the treatment effect.

17.1 Un-paired 't' Test

The above characteristic features are required especially for an unpaired or two independent sample 't' test (also called as parallel group test). Where as in a paired student 't' test, the two treatments are applicable on the same patient.

When two groups of patients (say) with un-equal number are subjected for treatment and the mean effect for their statistical significance is determined by the following equation:

$$t = \frac{difference}{standard\ error\ of\ difference}$$

and for calculation purpose, it is given by

$$t = \frac{\overline{x_{1i}} - \overline{x_{2i}}}{s} \sqrt{\frac{n_1 n_2}{n_1 + n_2}}$$

Where $\overline{x_{1i}}$ = mean of values of group 1, $\overline{x_{2i}}$ = mean of values of group 2, n_1 = number of observations in group 1, n_2=number of observations in group 2 and s = standard deviation is given by

$$s^2 = \frac{\{\sum x_{1i}^2 - \frac{(\sum x_{1i})^2}{n_1} + \sum x_{2i}^2 - \frac{(\sum x_{2i})^2}{n_2}\}}{(n_1 + n_2 - 2)}$$

Problem 1 on un-paired 't' test: Suppose one sample of four and another one sample of five are taken, respectively, from each of two lots of amobarbital capsules and the amount of amobarbital is determined in each capsule. It is desired to determine if there is a significant difference between the two samples. Conduct the test at 5 % level. The values of Sample 1 and Sample 2 are as follows:

Sample 1	Sample 2
10.1	9.8
13.6	9.6
12.5	11.4
11.4	9.1
	10.1

Solution: Let the null hypothesis H_o is defined as the average of sample 1 and sample 2 are equal. That is $H_o = \mu_1 = \mu_2$.

Let the alternate hypothesis is $H_a = \mu_1 \neq \mu_2$. This means that the test is two tailed since either of the sample means can be higher or lower than the other.

Now let us first calculate the standard deviation 's' so as to substitute in the student 't' test equation.

$$s^2 = \frac{\{\sum x_{1i}^2 - \frac{(\sum x_{1i})^2}{n_1} + \sum x_{2i}^2 - \frac{(\sum x_{2i})^2}{n_2}\}}{(n_1 + n_2 - 2)}$$

Tablet No	Sample 1(x_{1i})	Sample 2 (x_{2i})
1	10.1	9.8
2	13.6	9.6
3	12.5	11.4
4	11.4	9.1
5	-----	10.1
$\sum x_i$	47.6	50.0
$\sum x_i^2$	573.18	502.98
Mean	11.9	10.0
N	4	5

$$s^2 = \frac{\{573.18 - \frac{(47.6)^2}{4} + 502.98 - \frac{(50.0)^2}{5}\}}{(4 + 5 - 2)}$$

There for $s^2 = 1.3886$ and s $= 1.18$

Then

$$t = \frac{11.9 - 10.0}{1.18} \sqrt{\frac{4(5)}{4 + 5}}$$

Therefore 't' = 1.16 (1.49) = 2.40. This calculated 't' value has to be compared with theoretical 't' value. For a two tailed test, at 5 % probability, for a degree of freedom of 7, the theoretical 't' value is 2.365. In a 't' distribution curve, as calculated 't' value (2.4) is greater than theoretical 't' value (2.365), the calculated value falls in null hypothesis region which is rejected as there is statistical significant difference between the two samples. Since, the probability of these two samples being drawn from the same population is less than 0.05, we conclude that they were drawn from different populations (this conclusion may be wrong 5 times in 100).

Note: Several times, the difference in theoretical and calculated 't' values is very less. Under such circumstance, it is usually concluded that the sample size has to be increased (or re-drawn) for better conclusions.

17.2 Paired 't' Test

Unlike in two independent group student 't' test discussed earlier, in a paired 't' test, both the standard drug and test drug are tested on the same individual. In this test, the significance is determined by the ratio of average of the differences divided to the standard error. This ratio can be reduced by decreasing the denominator i.e., standard error. This can be achieved by increasing the sample size and decreasing the variability. In paired 't' test, the advantage is that the variability is less and this is due to less variation within the patient when compared among patients. The second advantage is that the test can be conducted with minimum patients i.e., if a paired 't' test has 24 patients, then un-paired 't' test has 48 patients. The disadvantage with paired 't' test is that the test is time consuming. The equation for calculating 't' value for a paired 't' test is

$$t = \frac{\overline{d}}{s} \sqrt{n}$$

Where, $\overline{d}$ = mean of the differences, $x_1 - x_2$ of the n pairs of observations.

$$s^2 = \frac{\left(\sum d_i^2 - \frac{(\sum d_i)^2}{n} \right)}{n - 1}$$

Problem 2 on paired 't' test: The duration of loss of the righting reflex (minutes) was measured in 16 mice following treatment with a barbiturate. The drug was administered in the morning and the afternoon on two different occasions; the order of giving the morning or the afternoon dose was randomized in each mouse. It was desired to test the null hypothesis that the duration of loss of the righting reflux is the same in the morning and the afternoon. The loss of righting reflux of the 16 mice was as follows:

Mouse No	AM (x_1)	PM (x_2)	Difference (d) = ($x_1 - x_2$)
1	75	73	2
2	86	89	-3
3	93	89	4
4	87	79	8
5	91	95	-4
6	87	81	6
7	76	77	-1
8	83	89	-6
9	87	82	5
10	95	91	4
11	91	87	4
12	86	86	0
13	83	78	5
14	76	69	7
15	82	78	4
16	93	88	5
			$\sum d_i = 40$
			$\sum d_i^2 = 354$
			$\bar{d} = 2.5$
			n = 16

Solution:

Let the null hypothesis H_0: $\delta = 0$, where δ is the hypothesized difference of the true means. It is hypothesized that the mean results of the two treatments are identical.

Substituting the values in paired 't' test equation i.e.,

$$s^2 = \frac{(354 - \frac{(40)^2}{16})}{16 - 1}$$

$s^2 = 16.9333$ and s = 4.11

Therefore,

$$t = \frac{\bar{d}}{s}\sqrt{n} = \frac{2.5}{4.11}\sqrt{16} = 2.43$$

At a probability of 5 percent (0.05) and degrees of freedom (df)= 15, the theoretical 't' value is 2.131. The calculated 't' value (2.43) is greater than theoretical 't' value (2.131). This indicates the probability of morning and afternoon values being the same is less than 0.05. This implies null hypothesis is rejected and we conclude loss of righting reflux for morning and afternoon values are different.

18 Chi-square Distribution

It was observed that binomial distribution becomes normal when the sample size is more. Likewise, when probability becomes small a binomial becomes a poisson distribution. Several distributions like chi-square (χ^2), F-distribution, student 't' distribution were derived from normal distribution. This clearly indicates large population parameters may fall into normal distribution but, as population data collection is not practical we have to depend on small samples that fall into either of the distribution except for normal distribution. Figure 18.1, illustrates the trend for a chi-square distribution

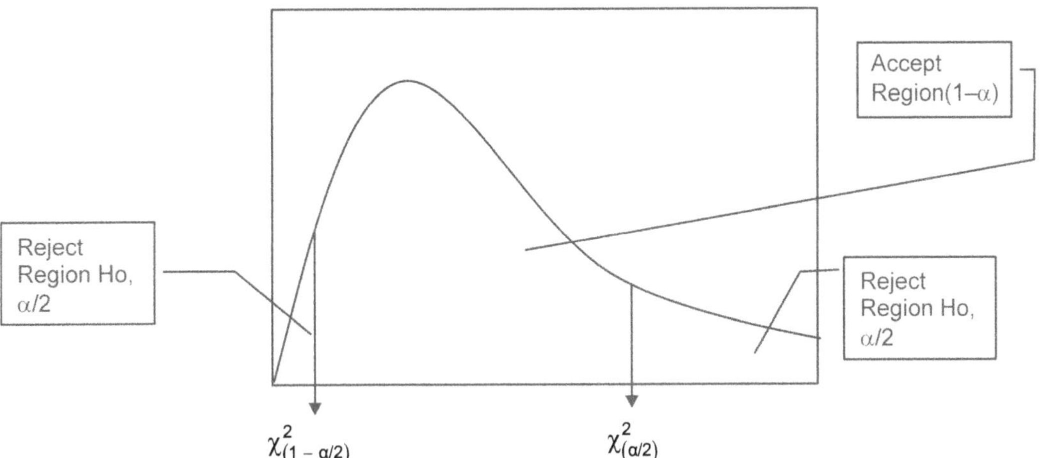

FIGURE 18.1 Chi-square Distribution (two tailed)

Experimental parameters that fall under the chi-square distribution are tested using chi-square test. The test is applied only when the individual observations of sample are independent which mean that the occurrence of one individual observation has no effect upon the occurrence of any. Chi-square is quite commonly used preliminary test to test the collected data is appropriate in collection or not and based on the result necessary changes can be made while collecting the data while doing the research. In other words, a chi-square test is used initially for testing data for significance and at a later stage suitable parametric or non-parametric statistic test can be conducted for drawing final conclusions.

This means that chi-square test is used not only for parametric but also for non-parametric. In addition to this the test is also suitable to categorical variables.

For degree of freedom up to 30, the confidence interval or the confidence limits for a chi-square distribution is given by

$$Z_c = \sqrt{2\chi_c^2} - \sqrt{2n-1}$$

Where, χ_c^2 is the test statistic and n is the sample size for the test statistic.

If the degree of freedom is more than 30, the Z_c is compared with the critical value with respect to normal distribution.

To test difference of two proportions from two independent samples, the chi-square test is used. A chi-square test is also used for any distribution. Chi-square test is used in statistics to designate when the sum of squares of standard deviations is a Gaussian distribution and is represented as

$$\chi^2 = \Sigma \left(\frac{x-\mu}{\sigma}\right)^2 \text{ or } \chi_c^2 = \frac{(n-1)s^2}{\sigma_0^2} \text{ or } \chi^2 = \Sigma \left[\frac{(O-E)^2}{E}\right]$$

Where, O = Observed frequency

E= Expected frequency

The calculated chi-square value is compared with tabled chi-square value. The tabled value of chi-square is referred to the table at a degree of freedom of (no. of columns-1) x (no. of rows – 1)

Problem 18.1, on chi-square test: Mydriatic action of ephedrine was tested on sixty subjects by instilling a 2% solution into the conjunctiva. Half of the subjects were European and the other half were non-European. The extent of the dilatation of the pupil produced in these two groups of subjects is as follows:

Race	Dilatation of pupil 1 mm or more	Dilatation of pupil less than 1 mm	Row totals
Europeans	23	7	30
Non-Europeans	3	27	30
Column totals	26	34	60

Solution:

Step 1: Let us assume the null hypothesis H_0 as there is no difference between mydriatic action (pupil dilatation) between European and non-Europeans.

Step 2: Let the alternate hypothesis be H_a as, there is difference between mydriatic action (pupil dilatation) between European and non-Europeans.

Step 3: The researcher has the intention to nullify the null hypothesis and performs the chi-square test.

Race	Dilatation of pupil 1 mm or more (Expected)	Dilatation of pupil less than 1 mm (Expected)	Row totals
Europeans	30 X 26/60 = 13	30 X 34/60 = 17	30
Non-Europeans	30 X 26/60 = 13	30 X 34/60 = 17	30
Column totals	26	34	60

Substituting the values in the equation i.e.,

$$\chi^2 = \sum \left[\frac{(O-E)^2}{E} \right]$$

Where, O = Observed frequency

E = Expected frequency

$\chi^2 = (23-13)^2/13 + (7-17)^2/17 + (3-13)^2/13 + (27-17)^2/17$

$\chi^2 = 100/13 + 100/17 + 100/13 + 100/17 = 7.67 + 5.88 + 7.69 + 5.88 = 27.14$

Step 4: Here the degrees of freedom (df) is (r-1)(c-1) = (2-1)(2-1) = 1. Hence, at degree of freedom of 1, the tabled chi-square value at 5% probability is 3.84. The calculated value is 27.14. As the calculated value is greater than theoretical value, the null hypothesis is rejected and alternate hypothesis is accepted.

Step 5: Hence, we can conclude that there is difference between the mydriatic action of European and non-European.

Step 6: As the number of mydriatic action (pupil dilatation) in European (23) is higher than non-European (3), this clearly indicates that Europeans are more sensitive to pupil dilatation for Ephedrine.

Problem 18.2, on chi-square test: A multicenter clinical trial on treatment of low back pain was conducted on 336 patients. Four types of treatments were used i.e., 'A' by manipulation, 'B' by manipulative physiotherapy, 'C' by use of a corset or brace, 'D' by analgesics. After 6 weeks the classes of treatment were assessed by physicians under the six categories of α: worse, β: unchanged; γ: slightly improved, δ: moderately improved, ε: markedly improved, ζ: completely relieved. The observed and expected distributions are as follows:

Class	Samples				Class totals
	A	**B**	**C**	**D**	
α (alpha)	10 (6.6)	3 (5.8)	4 (5.6)	7 (6.0)	24
β (beta)	12 (14.5)	12 (12.8)	13 (12.5)	16 (13.3)	53
γ (gamma)	5 (10.7)	12 (9.4)	8 (9.2)	14 (9.8)	39
δ (delta)	11 (11.2)	8 (9.9)	13 (9.6)	9 (10.3)	41
ε (epsilon)	28 (25.7)	26 (22.7)	21 (22.1)	19 (23.5)	94
ζ (zeta)	26 (23.2)	20 (20.5)	20 (20.0)	19 (21.3)	85
Sample totals	92	81	79	84	336

Solution:

Step 1: Let us assume as null hypothesis all the four treatments have no difference and the alternate hypothesis that the four treatments have significant difference.

Step 2: To conduct the chi-test, expected observation is calculated using the equation (class total x sample total/grand total).

Step 3: The calculated chi-test value is

$$\chi^2 = \sum \left[\frac{(O-E)^2}{E} \right]$$

Which is equal to 11.38.

Step 4: The tabled value of chi-test at degree of freedom of (4-1)(6-1)=15 and at probability of 10 % is 15.99 (for df 10) and 28.41 (for df 20).

Step 5: As the calculated value is lower than the tabled value, we accept the null hypothesis and conclude that there is no significant difference between the treatments.

19 F-Distribution (Variance Ratio) and ANOVA

19.0 Introduction

A student 't' test is used to compare two means, likewise an 'F' test is used to compare two variances. When the groups are more than two, Analysis of Variance (ANOVA) helps in comparing by one test instead of several multiple 't' (among means) and 'F' (among variances) tests. However, if the researcher wants to find among which two means and two variances, it is necessary to depend on 't' and 'F' tests respectively.

19.1 F-Distribution

Like t-test is used to compare two means, F-distribution developed by R. A. Fisher from χ^2 statistic has been developed for comparing two variances. A distribution of 'F' is as mentioned in Figure 19.1.

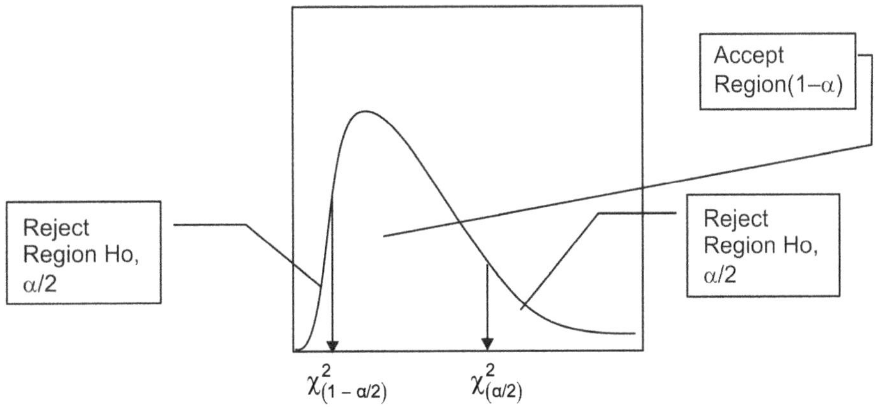

FIGURE 19.1 F-Distribution (two tailed)

Therefore, chi-square is represented by

$$\chi^2 = \sum[(x-\mu)^2/\sigma]=ns^2/\sigma^2$$

Where, x=individual parameter, μ=mean of parameter, σ=population standard deviation, s = sample standard deviation and s^2 = sample variance.

The value of $F = (s_1)^2/(s_2)^2$,

where $(s_1)^2$ is greater than $(s_2)^2$.

Hence F value can be represented as $F = \{[(\chi_1)^2/n_1]/(\chi_2)^2/n_2]\}$,

where n_1, n_2 are degrees of freedom.

For a small sample size, the chance of error while calculating variances is large. Hence, in order to minimize the error, a correction factor is included as mentioned below

$$F = [(s_1)^2/(s_2)^2] \times [N_1/(N_1 - 1)] \times [N_2/(N_2 - 1)]$$

Where N_1 and N_2 are sample sizes.

Problem 19.1, on F-test:

Patients were being selected for use in a trial of an antihypertensive drug. Of the 11 patients available, 5 were attending one clinic (clinic A) and 6 another (clinic B). The systolic blood pressures (mmHg) were as follows:

Patients in clinic A	190	195	200	205	210	---
Patients in clinic B	165	175	190	200	225	245

Find out whether there is any difference between the variances of the two groups.

Solution:

	N	$\sum Y$	$\overline{Y}$ (Y-bar)	$\sum Y^2$	$\sum(Y-\overline{Y})^2$	n	s^2
A	5	1000	200	200250	250	4	62.5
B	6	1200	200	244600	4600	5	920

Therefore

$$F = \left[\frac{(s_1)^2}{(s_2)^2}\right] \times \left[\frac{N_1}{(N_1 -1)}\right] \times \left[\frac{N_2}{(N_2 -1)}\right] = \left[\frac{(920\times6\times5)}{(62.5\times5\times4)}\right] = \frac{27600}{1250} = 22.08$$

Tabled 'F' value at 5% probability and degree of freedom of 5 in the numerator and degree of freedom of 4 in the denominator is 6.26 (approx.). Since, calculated 'F' value is greater than tabled value, we can conclude that the two variances are different and the two groups of patients are significantly different.

19.2 Analysis of Variance or ANOVA

When two or more means have to be compared, whether there is any difference among them, it is by Analysis of Variance statistical analysis it can be concluded. It is necessary to understand that if it has to be compared among two means, on can apply student 't' test. Hence, it is usual to compare more than two means by analysis of variance (ANOVA) technique.

Analysis of variance (ANOVA) is of several types i.e., one way ANOVA and the other by two way ANOVA etc., One way ANOVA is in analogy with un-paired 't' test (or two independent group 't' test or completely randomized design) whereas, a two way ANOVA goes in analogy with paired 't' test (or randomized blocks).

Let us imagine two generic drugs A and B have to be compared with a control drug. Three groups of equal number of patients were allotted as three treatment groups as A, B and Control. Analysis of variance (ANOVA) helps in minimizing the errors between treatments (groups) as well as errors occurring within the group.

An ANOVA tabled (standard) values are established on four factors i.e., source of variance, degrees of freedom, sum of squares and mean squares. Variances are observed between treatments, within a group (treatment) and in total terms; degrees of freedom (indirectly on sample size) indicating the variance occurring when small samples taken for test, sum of squares and finally the mean square which is determined by dividing sum of squares by degrees of freedom.

19.2.1 One-way ANOVA

One-way ANOVA is also called as randomized controlled design or randomized controlled experiment. In one-way ANOVA, the Total Sum of Squares (TSS) is addition of Between Sum of Squares (BSS) and Within Sum of Squares (WSS). It is necessary to understand that WSS (Within Sum of Squares) assess the errors occurring due to variations in the patients (subjects) etc.

In ANOVA, the comparison of variances is made by the F distribution formula i.e., the variance ratio i.e.,

$$F = \frac{Between\ Mean\ Square\ (BMS)}{Within\ Mean\ Square\ (WMS)}$$

In order to obtain Between Mean Square (BMS), it is given as division of Between Sum of Squares (BSS) by degree of freedom which is given by (t-1), where t indicates the number of treatment groups. For obtaining Within Mean Square (WMS), it is given as division of Within Sum of Squares (WSS) by degree of freedom which is given by (n-t), where n is the total number of observations as a whole in all the treatment groups and 't' is the number of treatment groups.

Hence,

$$F = \frac{Between\ Mean\ Square\ (BMS)}{Within\ Mean\ Square\ (WMS)} = \frac{BSS/(t-1)}{WSS/(n-t)}$$

Hence, it is necessary to find out BSS, WSS and TSS to calculate BMS, WMS and to finally calculate the F value.

The equations to determine the Total Sum of Squares (TSS), Between Sum of Squares (BSS) and Within Sum of Squares (WSS) are as follows:

$$Total\ SS\ (or\ TSS) = \sum x^2 - \frac{(\sum x)^2}{N}$$

$$Between\ SS\ (or\ BSS) = \frac{(\sum x_1)^2}{n_1} + \frac{(\sum x_2)^2}{n_2} + \frac{(\sum x_3)^2}{n_3} + \cdots + \frac{(\sum x_{10})^2}{n_{10}} - \frac{(\sum x)^2}{N}$$

$$Within\ regimens\ SS\ (or\ WSS) = TSS - BSS$$

After calculating the 'F' value, it is compared with the tabled 'F' value. In order to obtain the tabled 'F' value, it is necessary to refer on the horizontal side for degree of freedom (referring to greater mean square) and on the vertical side for degree of freedom (referring to smaller mean square). If the calculated 'F' value is greater than Tabled 'F' value then we reject the null hypothesis (which indicates all the means are same) and accept alternate hypothesis (which indicates at least two means are different).

Problem 19.2, on One-Way ANOVA:

Groups of three subjects each were given one of 10 food regimens and showed the weight gains (lb) and the detailed data is as mentioned in the Table below. These are un-paired data, and this type of study is referred to as a completely randomized experiment. Determine whether there is difference between food regimens or not.

Weight Gains in Ten Food Regimens									
A	B	C	D	E	F	G	H	I	J
2	1	2	4	9	3	6	7	4	4
3	2	4	8	8	8	5	6	4	6
2	0	1	7	11	6	6	6	7	6

Solution:

Weight Gains in Ten Food Regimens											
	A	B	C	D	E	F	G	H	I	J	(t=10 regimens)
	2	1	2	4	9	3	6	7	4	4	
	3	2	4	8	8	8	5	6	4	6	
	2	0	1	7	11	6	6	6	7	6	
											Sums
$\sum x_i$	7	3	7	19	28	17	17	19	15	16	$\sum x = 148$
$\sum (x_i)^2$	17	5	21	129	266	109	97	121	81	88	$\sum (x)^2 = 934$
n_i	3	3	3	3	3	3	3	3	3	3	N=30
$n_i - 1$	2	2	2	2	2	2	2	2	2	2	$\sum (n_i - 1)$= (or (n-t))=20
$\bar{x}_i$	2.3	1	2.3	6.3	9.3	5.7	5.7	6.3	5	5.3	---

$$Total\ SS\ (or\ TSS) = \sum x^2 - \frac{(\sum x)^2}{N} = 934 - (148)^2/30 = 203.87$$

$$Between\ SS\ (or\ BSS) = \frac{(\sum x_1)^2}{n_1} + \frac{(\sum x_2)^2}{n_2} + \frac{(\sum x_3)^2}{n_3} + \cdots + \frac{(\sum x_{10})^2}{n_{10}} - \frac{(\sum x)^2}{N}$$

$$Between\ SS\ (or\ BSS) = \frac{(7)^2}{3} + \frac{(3)^2}{3} + \cdots + \frac{16^2}{3} - \frac{(148)^2}{30} = 160.54$$

$$Within\ regimens\ SS\ (or\ WSS) = TSS - BSS = 203.87 - 160.54 = 43.33$$

$$F = \frac{Between\ Mean\ Square\ (BMS)}{Within\ Mean\ Square\ (WMS)} = \frac{BSS/(t-1)}{WSS/(n-t)} = \frac{160.54/(10-1)}{43.44/(30-10)} = \frac{17.81}{2.17}$$

$$= 8.22$$

At, p=0.01, the tabled value of 'F' is 3.45 at degree of freedom of 9 of the greater mean square (horizontal side of 'F' table) vs. degree of freedom of 20 of the lower mean square. As the calculated value is greater than the Table value, the probability of these 10 samples being drawn from the same population is less than 0.05 (actually, it is less than 0.01), it is concluded that they are not all the same (i.e., not all the means are equal).

Problem 19.3, on One-Way ANOVA:

Suppose that 15 tablets are available for the comparison of three assay methods, 5 tablets for each assay. The one-way ANOVA design would result from a random assignment of the tablets to the three groups i.e., five tablets are assigned to each group. The results of assays comparing the three analytical methods are as mentioned in the Table:

Results of Assays Comparing Three Analytical Methods		
Method A	Method B	Method C
102	99	103
101	100	100
101	99	99
100	101	104
102	98	102

Conduct a one-way ANOVA test and conclude whether all the methods are equivalent or not.

Solution:

Results of Assays Comparing Three Analytical Methods			
	Method A	Method B	Method C	
	102	99	103	
	101	100	100	
	101	99	99	
	100	101	104	
	102	98	102	
				Sums
$\sum x_i$	506	497	508	$\sum x = 1511$
$\sum (x_i)^2$	51210	49407	51630	$\sum (x)^2 = 152247$
n_i	5	5	5	N=15
$n_i - 1$	4	4	4	$\sum (n_i - 1) =$ (or (n-t)) = 12
$\overline{x}_i$	101.2	99.4	101.6	---

$$Total\ SS\ (or\ TSS) = \sum x^2 - \frac{(\sum x)^2}{N} = \left\{ 152247 - \left[\frac{2283121}{15}\right]\right\}$$

$$= \{152247 - 152208.06\} = 38.93$$

$$Between\ SS\ (or\ BSS) = \frac{(\sum x_1)^2}{n_1} + \frac{(\sum x_2)^2}{n_2} + \frac{(\sum x_3)^2}{n_3} - \frac{(\sum x)^2}{N}$$

$$Between\ SS\ (or\ BSS) = \frac{(506)^2}{5} + \frac{(497)^2}{5} + \frac{(508)^2}{5} - \frac{(1511)^2}{15}$$

$$= 152221.8 - 152208.06 = 13.73$$

$$Within\ regimens\ SS\ (or\ WSS) = TSS - BSS = 38.93 - 13.73 = 25.2$$

$$F = \frac{Between\ Mean\ Square\ (BMS)}{Within\ Mean\ Square\ (WMS)} = \frac{BSS/(t-1)}{WSS/(n-t)} = \frac{13.73/(3-1)}{25.2/(15-3)}$$

$$= \frac{6.865}{2.1} = 3.27$$

Hence, calculated 'F' value is 3.27 and tabled 'F' is 3.89 when taken degree of freedom of 2 on the horizontal side of the F-table (greater mean square) and degree of freedom of 12 on the vertical side of the F-table (smaller mean square). If the null hypothesis is assumed that the mean of method A = mean of method B = mean of method C, and as calculated F-value is smaller than the Tabled F-value, we cannot reject the null hypothesis and thus we say that all the means are equal and finally we conclude that all the methods A, B, C are equal.

19.2.1.1 Multiple Comparisons

In a student 't' test, one can compare two means and can judge whether there is significant difference between the two means. If the number of means are more than two, and are from independent samples (un-paired), then we employ one way ANOVA test. The limitation with the ANOVA test is that we know whether there is significant difference among the means. But, we do not know which two means are significantly different or vice-versa. For, this we have to conduct several times student 't' test for every two means and see. This can be overcome by using multiple comparison method. In this method, if the sample sizes are the same in each group, a single least significant difference (LSD) can be constructed using the formula:

$$LSD = t_{df,\alpha} \sqrt{s^2 \left[\frac{2}{N}\right]}$$

Where, t is the Tabled value of 't' with appropriate degree of freedom at the α level of significance. Any difference exceeding the LSD can be considered to be significant. The LSD test should be used only if the F test from the ANOVA is significant.

Problem 19.3.1, on Oneway ANOVA and Multiple Comparison using LSD:

An analytical method is tested by sending the same (blinded) sample to each of seven laboratories from the same company, located at different sites. Each of laboratories 1 through 6 has three analysts perform the analysis. Laboratory 7 reports only two results because only two analysts are available. The results are as follows.

Assay Results of Seven Laboratories							
Laboratory No/Sample No	1	2	3	4	5	6	7
1	9	11	6	10	5	7	12
2	8	9	9	10	3	7	10
3	7	13	9	7	4	7	---

Conduct a oneway ANOVA and a multiple comparison using least significant difference and conclude.

Solution:

Assay Results of Seven Laboratories								
Laboratory No/Sample No	1	2	3	4	5	6	7	
1	9	11	6	10	5	7	12	
2	8	9	9	10	3	7	10	
3	7	13	9	7	4	7	---	
								Sums
Σx_i	24	33	24	27	12	21	22	$\Sigma x = 163$
$\Sigma(x_i)^2$	194	371	198	249	50	147	244	$\Sigma(x)^2 = 1453$
n_i	3	3	3	3	3	3	2	$N = 20$
$n_i - 1$	2	2	2	2	2	2	1	$(n-t) = (20-7) = 13$
x_i bar	8.00	11.00	8.00	9.00	4.00	7.00	11.00	---

$$Total\ SS\ (or\ TSS) = \sum x^2 - \frac{(\sum x)^2}{N} = 1453 - \frac{(163)^2}{20} = 1453 - 1328 = 125$$

$$Between\ SS\ (or\ BSS) = \frac{\left(\sum x_1\right)^2}{n_1} + \frac{\left(\sum x_2\right)^2}{n_2} + \frac{\left(\sum x_3\right)^2}{n_3} + ... + \frac{\left(\sum x_n\right)^2}{n_n} - \frac{(\sum x)^2}{N}$$

$Between\ SS\ (or\ BSS)$
$$= \frac{(24)^2}{3} + \frac{(33)^2}{3} + \frac{(24)^2}{3} + \frac{(27)^2}{3} + \frac{(12)^2}{3} + \frac{(21)^2}{3} + \frac{(22)^2}{2}$$
$$- \frac{(163)^2}{20}$$

$$Between\ SS\ (or\ BSS) = 192 + 363 + 192 + 243 + 48 + 147 + 242 - 1328$$
$$= 1427 - 1328 = 99$$

$$Within\ regimen\ SS\ (or\ WSS) = TSS - BSS = 125 - 99 = 26$$

$$F = \frac{\text{Between Mean Square (BMS)}}{\text{Within Mean Square (WMS)}} = \frac{BSS/t-1}{WSS/n-t} = \frac{99/6}{26/13} = \frac{16.5}{2} = 8.25$$

Hence, calculated 'F' value is 8.25 and tabled 'F' is 2.915 when taken degree of freedom of 6 on the horizontal side of the F-table (degree of freedom on numerator) and degree of freedom of 13 on the vertical side of the F-table (degree of freedom on denominator). If the null hypothesis is assumed that there is no significant difference between the means of laboratory tests and since the calculated value is greater than the tabled F value, then null hypothesis is rejected. This indicates the means are not equal and there is a significant difference in the laboratory tests. This implies that at least two laboratory means are different and which two we do not know until every two means are tested with independent 't' test.

In the above circumstances, the one-way ANOVA test is significant enough saying that there is significant difference in the tests and to find out which two laboratory test are not significant, one can now apply a single least significant difference (LSD) test using the formula.

$$LSD = t_{df,\propto} \sqrt{s^2 \left[\frac{2}{N}\right]}$$

If we consider tabled 't' value at 5 % equal to 2.16, s^2 as within mean square, and at degree of freedom i.e.. total number of observation minus number of laboratories i.e., $20 - 7 = 13$, then

$$LSD = t_{df,\propto} \sqrt{s^2 \left[\frac{2}{N}\right]} = 2.16 * \sqrt{2\left[\frac{2}{3}\right]} = 2.16 * \sqrt{1.333} = 2.16 * 1.155 = 2.494$$

When we take the difference of means of laboratory 1 and laboratory 2, it is 11-8= 3, which is greater than LSD calculated value 2.49. This indicates there is significant difference in the tests of laboratory 1 and laboratory 2. Similarly, laboratory 1 and laboratory 5, it is 8-5 =3, which is greater than LSD calculated and there is a significant difference.

As the number of analysts in laboratory 7 are two, we compare laboratory 1 and 7 using two sample 't' test i.e.,

$$t = \frac{|\bar{x}_1 - \bar{x}_2|}{\sqrt{s^2 \left[\frac{1}{n_1} + \frac{1}{n_2}\right]}} = \frac{|11 - 8|}{\sqrt{2\left[\frac{1}{3} + \frac{1}{2}\right]}} = \frac{3}{\sqrt{2 * 0.833}} = \frac{3}{\sqrt{1.666}} = \frac{3}{1.291} = 2.32$$

As the calculated 't' value 2.32 is greater than tabled 't' value at 5 % probability i.e., 2.16, we conclude that there is a significant difference between the means of laboratory 1 and laboratory 7, hence there is a significant difference in the tests.

Yet another test called as Tukey's multiple range test is conducted using the formula

$$\text{Tukey's Test (i.e., q)} = \frac{Compute|Difference|}{\sqrt{\dfrac{s^2}{N}}}$$

$$Therefore, Compute|Difference| = q * \sqrt{\frac{s^2}{N}}$$

Yet Snedecor and Cochran suggested, significant values of q with respect to number of treatments, degree of freedom and α level. But, 'N' should be same in each group (or laboratory). Just in case we assume that all the laboratories have same 'N=3' value, then q = 4.88.

$$Then, Compute|Difference| = q * \sqrt{\frac{s^2}{N}} = 4.88 * \sqrt{\frac{2}{3}} = 4.88 * 0.8165 = 3.98$$

Hence, the difference in means exceeds the above computed difference, then the laboratory tests are significantly different. That is laboratory 1 and 2 if we take into consideration, the difference of mean values are $11 - 8 = 3$, which is less than computed difference and there is no significant difference in the tests of laboratory 1 and 2. Laboratory 5, is significantly different from all the other laboratories except for laboratories 1, 3 and 6. It has to be observed that the computed differences are different with the methods.

19.2.2 Two-way ANOVA

A two-way ANOVA design is analogous to paired 't' test. Let us consider three variations in acne products i.e., A, B, C and a control product are applied to sites on the backs of eight patients. The assignment of the four products to the four sites on the patient is random i.e., a random assignment of treatments to the four sites on each patient is done for each patient, using a random-number table. The products are applied, and after 24 hr, the degree of irritation is determined by assessing irritation subjectively on a scale of 1 to 10. A value of 1 means no irritation and a value of 10 means extreme irritation. The results are as follows: (problem 19.4, on two-way ANOVA)

Patient	Treatment			
	A	B	C	Control
1	7	5	5	4
2	4	3	5	2
3	8	9	7	6
4	8	6	4	5
5	7	7	4	2
6	6	7	5	4
7	5	6	4	5
8	4	7	5	4

In a two-way ANOVA, the variance occurring between treatments (columns), between patients (rows) and error sum of squares (or expected sum of squares) are determined to finally determine the 'F' ratio.

Step 1: Determination of Total Sum of Squares (TSS):

The total sum of square is determined by the following formula.

$$Total\ SS\ (or\ TSS) = \sum x^2 - \frac{(\sum x)^2}{N}$$

Patient	Treatment				
	A	**B**	**C**	**Control**	
1	7	5	5	4	
2	4	3	5	2	
3	8	9	7	6	
4	8	6	4	5	
5	7	7	4	2	
6	6	7	5	4	
7	5	6	4	5	
8	4	7	5	4	
$\sum x_i$	49	50	39	32	$\sum x = 170$
$\sum (x_i)^2$	319	334	197	142	$\sum(x)^2 = 992$

$$Total\ SS\ (or\ TSS) = \sum x^2 - \frac{(\sum x)^2}{N} = 992 - \frac{(170)^2}{32} = 992 - 903.125$$
$$= 88.875$$

Step 2: Determination of Between Treatments Sum of Squares (Between Treatments SS):

The formula to calculate the variance between treatments (or between columns) is as follows:

$$Between\ SS\ (or\ BSS) = \frac{(\sum x_1)^2}{n_1} + \frac{(\sum x_2)^2}{n_2} + \frac{(\sum x_3)^2}{n_3} - \frac{(\sum x)^2}{N}$$

$$Between\ Treatments\ SS = \frac{(49)^2}{8} + \frac{(50)^2}{8} + \frac{(39)^2}{8} + \frac{(32)^2}{8} - \frac{(170)^2}{32}$$
$$= 930.75 - 903.125 = 27.625$$

Step 3: Determination of Between Patients Sum of Squares (or Between Rows Sum of Squares) (Between Patients SS):

For this, the Table is transposed for convenience for easy understanding i.e.,

Treatments	Patients								
	1	**2**	**3**	**4**	**5**	**6**	**7**	**8**	
A	7	4	8	8	7	6	5	4	
B	5	3	9	6	7	7	6	7	
C	5	5	7	4	4	5	4	5	
Control	4	2	6	5	2	4	5	4	
$\sum x_i$	21	14	30	23	20	22	20	20	$\sum x = 170$
$\sum (x_i)^2$	115	54	230	141	118	126	102	106	$\sum(x)^2 = 992$

$$Between\ Patients\ SS = \frac{(\sum x_1)^2}{n_1} + \frac{(\sum x_2)^2}{n_2} + \frac{(\sum x_3)^2}{n_3} - \frac{(\sum x)^2}{N}$$

$$Between\ Patients\ SS = \frac{(21)^2}{4} + \frac{(14)^2}{4} + \frac{(30)^2}{4} + \frac{(23)^2}{4} + \frac{(20)^2}{4} + \frac{(22)^2}{4} + \frac{(20)^2}{4} + \frac{(20)^2}{4} - \frac{(170)^2}{32}$$

$$Between\ Patients\ SS = 937.5 - 903.125 = 34.375$$

Step 4: Determination of Expected Sum of Squares (or Error Sum of Squares or Error):

The formula for calculating

Error = TSS – Between Treatments SS – Between Patients SS

Error = 88.875 –27.625 – 34.375 = 26.875

Step 5: Calculation of F ratio:

$$F = \frac{Between\ Mean\ Square\ (BMS)}{Error} = \frac{Between\ Treatments\ SS/(t-1)}{Error/(no.\,of\ rows - 1)(no.\,of\ columns - 1)}$$

$$= \frac{27.625/(4-1)}{26.875/(8-1)(4-1)} = \frac{9.208}{1.279} = 7.199$$

Step 6: Inference and conclusion:

The calculated value of 'F' = 7.199 is greater than the Table value of 'F =3.072' at a degree of freedom of 3 on the horizontal side vs. a degree of freedom of 21 on the vertical side in the F-table. Hence, it can be concluded that at least two treatments are different. To find out in precise, every two treatments have to be compared by other methods and draw further conclusions.

19.2.3 Crossover ANOVA Design

Other than one-way and two-way ANOVA, Crossover ANOVA design is widely used. When a comparison is made among two-way ANOVA and crossover ANOVA design, the latter is considered as an improvement of the former. In the current design, an additional constraint is included i.e., order or balance. For instance, three products A, B, C were to be compared for their bioavailability and nine subjects each were included in three groups. The three different groups undergo the drug product treatment at different periods during a possible extraneous factor that may occur and interfere during a study period. In this design, the balancing order is to minimize possible extraneous variables as errors affecting the outcome differently in one period compared to another. Hence, all the treatments (administering drug product) are planned and affected equally in such a way that all the three drug products are given equal number of times in an order for every group in every period. Conversely, in one way or two way designs, one group gets one drug product at a period and later the same group gets another drug product during a different period. As illustrated below, Latin square design has a relation in the design of Crossover ANOVA. The illustration indicates, Crossover ANOVA design meets the class of paired-sample or two-way designs.

Crossover ANOVA Design			
Subject	Period I	Period II	Period III
1	B	C	A
2	A	C	B
3	B	A	C
4	C	B	A
5	A	B	C
6	C	A	B
7	B	A	C
8	C	B	A
9	A	C	B

Problem 19.4, on Crossover ANOVA Design:

Three drug formulations A, B and C were administered to nine subjects in a bioavailability study according to the crossover design and the area under the blood level curves were computed for each dosing, and the results are as mentioned below:

Crossover ANOVA Design				
Subject	Period I	Period II	Period III	Sum
1	B=107	C=102	A=99	308
2	A=100	C=106	B=89	295
3	B=98	A=90	C=128	316
4	C=71	B=54	A=63	188
5	A=92	B=111	C=107	310
6	C=113	A=115	B=91	319
7	B=169	A=187	C=195	551
8	C=88	B=95	A=77	260
9	A=122	C=168	B=155	445
Period Sum	I = 960	II=1028	III=1004	$\sum x = 2992$
Total Treatment Sum	A=945	B=969	C=1078	$\sum (x)^2 = 364720$
Total Treatment Average	A=105	B=107.7	C=119.8	

Solution:

Step 1: Determination of Total Sum of Squares (TSS):

The total sum of square is determined by the following formula.

$$Total\ SS\ (or\ TSS) = \sum x^2 - \frac{(\sum x)^2}{N}$$

$$Total\ SS\ (or\ TSS) = \sum x^2 - \frac{(\sum x)^2}{N} = 364720 - 331558 = 33162$$

Step 2: Determination of Between Subject Sum of Squares (Sub SS):

$$Sub\ SS = \frac{\sum row^2}{3} - \frac{(\sum x)^2}{N} = \frac{1084176}{3} - \frac{8952064}{27} = 361392 - 331558$$

$$= 29834$$

Step 3: Determination of Between Treatment Sum of Squares (Treatment SS):

$$Treatment\ SS = \frac{\sum treat.\,sum^2}{9} - \frac{(\sum x)^2}{N} = \frac{2994070}{9} - \frac{8952064}{27}$$

$$= 332674 - 331558 = 1116$$

Step 4: Determination of Order Sum of Squares (OrderSS):

$$Order\ SS = \frac{[I^2 + II^2 + III^2]}{9} - \frac{(\sum x)^2}{N} = \frac{[2986400]}{9} - \frac{8952064}{27}$$

$$= 331822 - 331558 = 264$$

Step 5: Determination of Expected Sum of Squares (or Error Sum of Squares or Error):

The formula for calculating

Error = TSS – Subject SS – Treatment SS – Order SS

Error = 33162 – 29834 – 1116 – 264 = 1948

Step 6: Calculation of F ratio:

The consolidated values are as follows:

Analysis of Variance Calculations				
Source of Variation	**Degrees of Freedom (df)**	**Sums of Squares (SS)**	**Mean Squares (= SS/df)**	**F-Ratio**
Between Subjects	8	29834	3729	
Between Treatments	2	1116	558	558/139 = 4.01
Order	2	264	132	
Error	14	1948	139	
Total	26	33162		

$$F = \frac{\text{Between Treatments Mean Square (Bet Subj MS)}}{\text{Error}}$$

$$= \frac{\text{Treatments SS} / \text{degree of freedom w. r. t to total treatments}}{\text{Error} / \text{degrees of freedom}}$$

$$= \frac{\frac{1116}{2}}{\frac{1947}{14}} = \frac{558}{139} = 4.01$$

Step 7: Inference and conclusion:

The calculated value 'F' = 4.01 is greater than the table value of 'F =3.7' at a degrees of freedom of 2 on the horizontal side vs. a degree of freedom of 14 on the vertical side in the F-table at 5% probability. Hence, it can be concluded that the treatments are different indicating the formulations are different.

19.2.4 Three-way ANOVA

Three-way ANOVA is also called as 'factorial ANOVA' or 'three-way between subjects ANOVA'. Three-way ANOVA design helps in understanding whether there is any interaction between three independent variables on one dependent variable which is continuous. The independent variables are called as 'factors' or 'between subject factors'. The experimental data generated with a purpose of conducting three-way ANOVA has to be ensured suitable for the test and proceed further. In order to ensure the data qualifies for conducting the three-way ANOVA, the data must cross six assumptions. The six assumptions are as follows:

i.   Dependent variable should be measured as a continuous variable (interval or ratio variable)

ii. Three independent variable should belong to two or more categorical independent groups (i.e., gender: male/female/, ethnicity: Caucasian/African American/Hispanic, profession: nurse/doctor/surgeon/pharmacist/therapist etc.)

iii. The observations are independent and are not related with other observations within a group or among groups.

iv. The data should not have any significant outliers.

v.   The dependent continuous variable should approximately have normal distribution for each combination of the groups of the three independent variables.

vi. Existence of homogenous variances for each combination of the groups of the three independent variables.

Problem 19.5, on Three-way ANOVA

A researcher wanted to examine a new class of drug that has the potential to lower cholesterol levels and thus help against heart attack. Due to the specific molecular mechanisms by which this new class of drugs works, the researcher hypothesized that the new class of drug might affect males and females differently, as well as those already at risk of a heart attack. There were three different types of drug within this new class of drug, but the researcher was unsure which would be more successful.

Therefore, the researcher recruited 72 participants split evenly between males and females. Males and females were further (equally) subdivided into whether they were at low or high risk of heart attack. Each of these subgroups then received one of the three different drugs. After one month on the different drugs, cholesterol concentration was measured. The researcher wants to understand how each factor (i.e., type of drug, risk of heart attack, gender) interacts to predict cholesterol concentration.

Participants' cholesterol concentration was recorded in the variables cholesterol, their gender (in gender), their risk of heart attack (in risk) and the drug they took (in the variable drug). In variable terms, the researcher wants to know if there is an interaction between gender, risk and drug on cholesterol.

Note: The data in the example is made up to illustrate the use of the three-way ANOVA (i.e., the data is fictitious).

Setup in SPSS Statistics

In this example, there are four variables: (1) the dependent variable, cholesterol, which is the cholesterol concentration (in mmol/L); (2) the independent variable, gender, which has two categories: "male" and "female"; (3) the independent variable, risk, which has two categories: "low" and "high"; and (4) the independent variable drug, which has three categories: "drug A", "drug B" and "drug C". The file setup in the Data View window is shown below:

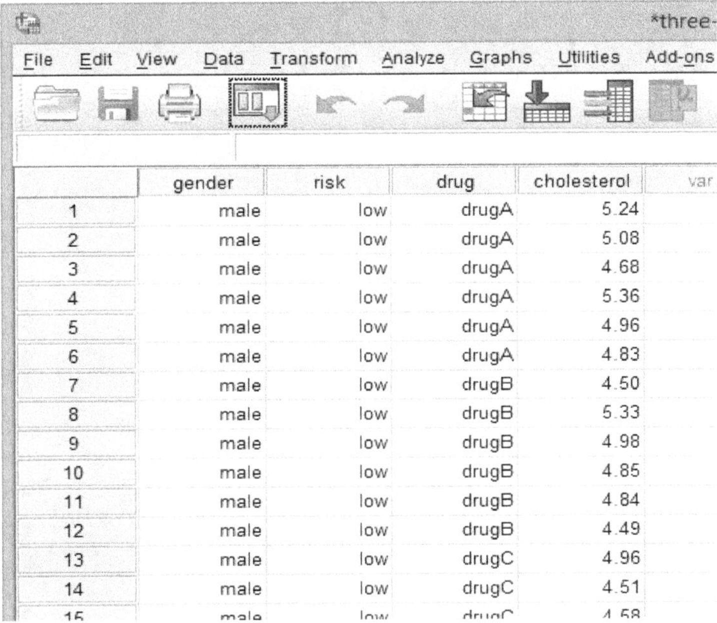

Test Procedure in SPSS Statistics

The six steps below show you how to analyze your data using a three-way ANOVA in SPSS Statistics when the six assumptions in the previous section, assumptions, have not been violated. At the end of these six steps, forthcoming steps show you how to interpret the results from the test.

Click **Analyze >General Linear Model >Univariate...** on the main menu, as shown below:

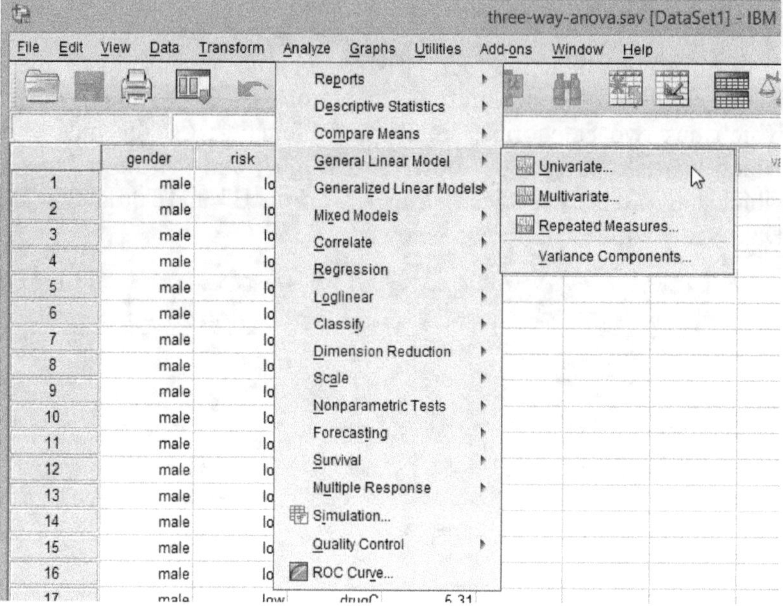

You will be presented with the **Univariate** dialogue box, as shown below:

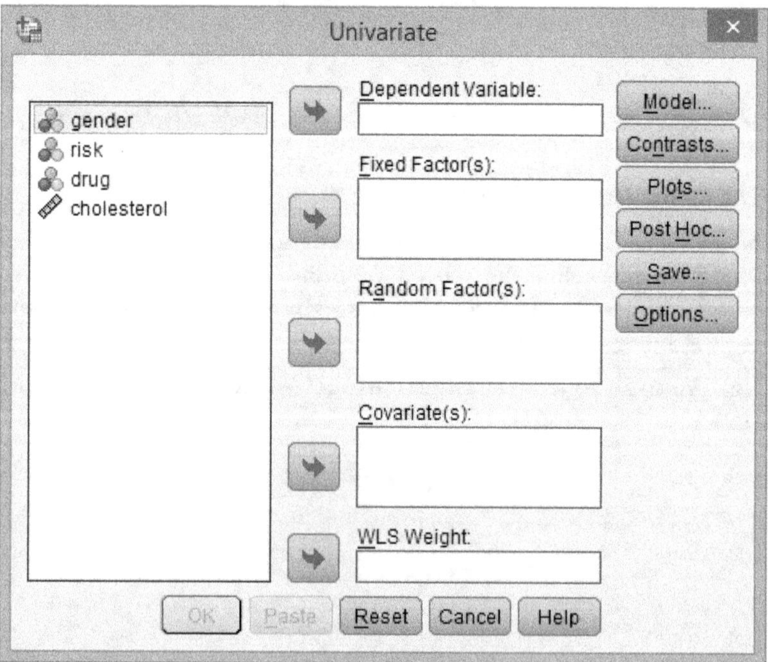

- Transfer the dependent variable, cholesterol, into the <u>D</u>ependent Variable box and the independent variables – gender, risk and drug – into the <u>F</u>ixed Factor(s) box, using the appropriate buttons. You will end up with a screen similar to the one below:

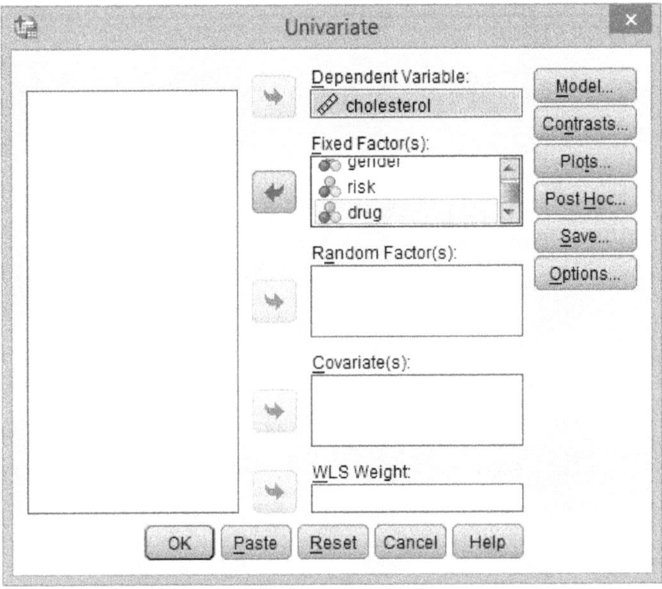

- Click the **Options...** button and you will be presented with the **Univariate: Options** dialogue box, as shown below:

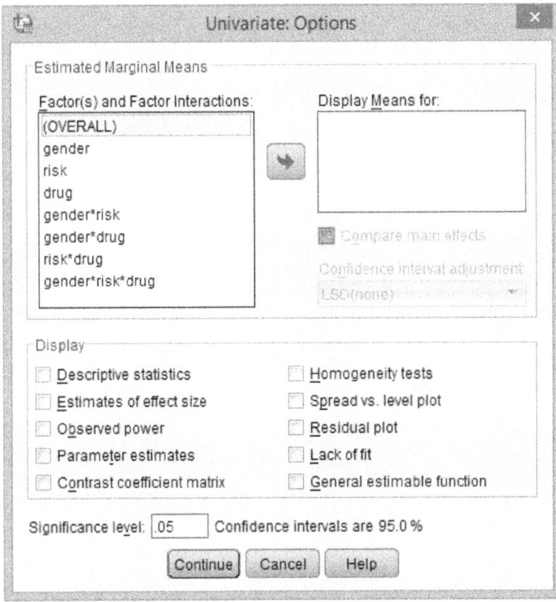

- Transfer the three-way interaction term, gender*risk*drug, from the Factor(s) and Factor Interactions box to the Display Means For box by highlighting it and clicking the button. Then select the Descriptive statistics and Homogeneity tests options in the –Display– area. You will end up with the screen shown below:

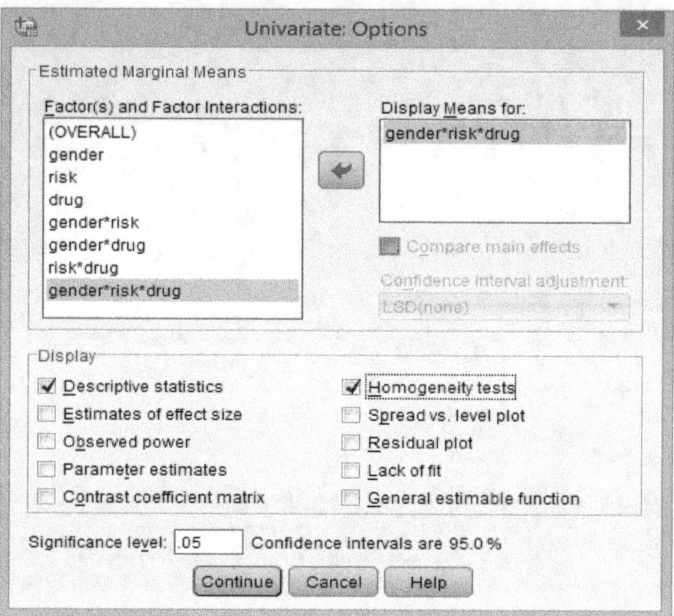

- Click the Continue button and you will be returned to the **Univariate** dialogue box.

- Click the OK button. This will generate the output.

Three-way ANOVA result

The primary goal of running a three-way ANOVA is to determine whether there is a three-way interaction between three independent variables (i.e., a gender*risk*drug interaction). Essentially, a three-way interaction tests whether the simple two-way risk*drug interactions differ between the levels of gender (i.e., differ for "males" and "females").

To determine whether you have a statistically significant three-way gender*risk*drug interaction, you need to consult the "**gender * risk * drug**" row in the **Tests of Between-Subjects Effects** table, as highlighted below:

Tests of Between-Subjects Effects

Dependent Variable: cholesterol

Source	Type III Sum of Squares	df	Mean square	F	Sig.
Corrected Model	12.374[a]	11	1.125	13.326	.000
Intercept	1893.979	1	1893.979	22436.576	.000
gender	1.367	1	1.367	16.196	.000
risk	7.825	1	7.825	92.699	.000
drug	1.235	2	.618	7.318	.001
gender * risk	.012	1	.012	.141	.708
gender * drug	.564	2	.282	3.338	.042
risk * drug	.120	2	.060	.713	.494
gender * risk * drug	**1.250**	**2**	**.625**	**7.406**	**.001**
Error	5.065	60	.084		
Total	1911.418	72			
Corrected total	17.439	71			

a. R Squared = .710 (Adjusted R Squared = .656)

The "**Sig.**" column presents the statistical significance level (i.e., p-value) of the three-way interaction term of the three-way ANOVA. You can see that the statistical significance level of the three-way interaction term is **.001** (i.e., $p = .001$). This value is less than .05 (i.e., it satisfies $p < .05$), which means that there is a statistically significant three-way gender*risk*drug interaction effect.

One can report this result as follows:

There is a statistically significant three-way interaction between gender, risk and drug, $F(2, 60) = 7.406$, $p = .001$.

20 Non-Parametric Statistical Tests

20.0 Introduction

Unlike parametric statistical tests where samples are expected to fulfill either of the continuous distributions such as normal, binomial, poisson, t-distribution, F-distribution, chi-square distribution, non-parametric tests depends on discontinuous distributions or where a distribution cannot be assumed. Such discontinuous distributions are mainly due to very small sample sizes and several times non-parametric tests are conducted for preliminary assessments and at a later stage for a more precise parametric tests. Non-parametric tests are usually called as distribution free statistics and in several circumstances it may be for continuous. In several circumstances, non-parametric tests are simple calculation based and involve with ordering, ranking of the data and do not depend on the assumption of normality.

In pharmaceuticals a parameter is an attribute of a human for a clinical condition or an attribute for a product. For instance, to estimate the diabetic status of a patient, the attribute (parameter) i.e., blood glucose level is estimated. In the same way, one of the attribute (parameter) for a tablet is thickness of the tablet etc. In most of the circumstances a parametric statistical test is conducted directly on the data collected, where as in a non-parametric statistical test, an analysis of the secondary data generated from actual data collected is made. Hence, non-parametric test possess less power and in some circumstances they are proved with high power. The various non-parametric statistical tests are the sign test, Wilcoxon signed rank test, Wilcoxon rank sum test (also called as Mann-Whitney U-test), Kruskal-Wallis test (one-way ANOVA), Friedman test (two-way ANOVA).

20.1 Runs Test for Randomness

The test is non-parametric and helps in experiments where the attribute observation is continuously observed. The test tells us whether the experimental error is taking place on random or not. As discussed earlier, errors occurring on random are amenable to statistical tests. A 'run' is defined as a series of uninterrupted, like observations. A run test can be conducted in two different approaches i.e., direct referring the number of runs with respect to sample size with standard table 'Critical Values for Number of Runs at the 5% Level of Significance' and the second approach is used when sample size is more than 40 or more and is by 'normal approximation to the distribution of runs'. Here, a sample is collected and the median of the attribute is calculated. Every product's attribute from the sample collected is compared with median. If the product's attribute is higher than the median value, a '+' sign is assigned for that single product of the sample collected. If the product's attribute is lower than the median value, a '-' is assigned for that single product of the sample collected. When all the individual samples' attribute is compared with median value and assigned with corresponding positive or negative noted on a paper, a pattern is observed (i.e., a series of like signs is called) as 'runs'. If the runs are occurring quite next by next (or often), the experimental observation is occurring not on random.

Let us image a tablet press punching tablets. Twenty tablets were weighted and it has been observed that the median is 200 mg (say). It has been observed that the first six tablets weighed more than 200 mg, the next five tablets weighed less than 200 mg, the next four tablets weighed more than 200 mg and the next five tablets weighed less than 200 mg. When a positive sign for higher weight than median and when a negative sign for lower weight than median is assigned, the pattern of all the twenty tablets is as follows:

$$++++++-----++++-----$$

Hence, from the above pattern, we can observe four runs occurring. As the runs are occurring one after the other quite often, it indicates that the tablet machine is automatically adjusting quite often, which is an error that is occurring on non-random basis.

In the current method of direct reference to standard table of 'Critical Values for Number of Runs at the 5% Level of Significance', the number of runs of 4 with respect to sample size of 20 is compared with standard values mentioned in the table. It has been observed that, for a two tailed, at sample size of 20, the lower number is 6 and the higher number is 15. If the number of runs is less than or equal to the lower value or greater than or equal to the upper value, the sequence is considered non-random at the 5% level of significance. Hence, with respect to the current experiment, 4 runs is less than the tabled lower number 6, indicating that the error is non-random.

Normal approximation to the distribution of runs:

The method is used when the sample size is 40 or more. The equation used is as mentioned below:

$$z = \frac{\left| r - \left(\dfrac{N}{2+1} \right) \right|}{\sqrt{\dfrac{N(N-2)}{4(N-1)}}}$$

Where, r is the number of runs and N is the sample size.

Problem 20.1 on Runs Test: A standard is analyzed every 20th sample in an automated analytical procedure. A record of the readings for the standard in chronological order derived from one day's assay results are shown in the below mentioned table. Conduct a runs test and give your conclusion.

Readings of a Standard Solution in Chronological Order (Optical Density)							
Sample	Reading	Sample	Reading	Sample	Reading	Sample	Reading
1	0.795	11	0.782	21	0.796	31	0.813
2	0.796	12	0.795	22	0.797	32	0.804
3	0.804	13	0.798	23	0.795	33	0.801
4	0.801	14	0.8	24	0.802	34	0.793
5	0.792	15	0.8	25	0.8	35	0.79
6	0.816	16	0.802	26	0.801	36	0.791
7	0.791	17	0.799	27	0.802	37	0.784
8	0.819	18	0.805	28	0.82	38	0.791
9	0.796	19	0.82	29	0.788	39	0.788
10	0.815	20	0.802	30	0.78	40	0.794

Solution:

Step 1: Let us assume as null hypothesis, that there is randomness in analytical procedure.

Step 2: Let us assume as alternate hypothesis, that there is no-randomness in analytical procedure.

Step 3: Let us consider the test is two tailed at 5% probability.

Step 4: Here, a non-parametric test and as preliminary, a runs test is considered.

Readings of a Standard Solution in Chronological Order (Optical Density)							
Sample	Reading	Sample	Reading	Sample	Reading	Sample	Reading
1	0.78	11	0.793	21	0.799	31	0.802
2	0.782	12	0.794	22	0.8	32	0.804
3	0.784	13	0.795	23	0.8	33	0.804
4	0.788	14	0.795	24	0.8	34	0.805
5	0.788	15	0.795	25	0.801	35	0.813
6	0.79	16	0.796	26	0.801	36	0.815
7	0.791	17	0.796	27	0.801	37	0.816
8	0.791	18	0.796	28	0.802	38	0.819
9	0.791	19	0.797	29	0.802	39	0.82
10	0.792	20	0.798	30	0.802	40	0.82
Note: The values are sorted from lowest to highest							

The median of even samples is given by average reading of 20th and 21st sample i.e., $0.798 + 0.799/2 = 0.7985$.

With reference to original data collected, the runs are as follows:

$$--++-+-+--+---+++++++---+++++--+++-------$$

Here, the number or runs is 15.

$$z = \frac{\left| 15 - \left(\dfrac{40}{2+1} \right) \right|}{\sqrt{\dfrac{40(40-2)}{4(40-1)}}} = \frac{6}{3.12} = 1.92$$

Step 5: At 5% probability, standard Z value is 1.96, for a two tailed. Here the calculated Z value is 1.92 is greater than tabled standard value, which has very narrow difference when compared with standard value. With respect to standard table i.e. Critical Values for Number of Runs at the 5% Level of Significance, at sample size of 40, the lower value is 14 and upper value is 27. Hence we can accept null hypothesis that there is randomness in the experimental procedure.

Step 6: As the test indicates randomness, statistics can be applied for the experimental procedure (automated analytical procedure).

20.2 Sign Test

The test is used to compare equality of two medians. The test is used to compare paired data and the test is in analogy with paired-t test. Sign test has less power when compared to signed-rank test. The test is used for continuous, ranked, continuous interval and ratio type data. The statistical test is based on binomial distribution, the normal approximation to the binomial. Hence, a non-parametric sign test can be chi-square or a normality approximation. Here, the paired data is compiled and difference is calculated. A positive difference indicates the second treatment has high value and vice-versa. If the difference between the two treatment values is zero, the value is not counted or neglected or ignored. The second step is to calculate the proportion of the 'wins' that is the number of positive signs, and is compared with the expected under the null hypothesis of the equality of treatments. Hence, in this test the difference of the treatments and the number of positive or negative signs are compared and the two treatments are judged. There are three different approaches of sign test and are as follows:

i. **Referring Standard Sign Test Table for significance:** Comparison of the two treatments by identifying the number of positive or negative signs needed for significance. Here, the standard sign test Table 20.1, is referred to judge, the significance either at 5% or at 1% levels.

TABLE **20.1** Standard Sign Test Table: Number of Positive or Negative Signs Needed for Significance for the Sign Test

Sample Size	Number of Positive or Negative Signs for Significance	
	5% Level	1% Level
6	6	---
7	7	---
8	8	8
9	8	9
10	9	10
11	10	11
12	10	11
13	11	12
14	12	13
15	12	13
16	13	14
17	13	15
18	14	15
19	15	16
20	15	17

ii. **Sign test based on normal approximation to the binomial**: In this case, the observed proportion is compared with expected using the following formula:

$$Z = \frac{|p_A - 0.5| - \frac{1}{2N}}{0.5/\sqrt{N}}$$

Or

$$Z = \frac{|p_A - 0.5| - \frac{1}{2N}}{\sqrt{pq/N}}$$

Where, p_A = observed proportion, p=theoretical probability of '+ve' sign, q=theoretical probability of '–ve' sign and N = sample size.

The simplified version of the above equation is

$$Z = \frac{|number\ of +'s - number\ of -'s| - 1}{\sqrt{number\ of +'s + number\ of -'s}}$$

iii. **Sign test based on chi-square test:** As discussed earlier, chi-square test is used to compare two proportions, the chi-square test is conducted based on the below mentioned formula and the calculated value is compared with the Tabled value from chi-square Table against degrees of freedom and the probability.

$$\chi^2 = \frac{(|b - c| - 1)^2}{b + c}$$

Where b= number of '+ve' signs and c=number of '–ve' signs.

Problem 20.2, on Sign Test: Tablets were taken from two different punches of a tablet press at various times during a run because a difference in weight was suspected. The weight of the tablets from corresponding punches is as mentioned in the Table. Conduct a sign test and ensure whether any adjustment has to be made on the tablet press.

Weight of Tablets from Tablet Press					
Time(pm)	Right	Left	Time (pm)	Right	Left
1:00	220	221	4:15	218	219
1:15	221	220	4:30	222	223
1:30	219	223	4:45	226	228
1:45	218	221	5:00	217	227
2:00	223	218	5:15	219	220
2:15	217	213	5:30	215	218
2:30	221	225	5:45	220	224
2:45	218	220	6:00	219	220
3:00	226	224	6:15	223	221
3:15	220	223	6:30	216	220
3:30	217	219	6:45	222	226
3:45	224	223	7:00	221	221
4:00	222	225			

Solution:

Here, the tablet press is one and the tablets are from two punches that are right and left. Hence, the data is paired with respect to right and left punches.

Step 1: Let us assume that the null hypothesis as there is no significant difference in tablet weights of the two punches of the tablet press. The alternate hypothesis is that there is significant difference between weights of right and left punches of the tablet press.

Step 2: As a preliminary test, sign test is planned for faster assessments. Hence, the differences in the tablets from the punches at the same time were calculated.

Weight of Tablets from Tablet Press							
Time(pm)	Right	Left	Difference	Time (pm)	Right	Left	Difference
1:00	220	221	+1	4:15	218	219	+1
1:15	221	220	-1	4:30	222	223	+1
1:30	219	223	+4	4:45	226	228	+2
1:45	218	221	+3	5:00	217	227	+10
2:00	223	218	-5	5:15	219	220	+1
2:15	217	213	-4	5:30	215	218	+3
2:30	221	225	+4	5:45	220	224	+4
2:45	218	220	+2	6:00	219	220	+1
3:00	226	224	-2	6:15	223	221	-2
3:15	220	223	+3	6:30	216	220	+4
3:30	217	219	+2	6:45	222	226	+4
3:45	224	223	-1	7:00	221	221	0
4:00	222	225	+3				

Step 3: From the above differences, there are 18 wins (i.e., +ve signs). Hence the observed proportion is p_A = number of positive signs / sample size (after ignoring ties) = 18/24 = 0.75

Step 4: Considering the normal assumption to binomial, the equation is

$$Z = \frac{|0.75 - 0.5| - \frac{1}{48}}{0.5 / \sqrt{24}} = \frac{|0.25| - 0.0208}{0.5 / 4.8989} = \frac{0.2292}{0.1020} = 2.2470$$

Step 5: For a normal distribution, Tabled 'z' value at 5% level is 1.96. Hence, calculated z-value is higher than the Tabled value and hence, null hypothesis is rejected.

Step 6: As the null hypothesis is rejected, the alternate hypothesis is accepted that there is significant difference between weights of right and left punches of the tablet press and hence, the operator has to adjust the punches.

If a simplified equation is used, then

$$Z = \frac{|number\ of + 's - number\ of - 's| - 1}{\sqrt{number\ of + 's + number\ of - 's}}$$

Then,

$$Z = \frac{|18 - 6| - 1}{\sqrt{18 + 6}} = \frac{11}{4.8989} = 2.2454$$

If a chi-square test method is used, then

$$\chi^2 = \frac{(|b - c| - 1)^2}{b + c}$$

Where b = number of +ve differences and c = number of –ve differences, then

$$\chi^2 = \frac{(|18 - 6| - 1)^2}{18 + 6} = \frac{121}{24} = 5.041$$

The Table value of chi-square value at number of signs i.e., positive and negative signs with degrees of freedom = 2-1=1 is, 3.84 at 5% level. As the calculated chi-square value is higher than the tabled, the null hypothesis is rejected.

Finally, when the simplest sign test is planned, consider either the positive or the negative number of values and refer to standard sign test Table. Here, there are 18 positive values (larger among the two signs) and with respect to standard sign test Table, for a sample size of 24 (after ignoring ties), at 5% level, theoretically there should be at least the number mentioned in the Table. For instance, standard sign test Table indicates for a sample size of 20, at 5% level the minimum number of a particular sign is 15. This indicates that if the positive value is more than 15, it indicates the positive sign is predominating over negative sign and this indicates that two medians being compared are not statistically same. This indicates that the tablets from two punches are not the same and hence the operator of the tablet press has to adjust the right or the left punch so that the tablets weights from the right or the left punch give statistically significant same weight of the tablets.

20.3 Signed Rank Test (also called as Wilcoxon Signed Rank Test)

Signed Rank Test is a more sensitive non-parametric test than the sign test. Signed Rank Test (also called as Wilcoxon Signed Rank Test) is in analogy to paired 't' test. Using signed rank test, one can test equality of the means or the medians that possess symmetrical distribution. In this case, the difference between the paired values, sign and total sum of each individual sign differences play a key role. The steps involved in conducting Wilcoxon Signed Rank Test for paired values is that, firstly the difference between the values, secondly if the two paired values are tie (or difference is zero) the sample pair is discarded from the data, thirdly the differences are ranked from the lowest to the highest (if two or more differences have same value, the ranking is the average), fourthly the ranked values are assigned with the corresponding positive or negative signs, fifthly the total sum of positive and the total sum of negative signs are calculated (called as rank sums or the T-value), sixthly among the rank sums the lowest sum (calculated T-value)is compared with the standard Wilcoxon Signed Rank Test table. If the calculated 'T' value is equal to or less than the Table 'T' value, the null hypothesis is rejected at the significance level of probability.

Problem 20.3, on Signed Rank Test (or Wilcoxon Signed Rank Test):

A comparison of the time of peak plasma concentration for two formulations, A and B are made and values are as mentioned below:

	Time to peak concentration (hr)	
Subject	A	B
1	2.5	3.5
2	3.0	4.0
3	1.25	2.5
4	1.75	2.0
5	3.5	3.5
6	2.5	4.0
7	1.75	1.5
8	2.25	2.5
9	3.5	3.0
10	2.5	3.0
11	2.0	3.5
12	3.5	4.0

Calculate Signed Rank Test and ensure whether there is difference between the two formulations.

Solution:

Step 1: Let us assume the null hypothesis that the two formulations A and B are the same with respect to time of peak plasma concentration. Let the alternate hypothesis is that the two formulations A and B are not the same with respect to time of peak plasma concentration.

Step 2: Calculate the difference of the paired data and is as mentioned below:

Subject	Time to peak concentration (hr)		
	A	**B**	**Difference (B-A)**
1	2.5	3.5	+1
2	3.0	4.0	+1
3	1.25	2.5	+1.25
4	1.75	2.0	+0.25
5	3.5	3.5	0
6	2.5	4.0	+1.5
7	1.75	1.5	-0.25
8	2.25	2.5	+0.25
9	3.5	3.0	-0.5
10	2.5	3.0	+0.5
11	2.0	3.5	+1.5
12	3.5	4.0	+0.5

Step 3: Ranking the Differences initially without sign, later giving average value to common differences and later designating the sign

Subject	Time to peak concentration (hr)					
	A	**B**	**Difference (B-A)**	**Rank**	**Assigned Rank**	**Assigned Rank with Sign**
1	2.5	3.5	+1	7	(7+8)/2=7.5	+7.5
2	3.0	4.0	+1	8	(7+8)/2=7.5	+7.5
3	1.25	2.5	+1.25	9	9	+9
4	1.75	2.0	+0.25	3	(1+2+3)/3=2	+2
5	3.5	3.5	0	Ignore	Ignore	Ignore
6	2.5	4.0	+1.5	10	(10+11)/2=10.5	+10.5
7	1.75	1.5	-0.25	1	(1+2+3)/3=2	-2
8	2.25	2.5	+0.25	2	(1+2+3)/3=2	+2
9	3.5	3.0	-0.5	4	(4+5+6)/3=5	-5
10	2.5	3.0	+0.5	5	(4+5+6)/3=5	+5
11	2.0	3.5	+1.5	11	(10+11)/2=10.5	+10.5
12	3.5	4.0	+0.5	6	(4+5+6)/3=5	+5

Step 4: Calculation of Rank Sums (or T values) of positive and negative signed ranks individually:

Signed Rank Sum of Positive Value = 7.5 + 7.5 + 9 + 2 + 10.5 + 2 + 5 + 10.5 + 5 = 59

Signed Rank Sum of Negative Value = 2 + 5 = 7

Step 5: Comparison of lowest Rank Sum Value with the standard T-Table for Signed Rank Test:

The lowest Signed Rank Sum among the positive and negative is the negative which is equal to 7. Hence calculated T value of 7 is compared with the standard T-Table for Signed Rank Test which is mentioned below:

Standard Values Leading to Significance for the Wilcoxon Signed Rank Test (Two-Sided Test)		
Sample Size, N	5% Level	1% Level
6	0	---
7	2	---
8	3	0
9	5	1
10	8	3
11	10	5
12	13	7
13	17	10
14	21	13
15	25	16
16	30	19
17	35	23
18	40	28
19	46	32
20	52	37

The Tabled 'T' value at 5% level at sample size of 11 is 10. As the calculated 'T' value (7) is less than the Tabled 'T' value (10) and when calculated 'T' value is equal to or less than Table 'T' value the null hypothesis is rejected. Hence, here the null hypothesis is rejected saying that the time of peak plasma concentrations are significantly not the same and hence formulation A and B are not the same. This indicates that alternate hypothesis is accepted implying formulation A and B are different.

When sample sizes larger than those shown in standard signed rank test Table are observed, a normal approximation is available to compare two population means using the Wilcoxon Signed Rank test i.e.,

$$Z = \frac{\left|R - \frac{N(N+1)}{4}\right|}{\sqrt{\frac{[N(N+\frac{1}{2})(N+1)]}{12}}}$$

Where, R = Sum of ranks (either the larger or smaller rank sum can be used) and N is the sample size (disregarding ties). The formula also works for smaller sample sizes. Hence for the above worked example,

$$Z = \frac{\left|59 - \frac{11(11+1)}{4}\right|}{\sqrt{\frac{[11(11+\frac{1}{2})(11+1)]}{12}}} = \frac{\left|59 - \frac{11(12)}{4}\right|}{\sqrt{\frac{[11(11.5)(12)]}{12}}} = \frac{|59 - 33|}{\sqrt{126.5}} = \frac{26}{11.2472} = 2.3116$$

Here, calculated value of 2.3116 is greater than 1.96 at 5% level and hence the null hypothesis is rejected indicating acceptance of alternate hypothesis.

20.4 Rank Sum Test (Wilcoxon Rank Sum Test or Mann-Whitney U Test or Mann-Whitney-Wilcoxon Test or Wilcoxon-Mann-Whitney Test)

Rank Sum Test is one another non-parametric test which is in analogy to un-paired 't' test. Here, the two treatments are given to two independent groups individually and to be compared. The test is applicable to be atleast the data is ordinal (i.e., the observations are ordered). Here, firstly the two groups data are pooled at one place, secondly ranking the direct data keeping in view of both the groups giving importance to signs while ranking (for instance -1 has lower rank than 0.5), thirdly where the values are same-average rank is designated, fourthly sum of ranks of individual groups is calculated and assigned as 'T' for n_1 observations in the smaller sample computed. Also calculate T' (T dash) = $[n_1(n_1 + n_2 +1)-T]$. Hence we have values of n_1, n_2, T and T' (T dash). Taking whichever is smaller T or T', it is compared with standard Tabled 'Rank Sum Table' and if the calculated value is equal to or less than the Tabled value, the null hypothesis is rejected at the significance level of probability. It can also be interpreted that, if rank sum of smaller sample is equal to or lower than smaller numbers (in standard table) or equal to or larger than larger number (in standard table), groups are significantly different at 0.05 level (i.e. null hypothesis is rejected).

The second approach of calculation of Rank Sum test (Wilcoxon Rank Sum test), where in normality approximation is considered and the formula is as mentioned below:

$$Z = \frac{[T - E(T)]}{\sqrt{S_T^2}}$$

Where E(T) = $N_1(N_1 + N_2 + 1)/2$ and $S_T^2 = \frac{N_1 N_2 (N_1 + N_2 + 1)}{12}$

Or

$$Z = \frac{[T - \frac{N_1(N_1 + N_2 + 1)}{2}]}{\sqrt{\frac{N_1 N_2 (N_1 + N_2 + 1)}{12}}}$$

Where N_1 = Smaller sample size, N_2 = Larger sample size and T = Sum of ranks for smaller sized sample.

Problem 20.4, on Rank Sum Test (Wilcoxon Rank Sum Test or Mann-Whitney U test):

Dissolution test using the original dissolution apparatus and a modified dissolution apparatus was conducted using tablets. Amount dissolved in 30 minutes was determined and the values are as mentioned below. Conduct a Rank Sum Test and ensure whether original and modified dissolution apparatus are performing the same.

Original Apparatus	Modified Apparatus
Amount Dissolved	Amount Dissolved
53	58
61	55
57	67
50	62
63	55
62	64
54	66
52	59
59	68
57	57
64	69
---	56

Solution:

Step 1: Let us assume null hypothesis that both the original dissolution and modified dissolution apparatus perform the same. Let us assume the alternate hypothesis that both apparatus are different in performance.

Step 2: Let all the data is pooled into one Table and for the entire data give ranking in such a way lower numbers are ranked from lower rank to the highest. If a negative value is observed (say -1, 0.5). Give rank 1 to -1 and give rank 2 to 0.5. Also ensure in assigning average rank for ties. Later, calculate the total sum of the ranks for individual apparatus.

Original Apparatus		Modified Apparatus	
Amount Dissolved	Rank	Amount Dissolved	Rank
53	3	58	11
61	14	55	5.5
57	9	67	21
50	1	62	15.5
63	17	55	5.5
62	15.5	64	18.5
54	4	66	20
52	2	59	12.5
59	12.5	68	22
57	9	57	9
64	18.5	69	23
---	---	56	7
Sum of Ranks	**105.5**	**Sum of Ranks**	**170.5**

Step 3: Now consider smaller sample size as N_1 and larger sample size as N_2. Here, smaller sample size is ($N_1 = 11$) and larger sample size is ($N_2 = 12$). When referred to standard Rank Sum table, N_1 on the horizontal side and N_2 on vertical side, for 5% level, the value is 99. As the Rank Sum (105.5) of original apparatus is not equal to and larger than Tabled, it is interpreted that dissolution test of tablets of original and modified apparatus are the same (or significantly same). This interpretation is with respect to standard rank sum table.

Step 4: It can be concluded that both original and modified apparatus are significantly the same.

The second approach of solving the problem is by normality approximation method that is.

$$Z = \frac{\left[T - \dfrac{N_1(N_1 + N_2 + 1)}{2}\right]}{\sqrt{\dfrac{N_1 N_2 (N_1 + N_2 + 1)}{12}}} = \frac{\left[105.5 - \dfrac{11(11 + 12 + 1)}{2}\right]}{\sqrt{\dfrac{(11)(12)(11 + 12 + 1)}{12}}} = \frac{26.5}{16.25} = 1.63$$

At 5% level, with respect to normal distribution, Z value = 1.96. As calculated Z-value (1.63) is less than standard Table value, it can be interpreted that null hypothesis is accepted, indicating that both original and modified dissolution apparatus are performing same.

It is necessary to understand that sign test, signed rank test, rank sum test have individual standard Tables for drawing conclusions after calculations and comparisons. In addition to this, a second approach is by normality approximation and conclusions are made based on calculated and Tabled 'Z' values. In certain circumstances, a non-parametric chi-square test is conducted and the calculated value is compared with the Tabled. The degree of freedom for non-parametric chi-square test is different from degree of freedom for parametric chi-square test. But, the same chi-square standard Table is used for both.

20.5 Non-Parametric One-way ANOVA (or Kruskal-Wallis Test)

The Kruskal-Wallis test is an extended version of 'rank sum test' for more than two treatments. Hence, the test is considered as un-paired test or more than two independent group test. The test helps in determining the equality of variances in the different groups. If significant differences are observed, it indicates that the averages of at least two of the comparative treatments are different. The test is flexible with different number of observations in each group. However, equal sample size in each group is desirable. Here, all the group data are combined into one Table. Secondly, ranks are assigned keeping in view all the data in all the groups and where there are ties, average rank is assigned. The ranks are then summed for the entire individual group. Smaller sample size (N1) rank sum (calculated sum of ranks in the group) is compared with the Tabled value and, if the calculated value is not equal to or lower than the Tabled value, the null hypothesis is rejected i.e., at least two of the groups are not the same.

The second approach is by Chi-square test and it is assumed that Kruskal-Wallis test is approximately distributed as chi-square test and the equation is as follows:

$$\chi^2_{k-1} = \left[\frac{12}{N\,(N+1)}\left(\sum \frac{R_i^2}{n_i}\right) - 3\,(N+1)\right]$$

Where, N is the total number of observations in all groups combined, R_i the sums of ranks in i^{th} group, n_i the number of observations in i^{th} group and k the number of groups. If the calculated chi-square value is greater than the Tabled value (degree of freedom is equal to no. of treatments or groups minus 1) indicates that null hypothesis is rejected.

Yet a correction factor is provided where ties, so that chi-square value is increased that in turn increases the degree of significance. The correction factor helps where chi-square just misses significance by making end result in statistically significant difference.

The equation for correction is as follows:

$$Correction = \frac{\chi^2}{1 - \sum \frac{(t_i^3 - t_i)}{(N^3 - N)}}$$

Where, t_i is the number of tied observation in group I and N is the total number of observations.

Once it has been identified that there is difference between at least two treatments, it is obvious to have clarification which two (or more) treatments that are different. For this, two treatments in question are checked for the difference in the rank sum. If the difference value is greater than the standard Table value that is indicated in 'critical differences for significance comparing all possible pairs of treatments for non-parametric one-way ANOVA' Table, it indicates that the two treatments are significantly different (say at 5% level). The limitation with this is that the two treatments must have same sample size. In contrast, a parametric 't' test may further be conducted in order to find the treatments that are different in detail.

Problem 20.5, on Kruskal-Wallis Test:

A pre-clinical test was conducted on rats, where in two doses of an experimental compound and a control were administered and observed for known sedation. The time for the animals to fall asleep after injection was recorded. If an animal did not fall asleep within 10 minutes of the drug injection, the time to sleep was arbitrarily assigned a value of 15 minutes. The experimental results are as mentioned in the below Table. Conduct a Kruskal-Wallis Test and draw conclusions.

"Time to Sleep" for a Control and Two Doses of an Experimental Compound (minutes)		
Control	**Low Dose**	**High Dose**
8	10	3
1	5	4
9	8	8
---	6	1
9	7	1
6	7	3
3	15	1
15	1	6
1	15	2
7	7	2

Solution:

Step 1: Let us assume the null hypothesis that there is no difference between control, low and high treatments and let us assume the alternate hypothesis that there is difference.

Step 2: Compiling all the data and then ranking the data as an entire pool. If ties, an average rank is established as illustrated. After rankings, Rank sums are made for the entire individual groups.

"Time to Sleep" for a Control and Two Doses of an Experimental Compound (minutes)					
Control	Rank	Low Dose	Rank	High Dose	Rank
8	22	10	26	3	10
1	3.5	5	13	4	12
9	24.5	8	22	8	22
---	---	6	15	1	3.5
9	24.5	7	18.5	1	3.5
6	15	7	18.5	3	10
3	10	15	28	1	3.5
15	28	1	3.5	6	15
1	3.5	15	28	2	7.5
7	18.5	7	18.5	2	7.5
Sum of Ranks	149.5	---	191.0	----	94.5

Step 3: Using chi-square equation i.e.,

$$\chi^2_{k-1} = \left[\frac{12}{N\,(N+1)} \left(\sum \frac{R_i^2}{n_i} \right) - 3\,(N+1) \right]$$

$$\chi^2_{3-1} = \left[\frac{12}{29(29+1)} \left(\frac{149.5^2}{9} + \frac{191^2}{10} + \frac{94.5^2}{10} \right) - 3(29+1) \right] = 6.89$$

Step 4: When calculated chi-square value of 6.89 is compared with Tabled chi-square value at (3-1=2) degree of freedom at 5% level is 5.99, it is found that calculated value is greater than Tabled and hence, there is at least two among control, low dose and high dose have significant difference in time for falling asleep.

Step 5: In order to find out which groups have significant difference, this particular example does not have all the sample size in groups the same. However, when compared among the two groups which have same sample size, the difference is (191-94.5)=96.5. With respect to the standard Table of "Critical difference for significance comparing all possible pairs of treatments for non-parametric one-way ANOVA" at 5% level for horizontal side of 3 (number of treatments) and for vertical side of n_i=10 (for each treatment) is 92. If the calculated difference is greater than the tabled 'critical difference', it indicates that there is significant difference at 5% level among the two treatments that have equal sample size. This can be concluded that there is significant difference between time of sedation of low dose and high dose.

20.6 Friedman Test (A Non-Parametric Two-way ANOVA)

Friedman test is a non-parametric two-way Analysis of Variance (two-way ANOVA) test. The test is applied when there are more than two treatment groups. If two treatment groups are available, one might have planned for Wilcoxon Signed rank test (which goes in analogy with paired data). When more than two treatment groups as paired data are available, as randomized block design, Friedman Test is conducted. For the test, the data should be non-parametric as ranked or interval or ratio type data. In Friedman test, the treatments are ranked within each block disregarding difference between blocks. In other words, the data in the group or column (block) are ranked from lowest to the highest and the entire data is not pooled while ranking. If tie values within the block, average ranking is allotted. After ranking, the rank sum in each group is calculated and is substituted in the equation. If sample sizes are sufficiently large, a Chi-square distribution can be used and the equation is as follows:

$$\chi^2_{(k-1)} = \{\frac{12}{rc(c+1)}\left[\sum R_i^2\right] - 3r(c+1)\}$$

Where, k= number of treatment groups, r = number of rows, c = number of columns, R_i = Sum of Ranks in the ith group (column) and (k-1) is the degrees of freedom.

Problem 20.6, on Friedman Test: In order to test the performance of a tablet punching machine of a four tablet presses, with regard to hardness, average hardness of 10 tablets was computed for five different tablet products manufactured on four presses. The tablets are a random selection of five typical tablet products. The presses were identically set for the same pressure for each tablet formulation. Conduct a Friedman Test with the below computed data and judge whether there is any difference among the presses.

Average Hardness of 10 Tablets for Five Different Tablet Formulations Prepared on Four Presses				
Tablet Formulation	**Tablet Press**			
	A	**B**	**C**	**D**
1	7.5	6.9	7.3	7.0
2	8.2	8.0	8.5	7.9
3	7.3	7.9	8.0	7.6
4	6.6	6.5	7.1	6.4
5	7.5	6.8	7.6	6.7

Solution:

Step 1: Let us assume as null hypothesis (H_0), to intentionally nullify that there are no differences in the hardness of the tablets or tablet presses.

Step 2: As an alternative hypothesis (H_A), let us assume that there exist difference between the hardness of the tablets or tablet presses.

Step 3: As the data is randomized block designed, paired and contains more than two treatments, Friedman test is applicable.

Hence, the data is ranked with respect to the formulation within the row in such a way the lowest to the highest. Hence, as per the data, the ranks are assigned and are as mentioned in the parenthesis.

Average Hardness of 10 Tablets for Five Different Tablet Formulations Prepared on Four Presses				
Tablet Formulation	**Tablet Press (Ranks in parenthesis)**			
	A	**B**	**C**	**D**
1	7.5 (4)	6.9 (1)	7.3 (3)	7.0 (2)
2	8.2 (3)	8.0 (2)	8.5 (4)	7.9 (1)
3	7.3 (1)	7.9 (3)	8.0 (4)	7.6 (2)
4	6.6 (3)	6.5 (2)	7.1 (4)	6.4 (1)
5	7.5 (3)	6.8 (2)	7.6 (4)	6.7 (1)
R_i	14	10	19	7

Substituting the values in the chi-square test,

$$\chi^2_{(k-1)} = \left\{ \frac{12}{rc(c+1)} \left[\sum_i R_i^2 \right] - 3r(c+1) \right\}$$

$$\chi^2_{(4-1)} = \left\{ \frac{12}{5 * 4(4+1)} \left[(14)^2 + (10)^2 + (19)^2 + (7)^2 \right] - 3 * 5(4+1) \right\} = 9.72$$

Step 4: Upon referring to chi-square standard Table, at 5% probability and degree of freedom {(no. of treatment groups -1) = 4-1 = 3}, is 7.81. Hence, calculated chi-square value (9.72) is greater than standard Table value (7.81). This further indicates that reject the null hypothesis and accept alternate hypothesis.

Step 5: Hence from the above test, we can conclude that there is significant difference in the hardness of the tablets from at least two punches. Whether it is two punches or more where there is significant difference in the tablet hardness needs further analysis of taking every two columns (punches).

Note: In Friedman test, if n is the number of blocks and k is the number of treatments, the data will be in the form n x k.

i. For small samples (k < 6 and n < 14) the calculated value is compared with critical value from standard Table. If the calculated value is greater than the critical value (from standard Table), reject the null hypothesis.

ii. For larger samples (k > 6 and n > 13) the calculated value is compared with critical value from Standard chi-square Table. If the calculated is greater than the standard chi-square value, reject the null hypothesis.

Hence, depending on the sample size, either we have to refer to critical value Table or the chi-square Table.

21 Sample Size Determination

21.0 Introduction

At this juncture, after several discussions of fundamentals, the current question is how many number of subjects to be used for an experimental study. For achieving this, several approaches can be used and the current discussion is simplified.

In several circumstances a researcher initiates experiments with empirical sample size and later scratches whether the sample size is correct or not.

Hence, a researcher should have cleancut sample size and the sample collected must have strong scientific rationality.

21.1 Based on Past Experimental Data

In this approach, a past research data reported lead to determination of sample size for the current study. The equation suitable under such circumstance is as follows:

$$n = [z_{\frac{\alpha}{2}} \times \frac{\sigma}{E}]^2$$

Where, n = sample size; $z_{\alpha/2}$ = confidence interval assumed (standard deviate), σ = standard deviation in a previously reported study, E (standard error) = Error acceptable in the mean value of the present study

For instance, if z = 1.96, σ = 24.9 (from past reported data), E = 5, then

$$n = [1.96 \times \frac{24.9}{5}]^2 = 95.2$$

Hence, at least 96 subjects can be planned for the study.

21.2 Based on Theoretical Assumptions and No Past Reported Data

In this approach, the type I error, type II error and the difference between the means are defined and based on the equation mentioned, the sample size is calculated.

$$N = \sigma^2[(z_\alpha + z_\beta)/d]^2$$

Where, z_α = accepted significance of type I error, z_β = accepted significance of type II error, d = the difference to be detected. For a two sided test, z_α and z_β are with respect to the areas of normal distribution curves. z_α is the standard deviate value 1.28, 1.96, 2.58 at 10%, 5% and 1% probabilities respectively (in directly are of normal distribution curve). When considered the upper tail, z_β is the standard deviate value 0.842, 1.28, 1.645 at $\beta = 0.2$, $\beta = 0.1$, $\beta = 0.05$ respectively. Here 'α' is the probability of type I error, and 'β' is the probability of type II error.

Problem 21.1, on sample size: For detecting mean tablet weight 3 mg or more different from the target weight, the chance of concluding that a difference of 3 mg or more exists and the α (5%) and β (0.1) are fixed and if the standard deviation is 10, calculate the sample size of tablets to be collected and tested to achieve the mentioned results.

Solution:

$$N = \sigma^2\left[(z_\alpha + z_\beta)/d\right]^2$$
$$N = 10^2[(1.96 + 1.28)/3]^2 = 117$$

Hence, at least a sample size of 117 tablets are to be collected from the batch for the expected result.

Note: For a binomial data, it is necessary to replace 'σ^2' with 'pq'.

Note: When the sample size is small and variance 'σ^2' is unknown, the 't' value changes with change in sample size and a guess work may lead to incorrect value. Guenther suggested to add a factor "$0.5(z_\alpha)^2$" to the calculated N value especially when variance is unknown.

Problem 21.2, on sample size: In order to compare two formulations, a researcher wishes to collect blood samples from subjects after treatment and study the area under the curves for the plots of blood level vs. time. Calculate the sample size required for initiating the research. The difference expected in the AUCs is ± 20 hour.mcg/ml. The power of the test planned is 90% at 5% level. The average area expected is about 100 and the standard deviation is estimated to be 25.

Solution:

For a single sample study, bioequivalence test is usually designed in such a way that each subject received each formulation on separate occasions with a paired design. Here, $z_\alpha = 1.96$ and $z_\beta = 1.28$

$$N = \sigma^2\left[(z_\alpha + z_\beta)/d\right]^2 = 25^2[(1.96 + 1.28)/20]^2 = 16.4$$

As the variance is un-known, add a factor "$0.5(z_\alpha)^2$" to N that is., $\{[0.5 \times 1.96^2] + 16.4\} = 18.3$.

Hence, a minimum of 19 subjects are required for conducting the study.

For a two sample study, the equation is

$$N = 2\sigma^2\left[(z_\alpha + z_\beta)/d\right]^2$$

and if the variance is unknown, add the factor.

Problem 21.3, on sample size: Two formulations containing the same drug are to be compared for time to dissolution of 50%. How many tablets of each formulation have to be used to achieve a power of 80% and 10% level of significance, in a two sided test. The true difference between the dissolution times of two formulations is expected to be 15 min. The standard deviation is 10. Given $Z_\alpha = 1.645$ and $Z_\beta = 0.842$.

Solution:

$$N = 2\sigma^2\left[(z_\alpha + z_\beta)/d\right]^2 = 2(10)^2[(1.645 + 0.842)/15]^2 = 5.5\,tablets$$

Add to obtained sample size $0.25 * Z_\alpha^2$

Then, $0.25 * 1.65_\alpha^2 + 5.5\,tablets$

Therefore total number of tablets to be taken are $0.7 + 5.5 = 6.2$ tablets

As variance is unknown, upon adding the factor, the N value is 6.2. Hence, seven tablets are sufficient enough for the study.

As a whole, when a sample size has to be estimated, appropriate equations with the available data are used. In an equation, if one value is unknown and the other values are known, then upon re-arranging we can calculate the sample size.

Problem 21.4, on Power: A bioavailability study in which the average of the ratios of AUC of a tablet formulation and solution formulation of the same drug are to be assessed and ratios of AUC should be equal to 1, on the average. The FDA is interested in knowing the power of such tests because small sample sizes that result in non significant differences may have little power. What is the power of the test with a sample size of 12 in which protection is to be provided against erroneous acceptance of alternatives for which the true ratio differs from 1 by 0.2 (20%) or more. The test is performed at 5% level and standard deviation is approximately 0.25. Calculate the power when the sample size of 12, which is small. Given, $Z_\alpha = 1.96$.

Solution:

i.   Subtract from sample size factor $(0.5 * z_\alpha^2)$ and later use the result as N.

      Therefore, $N = 12 - [0.5 * (1.96)^2] = 10.08$

ii.   Using equation, $Z_\beta = \left[d * \sqrt{N/\sigma^2}\right] - z_\alpha$

$$= \left[0.2 * \sqrt{10/0.25^2}\right] - 1.96 = 0.57$$

iii. For $Z_\beta = 0.57$, then $\beta = 0.285$

      (obtained from normal distribution area)

iv.   Power $= (1 - \beta) = 1 - 0.285 = 0.715$ (or 71.5 percent)

21.3 Online Version of Sample Size Calculator

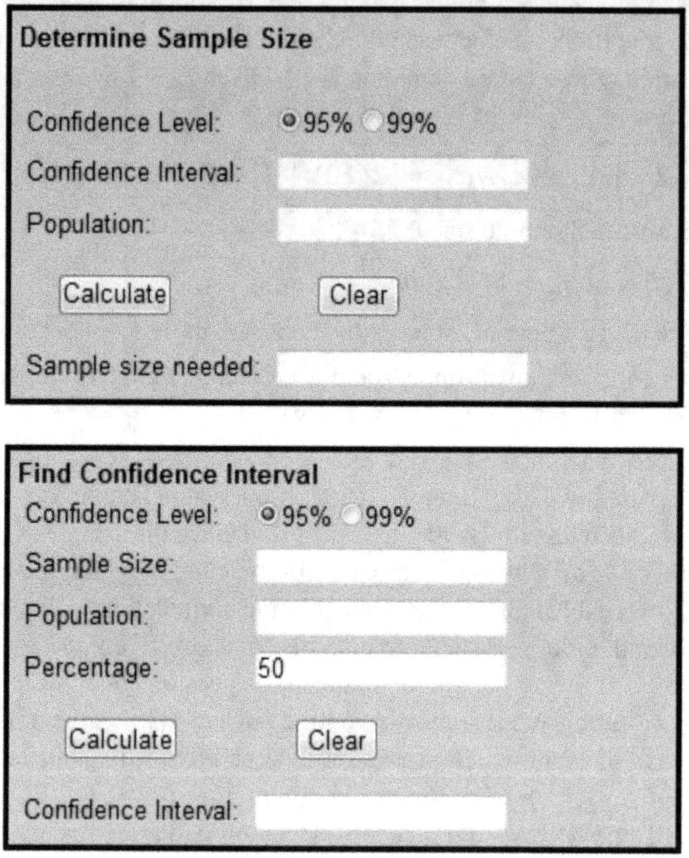

FIGURE 21.1 Sample Size Calculator

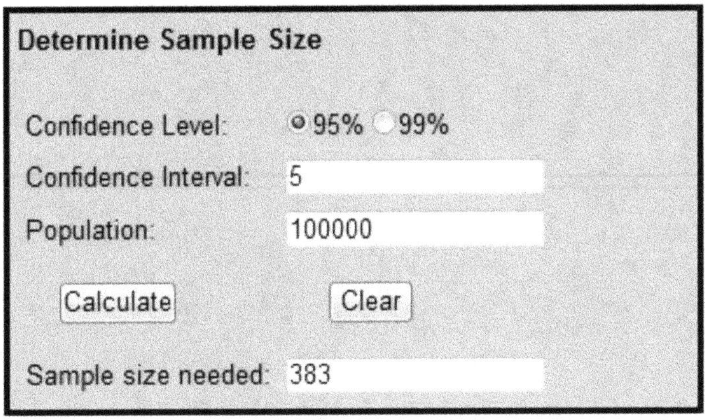

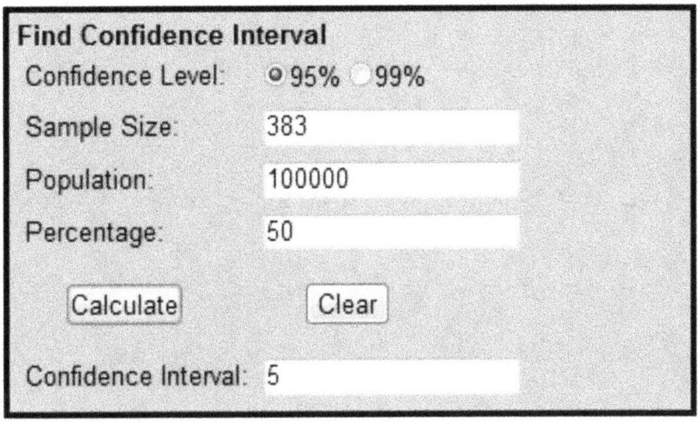

FIGURE 21.2 Sample Size Calculator upon giving Values

22 Introduction to Epidemiology

22.0 Introduction

The word Epidemiology was coined from a Greek terminology i.e., 'Epi' meaning on or upon, 'demos' meaning people and 'logos' meaning study of.

Epidemiology is defined as how often a disease occurs in defined groups of population and how. The objective of epidemiology is to study the etiology, plan and prevent the occurrence of a disease or a medical event, or a medical state or a medical condition. Secondly, Epidemiology can be defined as the measurement of disease outcomes in relation to a population at risk. Population at risk is defined as the group of people, healthy or sick, who would be counted as cases if they had the disease being studied.

Thirdly, Epidemiology is defined as the study of the distribution and determinants of health-related states or events in specified population. Here, distribution can be considered as the frequency or pattern of a health related state. A frequency can be considered as a number and its relation (or ratio) with respect to the population for a health related event. A pattern is the occurrence of health-related events by time; place and person i.e., annual, seasonal, daily, hourly, week day vs. week end; geographic variation, urban/rural differences, and location of work sites or schools and with respect to risk of illness, injury, disability such as age, sex, marital status, socio economic status etc., respectively. Determinant is a factor, event, characteristic, or cause that is responsible for occurrence of a health related event. Hence, epidemiologists assume that illness does not occur randomly in a population, but happens only when the right accumulation of risk factors or determinants exists in an individual. Therefore, fourthly, Epidemiology is defined as a frequency or pattern of a health related event in a population.

At this juncture, the distinguishing responsibilities of clinician and epidemiologist have to be well understood. In case of both clinician and epidemiologist a patient shall be counseled for his illness symptoms and is diagnosed for a disease and is then prescribed for cure of the condition. However, for a clinician the patient is seen as an individual but for an epidemiologist the patient is a representative of a community and he assess the incidence and prevalence of the health related state or condition.

22.1 Incidence

Incidence is defined as the proportion of cases in the population at a given time. In other words, incidence is the measure of probability of occurrence of a given medical condition in a population within a stipulated period of time.

22.2 Incidence Proportion

Incidence proportion is defined as the number of new cases within a specified period of time to the size of population initially at risk. This indicates that incidence proportion is a ratio of the cases to the number of years of the study duration.

22.3 Incidence Rate

Incidence rate is the number of new cases with respect to population at risk in a given period of time. The difference between incidence proportion and incidence rate is that the former is with respect to the total years (say) of study and in case of the latter it is with respect to a year (say). Incidence rate is also called as 'incidence density rate' or 'person-time incidence rate'.

For instance, incidence proportion is found to be 28 new cases per 1000 population per two years. This can be interpreted that incidence rate is 14 new cases per 1000 population per year. Thus using person-time rather than just time handles situations where the amount of observation time differs between people or when the population at risk varies with time. Thus incidence rate is observed constant over different periods of time. This can be witnessed with 28 new cases per 1000 population per two years with 14 new cases per 1000 population per year or 50 persons observed for 20 years.

Let us consider a study where a sample population of 225 people was monitored for occurrence of HIV over a period of 10 year period. During the survey, at time zero, the surveyor has identified 25 cases and after 5th year 20 new cases and on a later follow up i.e., after 10th year 30 new HIV cases. In this study, it can be stated that incidence proportion is 50/225/10 years and incidence rate is 5/225 person-one year. In case of prevalence (discussed at a later stage), it is the cases identified at the initiation of the study i.e., 25 cases and hence the final value of prevalence is 75 cases/ 225 = 0.33 or 33 percent by the end of the study. Hence, an incidence indicates risk of contracting the disease whereas prevalence indicates the widespread of the disease.

In the above case, when the study was made, the surveyor is identifying the new case only during the every five year observations. This does not indicate when exactly the disease has initiated. In order to calculate the incidence, it is assumed with respect to half time of the period (i.e., half-way point).

Let us now consider another study and at 5 years the number of new cases identified was 20 and we assume the patients have developed the HIV at 2.5 years ($0 + 5 = 5/2 = 2.5$ years) and hence contributing to 20 cases $\times$ 2.5 years = 50 person –years of disease free life.

At 10 years, the number of new cases identified was 30, but they did not have at 5 year study conducted earlier. Then the corresponding contribution is $30 \times (5 + 10 = 15/2 =)$ 7.5 years = 225 person-years of disease free life.

It was also identified that 150 people never developed HIV during the 10 years study period and the corresponding contribution is $150 \times 10 = 1500$ person-years of disease free life.

As a whole, a total of $1500 + 225 = 1775$ person-years of life is observed. When total number of new cases is divided by 1775, the value observed is 0.028 indicating 28 new cases of HIV per 1000 population per year. In other words, if you study a 1000 population for one year, it is expected for 28 new cases of HIV. Hence, it is believed that the incidence rate is a much accurate measure than prevalence.

22.4 Prevalence

It is defined as the proportion of disease found in a defined number of population. Hence in the above case study, 25 cases (at zero time) + 20 new cases (after 5 years) + 30 new cases (after 10 years) = 75 cases among the 225 sample are considered and the prevalence = $75/225 = 0.33$ or 33 percent.

Prevalence of a disease is classified into three types i.e., point, period and life time prevalence. In case of point prevalence, it is the proportion of new case identified during the point of time defined to the population specified. In case of period prevalence, it is the proportion of new cases identified during the period of time defined to the population specified. Where as in life time prevalence, the number of new cases identified during the life time of the people to the population specified. Hence, prevalence helps to know how many people have the disease right now. Whereas, incidence helps to know how many new cases the people acquire per year the disease? It is often considered that 12 month prevalence as period prevalence and is used in conjunction with lifetime prevalence. In case of point prevalence, the duration is a month or even less.

For a better understanding the differences between incidence and prevalence, let us consider a disease that takes long time to cure and was widespread in 2002 but dissipated in 2003. In this case the disease will have both high incidence and high prevalence in 2002, but in 2003 it will have a low incidence yet will continue to have a high prevalence. In contrast, a disease that has a short duration has low prevalence and high incidence. When the incidence is constant, prevalence is the product of disease incidence and average duration of disease i.e., prevalence = incidence X duration (average value). As per the equation mentioned, as incidence increases prevalence also increases and vice-versa. However, the relation does not hold for age-specific prevalence and incidence and the relation is expected to be complicated.

22.5 Other Terminology

Attributable Risk (AR): It is also called as Excess Risk (ER) and is defined as the difference between exposed population and un-exposed population. It is usually used in Cohort studies.

$$\text{Attributable risk (AR)} = (I_e - I_u),$$

where I_e = Incidence of exposed and I_u = Incidence of un-exposed.

In terms of percentage,

$$\text{AR percent} = (I_e - I_u)/I_e * 100$$

Population Attributable Risk (PAR): It is defined as reduction in incidence of a disease condition when entirely un-exposed with respect to the exposed pattern.

Etiologic Fraction: It is the proportion of cases where in exposure has played a casual role in disease development.

Excess Fraction: It is the proportion of cases that is occurring at a period of time among the exposed population and is in excess with respect to un-exposed.

It is necessary to understand that all excess cases are etiologic and not vice-versa.

For instance, a study was initiated to know the number of soldier with leukemia during a 20 year period after exposure to a nuclear bomb. When the study is conducted, several soldiers might have been identified with leukemia upon exposure and some soldiers might have been identified with leukemia even though they were not exposed.

Population Attributable Fraction (PAF): It is the percentage reduction in incidence rate of a disease, if the exposure was eliminated. Such measures help policy makers to develop public health interventions.

Combined Population Attributable Risk (Combined PAR): When a disease condition is based on a combination of risk factors, then a combined PAR is the sum of individual risk factor PAR leading to the same disease. Hence, combined PAR is usually lower than individual risk based PAR and this can be further interpreted as individual risk based PAR is leading to double counts of risks.

Absolute Risk: It is the risk of developing a disease over a period of time. Every individual have absolute risk of developing disease like cancer, heart attack etc.

Relative Risk (or Risk Ratio or RR): It is the risk of developing a disease when compared with exposed and un-exposed. For instance, development of a disease among smokers and non-smokers and here the stimulus is smoking and the outcome is cancer, which is a disease.

Relative risk can also be defined as the ratio of probability of occurrence of an event in the exposed to the probability of occurrence of an event in the un-exposed.

Odd ratios: For instance, if the probability of occurrence of cancer among smokers is 20% and probability of occurrence of cancer among non-smokers is 1%, the following table gives the number of people

Risk	Disease Status	
	Present	**Absent**
Smoker	a = 20	b = 80
Non-Smoker	c = 1	d = 99

Then relative risk (RR) = a/(a+b) / c/(c+d) = 20/100 / 1/100 = 20

When same case is considered in terms of odd ratios, when 'a' is very very small, a/(a+b) becomes a/b and when 'c' is very very small, c/(c+d) becomes c/d,

Then Odd Ratio (OR) = a/b/c/d = ad/bc

Hence, odd ratios have wider applications is statistics and are used.

23   Introduction to SAS, SPSS, Epi Info and Minitab

23.0   Introduction

The first inhibition for theoretical known statistics is lack of knowledge of using commercial statistical softwares. Commercial softwares are well accepted internationally and the data retrieved helps to draw directly the final conclusions upon inputting data to software. The current chapter introduces various commercial and non-commercial softwares. In the subsequent chapter an attempt is made to know the software from screen shots.

23.1   Statistics Analysis Systems (SAS)

23.1.1   Introduction

Statistics Analysis System, popularly known as 'SAS' was established in the year 1976 by North Carolina State University so as to analyze the data of Department of Agriculture, USA. In course of time, it has become popular due to its wide application in various platforms and usage by multiple vendors. It is believed that data collected speaks about facts and figures but, it seems to be more than that for business. Currently, SAS is one of the pioneers in data management, business intelligence and analytics. The company has customers in 148 countries and its software are being installed in over 83, 000 sites that includes business, government and universities. Ninety four of the top one hundred companies of 2016 Fortune Global 500 are SAS customers. In 2016, it has generated revenue of US $ 3.2 billion and in the year 2015, the company has reinvested 25% of the revenue on research and development (R&D).

23.1.2   Mission

SAS delivers proven solutions that drive innovation and improve performance and its values are approachable, customer driven, swift & agile, innovative and trustworthy.

23.1.3 Products Provided by SAS

#

- SAS® 9.4

A

- SAS® Anti-Advanced Analytics
- Advanced Analytics Lab for State and Local Government
- Analytics for Child Well-Being
- Analytics Platform
- Automotive
- SAS AppDev Studio
- SAS® Analytics Accelerator for Teradata
- SAS® Analytics for Containers
- SAS® Analytics for IoT
- SAS® Analytics Pro
- SAS® Analytics Pro for Midsize Business
- Money Laundering
- SAS® Asset Performance Analytics

B

- Banking & Financial Analytics
- Base SAS®
- Business Analytics
- Business Analytics Centers of Excellence Consulting Service
- Business Intelligence & Analytics Software
- SAS Bridge for Esri
- SAS® Banking Analytics Architecture
- SAS® BookRunner®
- SAS® Business Intelligence for Midsize Business
- SAS® Business Rules Manager

C

- Capital Markets Solutions
- Casino Floor Performance
- Casinos
- Commodity Classification
- Communications
- Consumer Goods Solutions
- Credit Scoring for SAS® Enterprise Miner™
- SAS® Capital Planning & Management
- SAS® Capital Planning & Management
- SAS® Capital Requirements for Market Risk
- SAS® Clinical Data Integration
- SAS® Cloud Analytics
- SAS® Collaborative Planning Workbench
- SAS® Contextual Analysis
- SAS® Cost and Profitability Management
- SAS® Credit Scoring for Banking
- SAS® Criminal Justice Data Integration and Analytics
- SAS® Curriculum Pathways®
- SAS® Customer Due Diligence
- SAS® Customer Intelligence
- SAS® Customer Intelligence 360
- SAS® Customer Link Analytics
- SAS® Cybersecurity

D

- Data Management Software
- Defense & Security Software
- SAS Data Management for Midsize Business
- SAS Data Surveyors
- SAS Desktop Data Mining for Midsize Business
- SAS® Data Governance

- SAS® Data Integration for Midsize Business
- SAS® Data Loader for Hadoop
- SAS® Data Management
- SAS® Data Management Consulting
- SAS® Data Quality
- SAS® Data Quality Accelerator for Teradata
- SAS® Data Quality for Midsize Business
- SAS® Decision Management
- SAS® Decision Manager
- SAS® Demand Forecasting for Retail

E

- Education Analytical Suite
- SAS® Econometrics
- SAS® Energy Forecasting
- SAS® Enterprise Analytics for Education
- SAS® Enterprise BI Server
- SAS® Enterprise Case Management
- SAS® Enterprise GRC
- SAS® Enterprise Guide®
- SAS® Enterprise Miner™
- SAS® Episode Analytics
- SAS® Episode Analytics
- SAS® EVAAS® for K-12
- SAS® Event Stream Processing
- SAS® Expected Credit Loss

F

- Foundation Tools
- SAS® Factory Miner
- SAS® Federation Server
- SAS® Field Quality Analytics
- SAS® Financial Management
- SAS® Firmwide Risk for Solvency II

- SAS® for Enterprise Fraud & Financial Crimes
- SAS® for Marketing Performance Management
- SAS® for Patron Value Optimization
- SAS® Forecast Analyst Workbench
- SAS® Forecast Server
- SAS® Forecasting for Desktop
- SAS® Forecasting for Midsize Business
- SAS® Fraud Framework
- SAS® Fraud Framework for Government
- SAS® Fraud Framework for Health Care
- SAS® Fraud Framework for Insurance
- SAS® Fraud Management
- SAS® Fraud Network Analysis

G

- Government Solutions
- SAS® Grid Manager

H

- Health Care Analytics & Big Data Solutions
- Health Insurance
- High-Performance Analytics
- High-Tech Manufacturing
- Higher Education Solutions
- Hotel Analytics
- SAS® High-Performance Data Mining
- SAS® High-Performance Econometrics
- SAS® High-Performance Optimization
- SAS® High-Performance Risk
- SAS® High-Performance Statistics

S

- SAS/ACCESS® Interface to Hadoop
- SAS/ACCESS® Interface to Impala
- SAS/ACCESS® Software
- SAS/AF
- SAS/CONNECT
- SAS/EIS
- SAS/ETS®
- SAS/FSP
- SAS/GRAPH
- SAS/IML®
- SAS/OR®
- SAS/QC®
- SAS/SECURE
- SAS/SHARE
- SAS/STAT®
- SAS® Scalable Performance Data Server
- SAS® Scoring Accelerator
- SAS® Security Intelligence
- SAS® Sentiment Analysis
- SAS® Service Parts Optimization
- SAS® Simulation Studio
- SAS® Size Optimization: SAS® Size Profiling and SAS® Pack Optimization
- SAS® Solutions for Hadoop

- SAS® Stress Testing Workbench
- SAS® Studio
- SAS® Supply Chain Intelligence
- Service Offerings for Grid
- Service Offerings for Hadoop
- Spend Analysis
- Sports Analytics

T

- SAS® Text Miner
- Travel & Transportation Software

U

- SAS® Underwriting Risk Management for P&C Insurance
- SAS® University Edition
- Utilities Solutions

V

- SAS® Visual Analytics
- SAS® Visual Analytics for UN Comtrade
- SAS® Visual Data Discovery
- SAS® Visual Data Mining and Machine Learning
- SAS® Visual Forecasting
- SAS® Visual Investigator
- SAS® Visual Statistics
- SAS® Viya™

Overall SAS provides enterprise solutions, sell software products, analyze data and provide consulting services. The key strategies of SAS and its products are to develop advanced analytics, establish customer intelligence, maintaining risk management, developing business intelligence so as to develop forecast so that which product is in demand in future, establish data management and makes the organisation (or customer) cautious from fraud and security intelligence as per the company's requirements.

23.1.4 Application of the SAS Software

Even though statistical software operates with its own computer language systems, software provides a provision for input of data from computer system and provides various options of selecting required fields of data and analyzing the data with inbuilt mathematical calculations and finally providing the output data of the required statistic at the desired significance level. Based upon the output data generated, one can conclude whether the scientific study is significant or not. In addition to this, SAS helps with various tools in presenting the data for making better interpretations and conclusions.

It is necessary to understand that statistical software becomes easy at the profession level upon understanding how data generated is calculated for a statistical test and how the data output is generated by the software. As a whole, statistical software only helps when a researcher is well understood with manual calculations of the statistical test with the corresponding equations upon knowing the standard distribution curves and their significance.

23.2 Statistical Package for Social Sciences (SPSS)

23.2.1 Introduction

SPSS, a product of IBM (International Business Machines Corp.,), is a data, trend, forecast, statistical management software wherein input of the data collected when subjected to the software helps in analyzing, draw conclusions with appropriate interpretations of the data. SPSS software system helps in statistical analysis and reporting, predictive modeling and reporting, decision management, deployment and finally helps in big data analytics. Like several other software SPSS takes data stored in the computer system and based on the requirements the necessary available statistical application can be executed.

Hence, in order to understand the output given by the SPSS software, one has to get acquainted with all the statistical methods available both theoretically and practically. By making manual mathematical calculations and referring to standard normal, binomial, student, chi-square, F-distribution Tables one can judge whether the statistical test is significant or not. This indicates that one should be in a position to interpret the data given by the SPSS software. Like several other software, SPSS is helpful for different sectors of business as well as research.

23.2.2 Products

1. IBM SPSS Modeler

Product versions:

    IBM SPSS Modeler Gold

    IBM SPSS Modeler on Cloud

    IBM SPSS Modeler Premium

    IBM SPSS Modeler Professional

    IBM SPSS Modeler Server

    IBM SPSS Modeler for Linux on System Z

2. **IBM SPSS Statistics**

   Product versions:

   > IBM SPSS Advanced Statistics
   >
   > IBM SPSS Amos
   >
   > IBM SPSS Bootstrapping
   >
   > IBM SPSS Categories
   >
   > IBM SPSS Complex Samples
   >
   > IBM SPSS Conjoint
   >
   > IBM SPSS Custom Tables
   >
   > IBM SPSS Data Preparation
   >
   > IBM SPSS Decision Trees
   >
   > IBM SPSS Direct Marketing
   >
   > IBM SPSS Exact Tests
   >
   > IBM SPSS Forecasting
   >
   > IBM SPSS Missing Values
   >
   > IBM SPSS Neural Networks
   >
   > IBM SPSS Regression
   >
   > IBM SPSS Statistics Base
   >
   > IBM SPSS Statistics Campus
   >
   > IBM SPSS Statistics Faculty Pack
   >
   > IBM SPSS Statistics GradPack
   >
   > IBM SPSS Statistics for Linux on System z
   >
   > IBM SPSS Statistics Premium
   >
   > IBM SPSS Statistics Professional
   >
   > IBM SPSS Statistics Programmability Extension
   >
   > IBM SPSS Statistics Server
   >
   > IBM SPSS Statistics Standard
   >
   > IBM SPSS Text Analytics for Surveys

3. **IBM SPSS Analytic Server**

4. **IBM SPSS Collaboration and Deployment Services**

   IBM SPSS Statistics, claims as follows:

   Why use IBM SPSS Statistics?

IBM SPSS Statistics is the world's leading statistical software. It enables you to quickly dig deeper into your data, making it a much more effective tool than spreadsheets, databases or standard multi-dimensional tools for analysts. SPSS Statistics excels at making sense of complex patterns and associations — enabling end users to draw conclusions and make predictions. It has a feature of handling tasks fast like data manipulation and statistical procedures in a third of the time of many non-statistical programs.

23.2.3 IBM SPSS Statistics Editions

Get the analytical power you need for better decision-making

IBM® SPSS® Statistics delivers a powerful set of statistical that enable the organization to make the most of the valuable information from data provided. By digging deeper into the data, one can discover information to improve decision-making—ultimately expanding markets, improving research outcomes, ensuring regulatory compliance, managing risk and maximizing ROI to name a few.

SPSS Statistics features robust and sophisticated functionality and procedures that address the entire analysis lifecycle:

- It includes procedures to account for missing data that otherwise could negatively impact the validity of your results.

- It supports all common data sources used by enterprise organizations.

- Statistical functions and procedures are kept apart from the data, reducing the risk of errors.

- Open technologies allow for the use of external programming languages, so you can add or customize additional functionalities.

- Various modular offerings support different types of analyses. SPSS Statistics comes in three editions to meet all the analysis requirements of your organization:

  IBM SPSS Statistics Standard—Essential analytical tools for the most common projects

  IBM SPSS Statistics Professional — A comprehensive set of features and tools to address the challenges of the entire analytic lifecycle

  IBM SPSS Statistics Premium — Designed for enterprise businesses with extensive needs across all advanced analytics efforts

23.2.3.1   SPSS Statistics standard edition capabilities

- Linear models
- Nonlinear models
- Simulation modeling
- Geospatial analytics
- Custom tables

IBM SPSS Statistics Standard

Whether you are a statistician or other analytics professional or have to analyze data as part of your business responsibilities, SPSS Statistics Standard offers the essential statistical procedures you need to increase the reliability of your analysis, so you reach more dependable conclusions. If you need an analytical package that combines the most common statistical procedures and functions that most analysts use on a day-to-day basis, choose SPSS Statistics Standard.

Cover the essentials with complement of core analytical capabilities

SPSS Statistics Standard is used in a number of fields to address fundamental business and research questions. With SPSS Statistics Standard, one can get a quick look at your data, formulate hypotheses for additional testing and then carry out a number of procedures to help clarify relationships between variables, create clusters, identify trends and make predictions.

Key capabilities include:

- **Linear models**— Make your analysis more accurate and reach more dependable conclusions.
- **Nonlinear models**—Have the ability to apply more sophisticated models to the data.
- **Simulation modeling**— Build better models and assess risk when inputs are uncertain using Monte Carlo simulation techniques.
- **Geospatial analytics**— Explore the relationship between data elements that can be tied to a specific location.
- **Customized tables**— Quickly slice and dice your data for easy analysis and reporting.

Linear models

SPSS Statistics Standard features a variety of regression and advanced statistical procedures designed to fit the inherent characteristics of data describing complex relationships, including:

- General linear models (GLM)
- Generalized linear mixed models (GLMM)
- Hierarchical linear models (HLM)
- Generalized linear models (GENLIN)
- Generalized estimating equations (GEE)

Nonlinear models

One can also apply more sophisticated models to the data using a wide range of nonlinear regression models, using these procedures:

- **Multinomial logistic regression (MLR)** — Predict categorical outcomes with more than two categories
- **Binary logistic regression**— Easily classify your data into two groups
- **Nonlinear regression (NLR) and constrained nonlinear regression (CNLR)**— Estimate parameters of nonlinear models
- **Probit analysis**— Evaluate the value of stimuli using a logit or probit transformation of the proportion responding

Simulation modeling

Simulation in SPSS Statistics Standard is designed to account for uncertainty in inputs to predictive models. Using this approach, uncertain inputs are modeled with probability distributions, and simulated values for those inputs are generated by drawing from those distributions. One can perform simulation even if one has categorical inputs in the data. Simulation features include the ability to produce heat maps and use Automatic Linear Modeling as a starting point for running simulations.

Geospatial analytics

SPSS Statistics can help to explore the relationship between data elements that are tied to a specific location. By fitting linear models for measurements taken over time at locations in 2D/3D space, one can predict "hot" areas and how those areas may change over time. Some of the business applications for this feature include building management and branch performance analysis.

Similarly, the Generalized Spatial Association Rule (GSAR) helps to discover associations between spatial and non-spatial attributes, so one can find hidden patterns and obtain richer insights than with traditional analysis methods alone. GSAR enables to use historical data such as location, type of event and the time the event occurred to describe the occurrences of events, which can be useful in areas such as crime pattern analysis and epidemic surveillance.

Customized tables

SPSS Statistics Standard enables to quickly "slice and dice" the data. Then one can create customized tables to help better understand the data and easily report the results.

23.2.3.2 SPSS Statistics professional edition capabilities

- Linear models
- Nonlinear models
- Simulation modeling
- Geospatial analytics
- Custom tables
- Data preparation
- Missing values and data validity
- Decision trees
- Forecasting

IBM SPSS Statistics Professional

Like SPSS Statistics Standard, SPSS Statistics Professional includes advanced statistical procedures to ensure the accuracy of analyses and table features to help better understand data and easily report results. But SPSS Statistics Professional goes much further — helping with issues of data quality and data complexity, and providing automation and forecasting capabilities to name a few.

Tools to address the challenges of the entire analytic lifecycle

If one routinely perform many types of in-depth and non-standard analyses and need to save time by automating data preparation tasks, SPSS Statistics Professional would be a good fit. SPSS Statistics Professional helps both professional analysts and business users easily accomplish tasks at every phase of the analytical process. Fully integrated SPSS Statistics capabilities enable one to step seamlessly from one task to the next.

SPSS Statistics Professional includes these capabilities:

- **Linear models**— Make your analysis more accurate and reach more dependable conclusions to drive decision-making.

- **Nonlinear models**—Have the ability to apply more sophisticated models to the data.

- **Simulation modeling**— Build better models and assess risk when inputs are uncertain using Monte Carlo simulation techniques.

- **Geospatial analytics**— Explore the relationship between data elements that can be tied to a specific location.

- **Customized tables**— Quickly slice and dice your data for easy analysis and reporting.

- **Data preparation**— Save time and improve the accuracy of your analysis.

- **Missing values and data validity**— Use a scientific approach to handling missing data.

- **Decision trees**—Better identify groups, discover relationships between groups and predict future events.

- **Forecasting**— Analyze time-series data to support decision-making.

Data preparation

SPSS Statistics Professional helps to streamline the data preparation stage of the analytical process — saving time and ensuring greater accuracy. Perform data checks based on each variable's measure level, quickly find multivariate outliers by searching for unusual cases based upon deviations from similar cases and preprocess data prior to model building with an optimal binning procedure.

Missing values and data validity

SPSS Statistics Professional includes critical tools for addressing data validity and missing values:

- Uncover missing data patterns by examining data from several different angles, using one of six diagnostic tests, and quickly generate a report highlighting serious missing data problems.

- Use the multiple imputation procedure to replace missing data values to better understand patterns of "missingness" in dataset and enable to replace missing values with scientific estimates.

Categorical and numerical data

Obtain clear insight into complex categorical and numeric data, as well as high-dimensional data. SPSS Statistics Professional includes procedures to visually interpret datasets and see how rows and columns relate in large tables of scores, counts, ratings, rankings or similarities. It includes a variety of advanced statistical operations on categorical data to turn qualitative variable into quantitative ones. One can also use perceptual maps and biplots to graphically display underlying relationships using dimension reduction techniques to clarify complex relationships in data for better decision making.

Decision trees

Create classification and decision trees to help better identify groups, discover relationships between groups and predict future events. Decision trees present categorical results in an intuitive manner, allowing exploring results and visually determining how model flows, and then clearly explain categorical results to non-technical audiences. One can also find specific subgroups and relationships that might not uncover using more traditional statistics.

Forecasting

Predict trends and develop forecasts quickly and easily with advanced statistical techniques to work with time-series data. Regardless of your level of experience, you can analyze historical data, predict trends faster and deliver information in ways that your organization's decision makers can understand and use.

Key features:

- Save models (e.g., XML) to a central file so that forecasts can be updated when data
- changes, without having to re-set parameters or re-estimate the model.
- Write scripts so that models can be updated with new data automatically.

In addition, Temporal Causal Modeling (TCM) enables to feed a large amount of time series data into SPSS Statistics to find out which series are causally related. For example, one may want to use this procedure to analyze stock price data, which is temporal in nature and dependent on the values of sets of variables at various points over time.

23.2.3.3 SPSS Statistics premium edition capabilities

- Linear models
- Nonlinear models
- Simulation modeling
- Geospatial analytics
- Custom tables
- Data preparation
- Missing values and data validity
- Categorical and numeric data

- Decision trees
- Forecasting
- Structural equation modeling
- Bootstrapping
- Advanced sampling assessment and testing
- Direct marketing and product decision-making procedures
- High-end charts and graphs

IBM SPSS Statistics Premium

No matter the focus of analysis, IBM SPSS Statistics Premium will significantly improve productivity and help achieve superior results for specific projects and business goals.

Be ready for any analytical project throughout your enterprise

SPSS Statistics Premium includes all the feature functionalities of the SPSS Standard and SPSS Professional editions... and much more. It adds advanced analytical techniques such as structural equation modeling (SEM), in-depth sampling assessment and testing, as well as procedures specifically geared for direct marketing. If one wants to be prepared to perform any type of analysis with the most sophisticated procedures available, SPSS Statistics Premium is the right choice.

SPSS Statistics Premium includes these features and functionality:

- **Linear models** – Make your analysis more accurate and reach more dependable conclusions to drive decision-making.
- **Nonlinear models** – Have the ability to apply more sophisticated models to data.
- **Simulation modeling** – Build better models and assess risk when inputs are uncertain using Monte Carlo simulation techniques.
- **Geospatial analytics** – Explore the relationship between data elements that can be tied to a specific location.
- **Customized tables** – Quickly slice and dice your data for easy analysis and reporting.
- **Data preparation** – Save time and improve the accuracy of your analysis.
- **Missing values and data validity** – Use a scientific approach to handling missing data.
- **Decision trees** – Better identify groups, discover relationships between groups and predict future events.
- **Forecasting** – Analyze time-series data to support decision-making.
- **Structural equation modeling** – Gain additional insight into causal models.
- **Bootstrapping** – Ensure models are stable and reliable

- **Advanced sampling assessment and testing** – Find the right sample size and determine the exact test for small samples.

- **Direct marketing and product decision-making procedures** – Quickly perform RFM analysis and better understand consumer preferences.

- **High-end charts and graphs** – Gain new ways to portray and communicate analytics to others.

Structural equation modeling

Structural equation modeling (SEM) can help to gain additional insight into causal models and explore the interaction effects and pathways between variables. SEM lets one more rigorously test whether the data supports your hypothesis. One can create more precise models than if used standard multivariate statistics or multiple regression models alone.

Bootstrapping

Bootstrapping provides an efficient way to ensure that the models are stable and reliable. It estimates the sampling distribution of an estimator by re-sampling with replacement from the original sample. With bootstrapping, one can reliably estimate the standard errors and confidence intervals of a population parameter, including the mean, median, proportion, odds ratio, correlation coefficient, regression coefficient and numerous others.

Who uses SPSS Statistics?

Businesses use it for...

- Sales and marketing forecasting and budgeting
- Database and direct marketing
- Product attribute testing

Higher education uses it for...

- Enrollment management
- Alumni development
- Research

School districts use it for...

- Student assessment
- Program assessment
- Planning and budgeting

Government agencies use it for...

- Fighting crime and protecting public safety
- Promoting public health
- Fighting fraud, waste and abuse
- Human capital management

Medical facilities use it for...

- Evidence-based medicine
- Treatment outcome analysis
- Behavioral and biomedical research

Advanced sampling assessment and testing

Find the right sample size for research in minutes and test the possible results before one begin the study. Compare the effects of different study parameters and determine the exact test needed to more accurately work with small samples and analyze rare occurrences in large databases.

Direct marketing and product decision-making procedures

Quickly perform various kinds of analyses, including recency, frequency and monetary value (RFM) analysis, cluster analysis and prospect profiling. Increases understanding of consumer preferences to more effectively design, price and market successful products — maximizing campaign effectiveness and return on investment.

High-end charts and graphs

Develop and create new visualizations — from basic, simple charts to advanced, highly compelling graphics— that enable new ways to portray and communicate analytics to others. View analytical output on multiple smart devices simultaneously for better decision-making anytime, anywhere.

Capabilities for "deep dive" analyses — no matter your focus

SPSS Statistics Premium helps data analysts, planners, forecasters, survey researchers, program evaluators and database markets — among others — to easily accomplish tasks at every phase of the analytical process. No matter what type of analysis one do, one has a broad array of fully integrated Statistics capabilities for specialized analytical tasks across the enterprise.

Data analysts have the statistical and analytical capabilities to maximize productivity at every point of the analytic process.

- Quickly detect anomalies and identify unusual cases that tend to skew overall results.
- Address dirty data, and complete datasets by replacing missing values with imputed estimates.
- Perform Monte Carlo simulation to assess risk and uncertainty in data.
- Test and ensure analytical procedures by quickly estimating the sampling distribution of an estimator.
- Discover if random effects introduce correlations.
- Summarize and clearly communicate the findings.

Planners and forecasters can plan and implement more successful strategies — analyzing time series data efficiently and accurately.

- Support data-driven decision-making with sophisticated analytics.

- Easily identify the right sample size.
- Make better predictions using powerful regression procedures.
- Build expert time-series forecasts in a flash.

Survey researchers have the tools to learn more about survey data, faster and more accurately.

- Go further than simple row-and-column math and summaries.
- Find patterns and associations.
- Present results as "decision trees" or crosstab tables.
- Create custom tabular reports for a variety of audiences — including those without a statistical background.

In **program evaluation**, needs assessment, process analysis, impact analysis and cost/benefit analysis involve the analysis of diverse and quantitative datasets that can obscure the effectiveness of programs? SPSS Statistics Premium gives researchers and analytic professionals the tools for the many phases of program evaluation.

- Easily access, manipulate and analyze a multitude of data types, including numerical and categorical.
- Capture a more accurate understanding of data when working with large-scale surveys.
- Employ specialized statistical techniques to account for the errors associated with sampling and sample design.
- Accurately model linear and non-linear relationships with or without categorical data.
- Discover if random effects introduce correlations within program data.
- Quickly summarize research and report findings with frequencies, crosstabs, and other descriptive statistics.

Database marketers have many responsibilities. Maximizing marketing programs and campaigns for efficiency and impact, understanding prospects and customers and removing unique cases to produce statistically significant response rates — the list is extensive. SPSS Statistics Premium lightens the load for the database marketer, as well as that of the supporting analysts.

- Streamline the process of validating sales and marketing data before analyzing it.
- Classify prospects and customers based on identifying characteristics, including RFM analysis.
- Test the results of existing campaigns against new campaigns and analyze control package tests.
- Detect anomalies and identify unusual cases and responses that can skew overall results.
- Create responder profiles and generate propensity to purchase scores.
- Model relationships that likely contains categorical data.

- Summarize findings with frequencies, crosstabs and other descriptive statistics.

23.2.4 About IBM Business Analytics

IBM Business Analytics software delivers data-driven insights that help organizations work smarter and outperform their peers. This comprehensive portfolio includes solutions for business intelligence, predictive analytics and decision management, performance management, and risk management.

Business Analytics solutions enable companies to identify and visualize trends and patterns in areas, such as customer analytics, that can have a profound effect on business performance. They can compare scenarios, anticipate potential threats and opportunities, better plan, budget and forecast resources, balance risks against expected returns and work to meet regulatory requirements. By making analytics widely available, organizations can align tactical and strategic decision-making to achieve business goals.

23.3 Epi Info

23.3.1 Introduction to CDC (Centers for Disease Control and Prevention)

The CDC Organisation is one of the major operating components of the Department of Health and Human Services. CDC works 24/7 to protect America from health, safety and security threats, both foreign and in the U.S. Whether diseases start at home or abroad, are chronic or acute, curable or preventable, human error or deliberate attack, CDC fights disease and supports communities and citizens to do the same.

CDC increases the health security of the nation. As the nation's health protection agency, CDC saves lives and protects people from health threats. To accomplish the mission, CDC conducts critical science and provides health information that protects the nation against expensive and dangerous health threats, and responds when these arise.

23.3.2 Role of CDC

The roles of CDC are,

- Detecting and responding to new and emerging health threats
- Tackling the biggest health problems causing death and disability for Americans
- Putting science and advanced technology into action to prevent disease
- Promoting healthy and safe behaviors, communities and environment
- Developing leaders and training the public health workforce, including disease detectives
- Taking the health pulse of the nation

CDC protects the nation and the world by:

- Detecting, responding to, and stopping new and emerging health threats.

- Preventing injuries, illnesses, and premature deaths.
- Discovering new ways to protect and improve the public's health through science and advanced technology.

23.3.3 Strategies of CDC

Strategic Priority #1: Improve health security at home and around the world.

CDC's expertise in preparedness, rapid detection, and response saves lives and safeguards communities from health threats. CDC is employing faster, more advanced ways to find, stop, and prevent infectious disease outbreaks here and abroad. The spread of infectious diseases in the U.S. not only causes suffering and death, it also has a substantial impact on healthcare costs and the economy. Food borne illnesses alone account for roughly 48 million illnesses and more than $15.5 billion in costs per year. About 2 million people become infected with antibiotic-resistant bacteria each year, and roughly 23,000 die of these infections. Each year, 75,000 Americans with healthcare-associated infections die while hospitalized. Building a skilled workforce, using proven intervention strategies, and strengthening laboratory networks across the U.S. and throughout the world provide the strong systems needed to protect the public's health.

Increase access to high-quality laboratory testing, including the use of advanced molecular detection (AMD) technologies.

- By employing new, cutting-edge AMD technologies in CDC and partner laboratories across the country and around the world, CDC now have the ability to more quickly detect, identify, and respond to emerging and antibiotic-resistant infectious disease outbreaks.

- As technologies advance, CDC continues to help state and local laboratories—which are at the frontlines in preparing for and responding to health threats—to implement modern, high-quality testing for infectious diseases.

- CDC's Environmental Health Laboratory provides service, standardization, and quality assurance to laboratories testing for newborn disorders, life-threatening diseases, nutrition status, and environmental exposures.

- CDC's laboratories serve as global reference centers solving new disease mysteries and preparing for annual influenza vaccines. CDC has 23 programs designated as WHO global collaborating centers, providing expertise and capabilities to protect Americans at home from threats abroad.

Enhance Global Health Security by building and sustaining capacity to detect and respond to disease threats such as polio, influenza, Ebola, the Middle East Respiratory Syndrome (MERS) virus, and insect-borne threats such as the Zika virus.

CDC is accelerating progress toward a world safe and secure from infectious disease threats and promoting global health security by increasing countries' capacity to:

- **Prevent** and reduce the likelihood of outbreaks—natural, accidental, or intentional.

- **Detect** threats early to save lives.
- **Respond** rapidly and effectively using multi-sector, international coordination and communication.

Enhance state and local abilities to prevent, detect, and respond to health threats.

- CDC supports state and local preparedness systems to increase molecular diagnostic testing capacity.
- CDC's select agent registry keeps Americans safer by tracking possession and use of pathogenic and toxic agents to prevent accidental or intentional misuse.
- By developing new tools such as the medical countermeasure operational readiness review, CDC make sure states can rapidly dispense medicines to reduce disease and death during a crisis.
- CDC National Syndromic Surveillance Program (NSSP)—a partnership among local, state, and national public health programs—enables partners to detect and characterize disease outbreaks, other hazardous events, or conditions of public health concern to strengthen regional and national situational awareness.
- CDC supports state and local rapid, population-based surveillance of microcephaly and other adverse outcomes possibly linked to Zika virus infection.

Some recent strategic priority accomplishments:

- The 2014–2016 Ebola epidemic in West Africa demonstrated the importance of readiness and remaining prepared for Ebola and other health threats to the United States. More than 4,000 CDC staff protected people in the U.S. and helped stop the spread of Ebola in Guinea, Sierra Leone, and Liberia through surveillance, contact tracing, laboratory testing, community engagement, infection prevention and control, and vaccine evaluation. CDC's field laboratory in Bo, Sierra Leone, operated for 421 days in a row, testing more than 27,000 specimens. At the height of the response, more than 200 CDC staff worked in the field in West Africa and 400 staff worked on Ebola at CDC's Atlanta headquarters. CDC investments in health infrastructure also prevented widespread transmission in other West African countries. For example, the substantial investment for polio eradication programs in Nigeria ensured that responders there were prepared for Ebola, enabling Lagos to rapidly stop its outbreak. If Ebola had not been stopped in Lagos, it likely would have spread for months or years to other parts of Nigeria and Africa, killing hundreds of thousands of people and setting back a decade of progress in saving lives.
- CDC also played a critical role protecting the United States from Ebola by aiding state and local health departments in their preparedness activities. Together with international, federal, and state partners, CDC established airport risk assessments for travelers leaving affected countries and entering the U.S., monitored travelers and other potentially exposed persons for 21 days, and helped hospitals across the country prepare to manage possible

cases of Ebola or other hemorrhagic disease through intensive training and preparedness activities.

- CDC continues to work to improve laboratory safety. In the past 10 years, CDC performed 2,072 laboratory inspections and restricted 338 people from accessing select agents and toxins.

- Lifesaving medical countermeasures from CDC's Strategic National Stockpile can be delivered in 12 hours or less to anywhere in the U.S. For example, CDC provided 50 vials of botulinum antitoxin to the Ohio Department of Health within 10 hours for an outbreak in April 2015.

- Since adoption of advanced molecular detection technologies, including whole genome sequencing (WGS), CDC is able to solve outbreaks more quickly and prevent illness and death that would have otherwise occurred.

- For example, more than 95% of tuberculosis isolates in the nation were tested for drug resistance, and molecular testing identified multiple outbreaks.

- During the past 10 years, CDC has deployed 294 pathogen- specific tests in 59 countries, helping to find and stop spread of disease at the source. In addition, CDC and in-country collaborators discovered 61 pathogens that were new to the region in which they were discovered and 12 new pathogens identified for the first time anywhere in the world.

- CDC supports more than 50 partner countries as well global partners to rapidly identify and share novel influenza strains. Sharing strains improves vaccine virus selection and enhances pandemic preparedness and provides the basis for response capacity for other infectious diseases such as MERS and Ebola.

- Since CDC and partners began to work towards eradication, polio cases have decreased from more than 350,000 per year in 1988 to 74 in 2015 and 19 through the first half of 2016. Following CDC surges in India and then Nigeria, India was declared polio-free in March 2014, and Africa completed a year with no wild poliovirus cases when Nigeria was verified to be polio-free in 2015, leaving only Afghanistan and Pakistan with continuing transmission.

- Provided more than 107 million rapid diagnostic tests and 243 million treatments for malaria since 2006 as part of the President's Malaria Initiative.

- In 2016, CDC rapidly identified the link between Zika virus and microcephaly in newborns and implemented prevention strategies appropriate to different parts of the United States.

Strategic Priority #2: Better prevent the leading causes of illness, injury, disability, and death.

The stakes are high—the top 10 leading causes of death account for nearly 75% of all deaths in the U.S., with cardiovascular disease, stroke, and cancer accounting for more than half of all deaths and more than $472 billion in healthcare costs.

Provide timely, quality data on priority health and health- care issues at the national, state, and local levels to better monitor and improve the health of Americans.

- CDC's gold-standard health surveys and public-use data sets provide accurate, timely, and comprehensive information on health and healthcare issues.

- CDC continue to lead the nation in conducting high- quality research related to the public's health, including population health surveillance and epidemiology at national and state levels and building the science basis for decision-making on public health programs, policies, and services.

- CDC is building and improving information systems, which will enable enhanced data exchange to improve internal and external information sharing.

- CDC is a trusted source of information for consumers and healthcare professionals through a variety of communication platforms including scientific publications, emergency health alerts for practicing clinicians, a comprehensive internet presence, and news and social media outreach.

Work with communities to prevent injury, disease, and disability.

- Vaccination programs, including the Vaccines for Children Program (VFC) provide half of all childhood vaccines in the U.S., in addition to epidemiology and laboratory capacity to detect and respond to vaccine preventable diseases. Childhood immunization saves \$3 in direct costs and \$10 in direct and indirect costs for every \$1 spent.

- CDC prevent heart attacks, strokes, cancer, diabetes, and other diseases that are the leading causes of illness and premature death by helping reduce tobacco use, improve physical activity and nutrition, and reduce obesity. For example, CDC's scientific research shows increasing access to tobacco-free environments, improving access to fluoridated water, and providing children with healthier food options in schools result in better health. CDC also works to ensure that tools for healthy living are accessible for people with disabilities.

- CDC's proven approaches to injury and violence prevention help reduce deaths due to motor vehicle crashes, still a leading cause of death and injuries in the U.S., with effective interventions to increase use of restraints and reduce speeding and alcohol-impaired driving. CDC focus on vulnerable populations, including American Indians and Alaska natives and older Americans. CDC also apply scientific expertise to help reduce deaths from the opioid overdose epidemic by supporting states to implement effective strategies, and equipping healthcare providers with the tools they need to improve safe opioid prescribing.

- CDC work to help children thrive by preventing child abuse and neglect, improving asthma management, increasing early identification of developmental disabilities such as autism spectrum disorder, improving treatment of children with Attention Deficit and Hyperactivity Disorder (ADHD), and preventing harms that include birth defects from maternal exposures such as medication use during pregnancy.

- CDC prevent work-related injuries, illnesses, and fatalities due to hazardous exposures and falls.

Support doctors, nurse practitioners, nurses, pharmacists, and other health professionals by increasing workforce capacity at the state and local levels.

CDC help build and train the public health workforce through financial and technical support to states and localities. Fellow-ship programs such as the Public Health Associate Program (PHAP), the Laboratory Leadership Service(LLS), and the Epidemic Intelligence Service (EIS) assign more than 500 CDC- trained public health workers and disease detectives to state, local, tribal, and territorial health departments.

Some recent strategic priority accomplishments:

- Most vaccine-preventable disease case counts are at their lowest levels ever, with greater than 90% coverage for many vaccines. Vaccination of children born in the U.S. between 1994 and 2013 prevented 322 million illnesses, avoided 732,000 deaths, and will save nearly $1.4 trillion in societal costs. Influenza vaccination alone prevented 1.9 million illnesses and 67,000 hospitalizations during the 2014–2015 flu seasons.

- Although more than 35 million Americans still smoke cigarettes, adult cigarette-smoking rates decreased to a new low of 15.1% in 2015, representing an estimated 10 million fewer smokers than in 2009.

- The Tips from Former Smokers (TIPS) campaign has helped at least 400,000 smokers quit for good since 2012. TIPS costs just $393 to save a year of life and less than $3,000 per life saved; it is a public health best buy.

- There was a 9% decrease in HIV diagnoses between 2010 and 2014.

- Providers using CDC's new HIV testing algorithm can detect acute infection just 4 days after RNA positivity.

- CDC released its STEADI (Stopping Elderly Accidents, Deaths, and Injuries) Initiative, which gives healthcare providers evidence-based tools and guidance needed to address and prevent falls among their patients.

- CDC data and research paved the way for a 2016 U.S. Food and Drug Administration (FDA) decision to permit fortification of corn masa flour with folic acid, which could reduce neural tube defects—severe birth defects of the brain and spine—particularly among the nation's Hispanic population.

- CDC's National Institute for Occupational Safety and Health (NIOSH) conducted a health-hazard evaluation study that found a high rate of carpal tunnel syndrome among workers at a poultry-processing plant that employed workers from an underserved population. These findings led to safer working conditions and updated industry guidelines.

- Encouraging widespread adoption of directly observed therapy for tuberculosis and increased support to local health departments have helped prevent tens of thousands of tuberculosis cases in the United States since 1993.

- EIS officers conduct more than 200 investigations per year, ranging from assessing the effectiveness of a vaccination campaign to preventing meningococcal disease in university students to determining risk factors for healthcare-associated infections.

- More than 350 Public Health Associate Program (PHAP) associates are assigned to public health agencies in 44 states, one territory, and the District of Columbia in addition to 34 Career Epidemiology Field Officers (CEFOs) in 27 state, territorial, or local public health programs.

Strategic Priority #3: Strengthen public health and healthcare collaboration.

CDC has a unique opportunity to increase the value of nation's health investments by better aligning public health and healthcare.

Leverage partnerships with clinicians and healthcare organizations to decrease healthcare-associated and antibiotic-resistant infections and prevent prescription drug overdoses.

- CDC has invested in practical and proven efforts to counter the threat of untreatable antibiotic-resistant infections.

- In 2014, the Chicago Prevention Epicenter completed a multicenter evaluation of a new prevention package in four long-term acute care hospitals, demonstrating a 56% reduction in deadly antibiotic-resistant carbapenem resistant Enterobacteriaceae (CRE) infections.

- Our 6/18 Initiative increases use of proven prevention practices. CDC provides partners with rigorous evidence and practical information on implementation to address high-burden health conditions and associated interventions to inform their decisions so they have the greatest health and cost impact. Multiple state Medicaid programs, commercial payers, and large employers are adapting their covered benefits to provide access to specific 6/18 interventions.

- The CDC Guideline for Prescribing Opioids for Chronic Pain provides recommendations for the prescribing of opioid pain medication for patients 18 or older in primary care settings outside of active cancer treatment, palliative care, and end-of-life care. Improving the way opioids are prescribed through clinical practice guidelines can ensure patients have access to safer, more effective chronic pain treatment while reducing the number of people who overdose or die of these drugs, as well as reducing rates of neonatal opioid withdrawal syndrome.

Increase ability of public health and healthcare systems to reduce disease threats and improve health by increasing prevention through the use of community, clinical, and laboratory services.

- CDC cancer programs increase access to recommended preventive screening to reduce mortality.

- Partnerships among community and clinical care providers help improve blood pressure and cholesterol control and help people stop smoking.

- CDC community and school-based programs reduce the risk that teens develop HIV, STDs, and unintended pregnancy.

Use emerging data sources, existing surveys, and innovative information delivery to inform clinical care systems to improve population health.

- CDC links national surveys with Medicaid enrollment and claims records collected from the Centers for Medicare and Medicaid Services (CMS) to better understand and improve changes in health status and healthcare use, including among low-income families with children, the elderly, and people with disabilities.

- Through the National Health Interview Survey (NHIS), CDC increased the number of states with accurate estimates of health insurance coverage, from 32 states in 2011 to all 50 states and Washington, D.C., in 2014.

- CDC has expanded the number of states and territories in the National Violent Death Reporting System (NVDRS) and has used this data to identify circumstances and prevention strategies for suicide.

- In FY 2015, CDC Vital Signs electronic media had a total potential reach of 6.6 million people.

- Annual mortality data are being reported more quickly than ever. CDC released final 2014 mortality data in early December 2015 and preliminary 2015 data in June 2016. In 2015, CDC received 38% of death records within 10 days of the event, a proportion which more than doubled since 2013.

- Specialized websites, such as the Community Health Improvement Navigator and Sortable Stats assist states, local communities, tribes, and territories with data, useful information and tools.

Some recent strategic priority accomplishments:

- The combination of CDC data systems, guidelines, and programs has contributed to significant reductions of healthcare-associated infections, including a 50% reduction in central line-associated bloodstream infections between 2008 and 2014.

- As of 2015, the Million Hearts® Hypertension Control Challenge recognized nearly 60 public and private healthcare practices and systems that reach more than 12 million adult patients in 29 states for achieving blood pressure control for at least 70% of their patients with hypertension.

- By September 30, 2015, the World Trade Center (WTC) Health Program had enrolled 73,199 eligible responders and survivors. In FY 2015, the WTC Health Program paid claims for eligible treatment, including medication, for more than 22,100 of these responders and survivors.

- Provided timely guidance to healthcare providers and the public in the U.S. and globally to prevent Zika virus infection and its effects, including immediately communicating with the American and global public about the importance of travel avoidance for pregnant women to avoid Zika virus infection following determination of its effects on pregnancy.

Introduction to Epi Info Software

Epi Info™ is a public domain suite of interoperable software tools designed for the global community of public health practitioners and researchers. It provides for easy data entry form and database construction, a customized data entry experience, and data analyses with epidemiologic statistics, maps, and graphs for public health professionals who may lack an information technology background. Epi Info™ is used for outbreak investigations; for developing small to mid-sized disease surveillance systems; as analysis, visualization, and reporting (AVR) components of larger systems; and in the continuing education in the science of epidemiology and public health analytic methods at schools of public health around the world.

23.4 Minitab

In order to teach students, in the year 1972, three Penn State Professors for the first time created 'Minitab' statistical software. Initiated with an objective of learning of the statistical concepts, the software gathered its importance at the schools for data analysis and interpretations. Currently, the software is widely used for business and research for statistical analysis. The software is provided by "Minitab Inc" along with its subsidiary as Minitab Ltd., Minitab Sarl and Minitab Pvt. Ltd.

The organization provides statistical training, services, consulting along with custom developments for a specific purpose use.

The key products of "Minitab Inc" are Minitab 18, Quality Trainer and Companion. 'Minitab 18' is a software for analyzing data, 'Quality Trainer' is a software for learning the concepts and finally 'Companion' is a software that provides tools for creating and executing quality improvement projects in one application.

Yet other products are 'Minitab Express' a software for academic purpose with an objective of introducing various concepts, 'Qeystone' a software for managing and monitoring process improvement initiatives.

As a whole the software helps in developing hypothesis, analyzing, describing, plotting, sampling, interpreting the distribution of the data and finally providing with the confidence intervals.

24 Applications of SPSS, Epi Info and Minitab Softwares (Screen Shots)

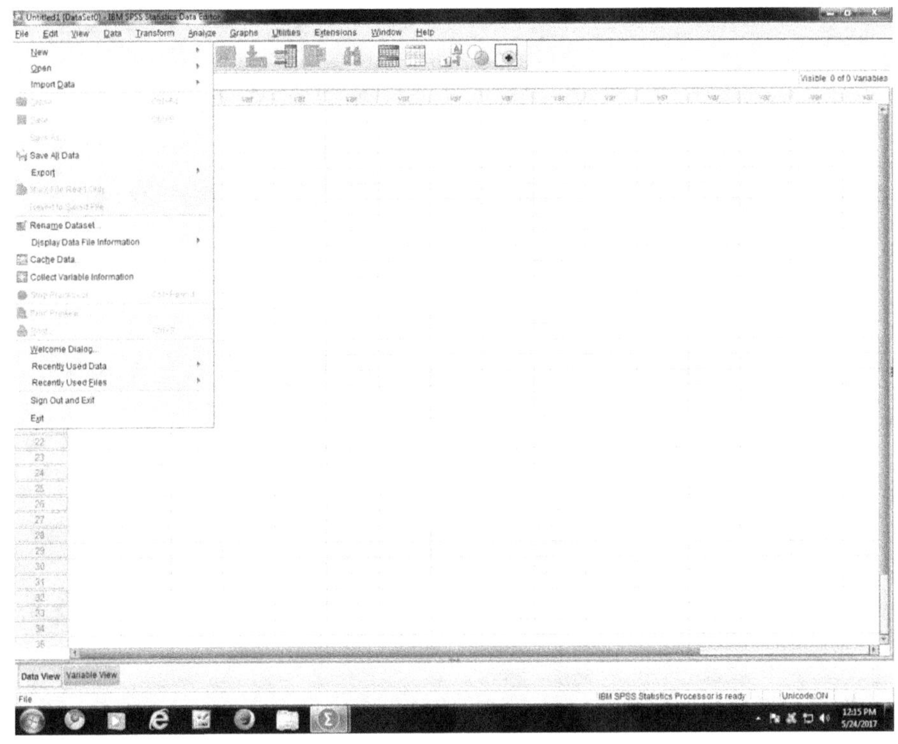

FIGURE 24.1 SPSS Software Screen Shot 1

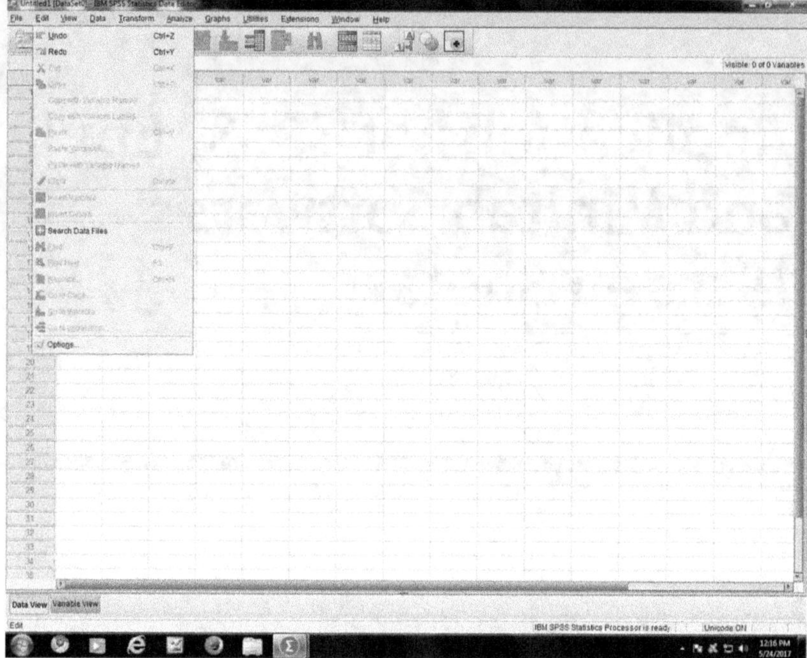

FIGURE 24.2 SPSS Software Screen Shot 2

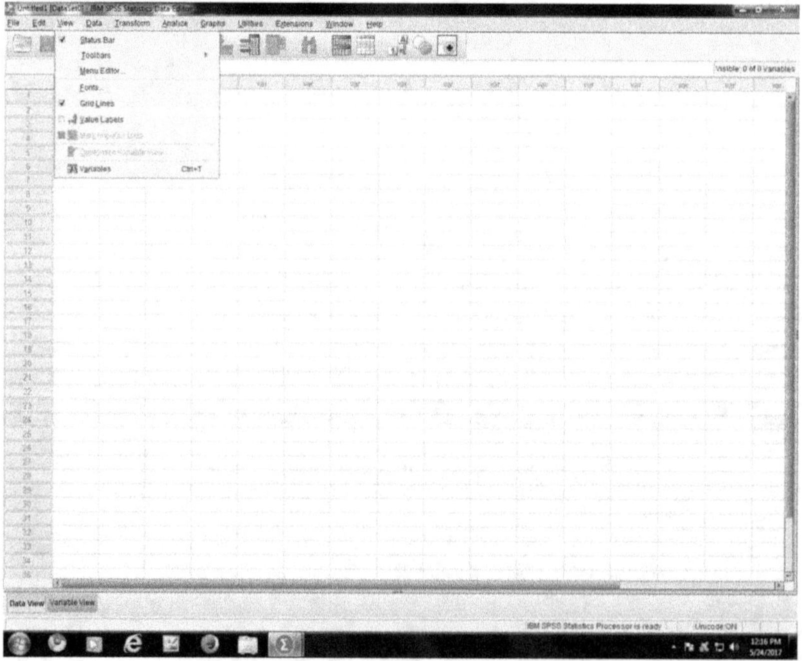

FIGURE 24.3 SPSS Software Screen Shot 3

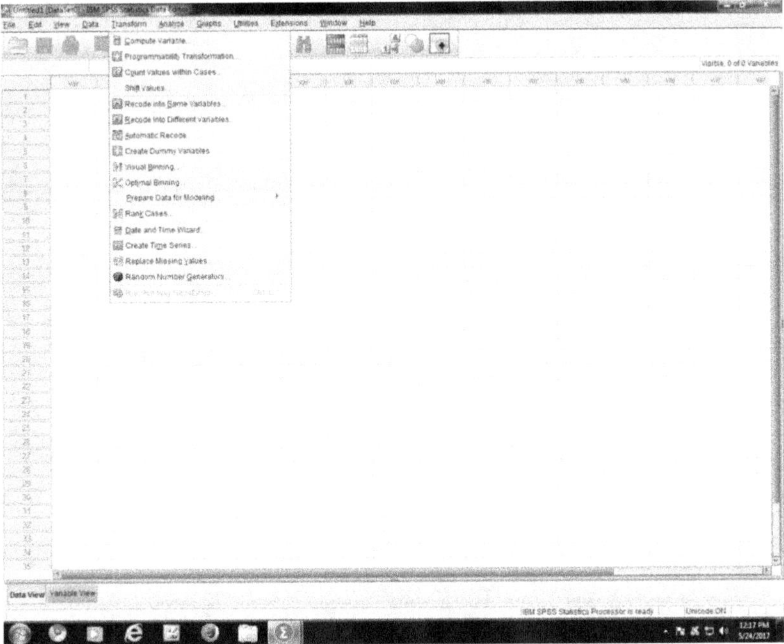

FIGURE 24.4 SPSS Software Screen Shot 4

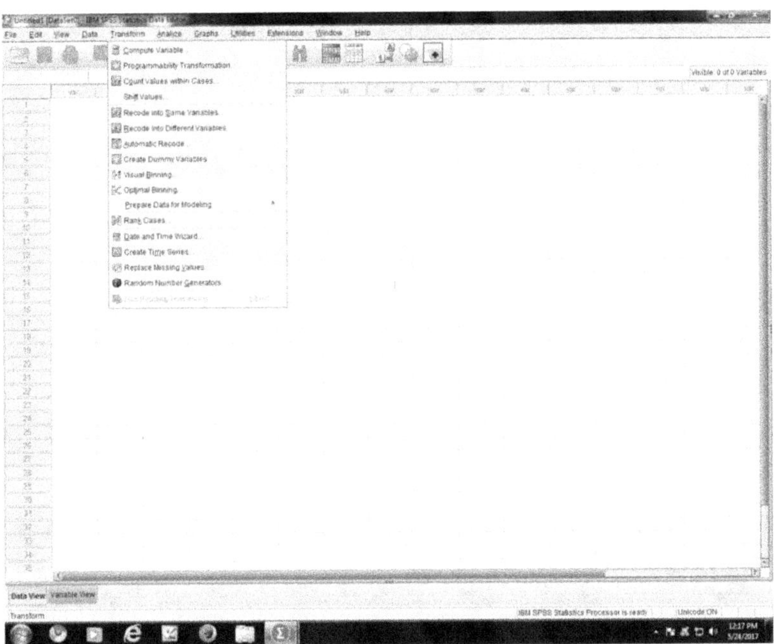

FIGURE 24.5 SPSS Software Screen Shot 5

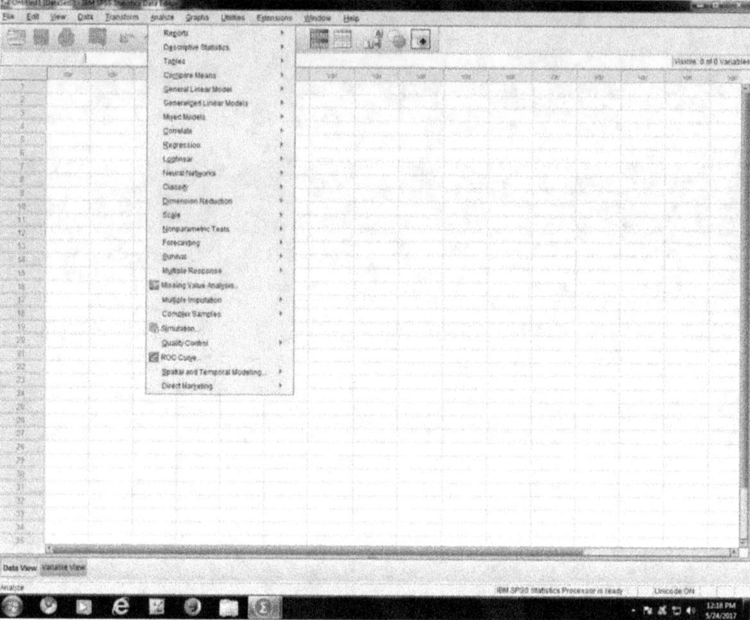

FIGURE 24.6 SPSS Software Screen Shot 6

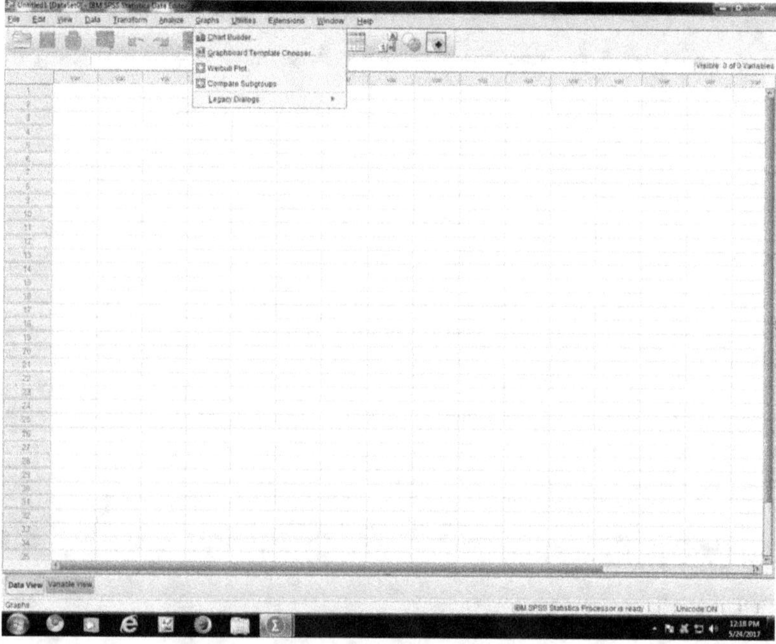

FIGURE 24.7 SPSS Software Screen Shot 7

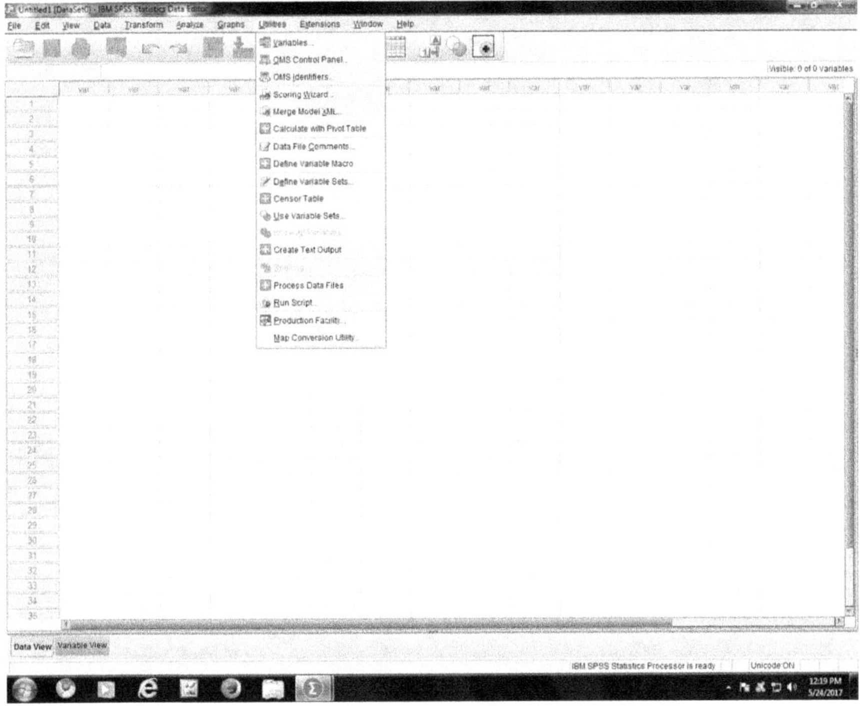

FIGURE 24.8 SPSS Software Screen Shot 8

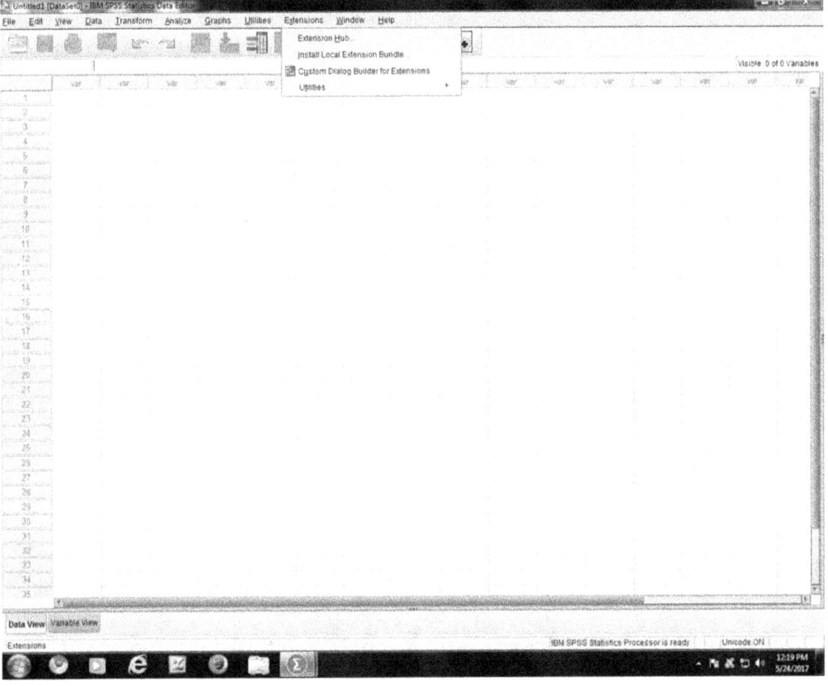

FIGURE 24.9 SPSS Software Screen Shot 9

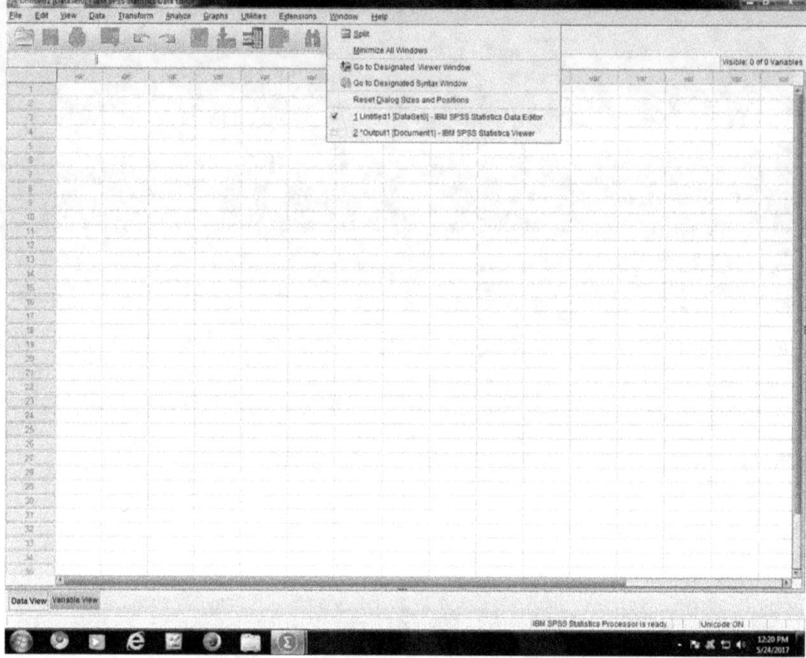

FIGURE 24.10 SPSS Software Screen Shot 10

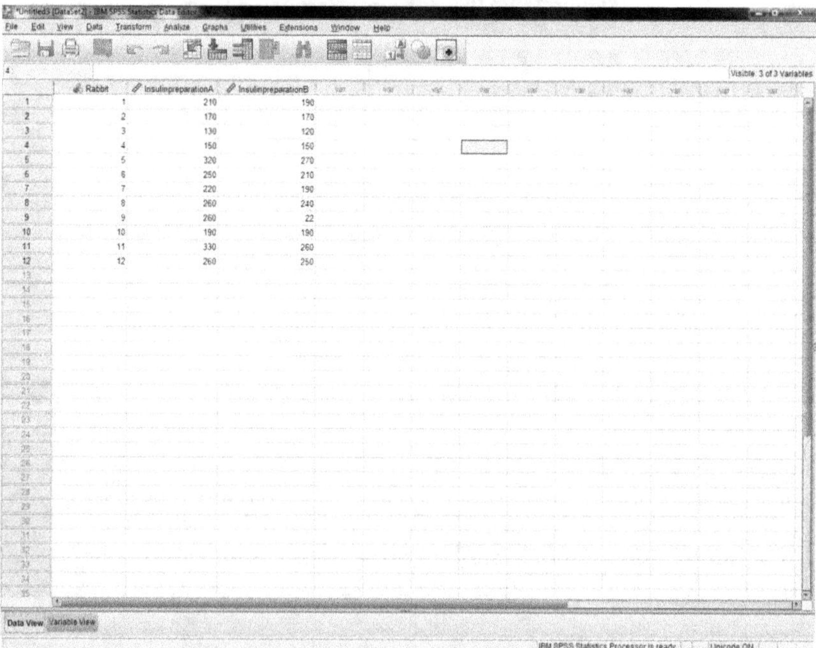

FIGURE 24.11 SPSS Software Application Paired 't' test Screen Shot 1

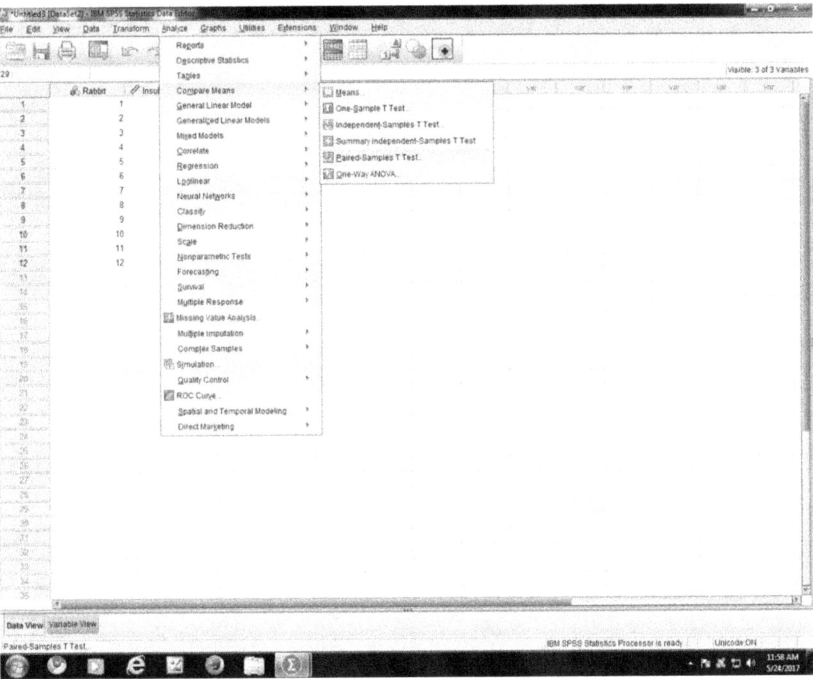

Figure 24.12 SPSS Software Application Paired 't' test Screen Shot 2

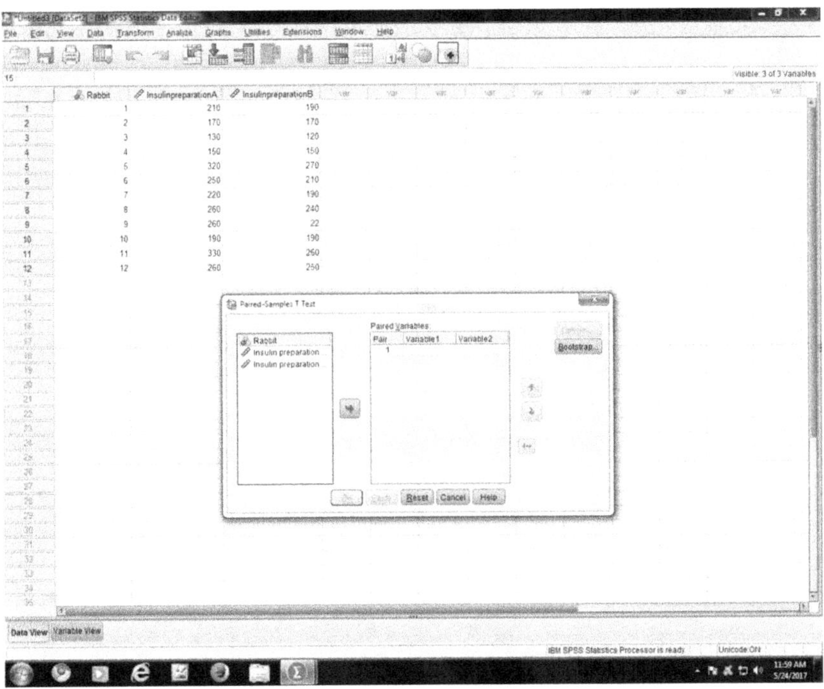

Figure 24.13 SPSS Software Application Paired 't' test Screen Shot 3

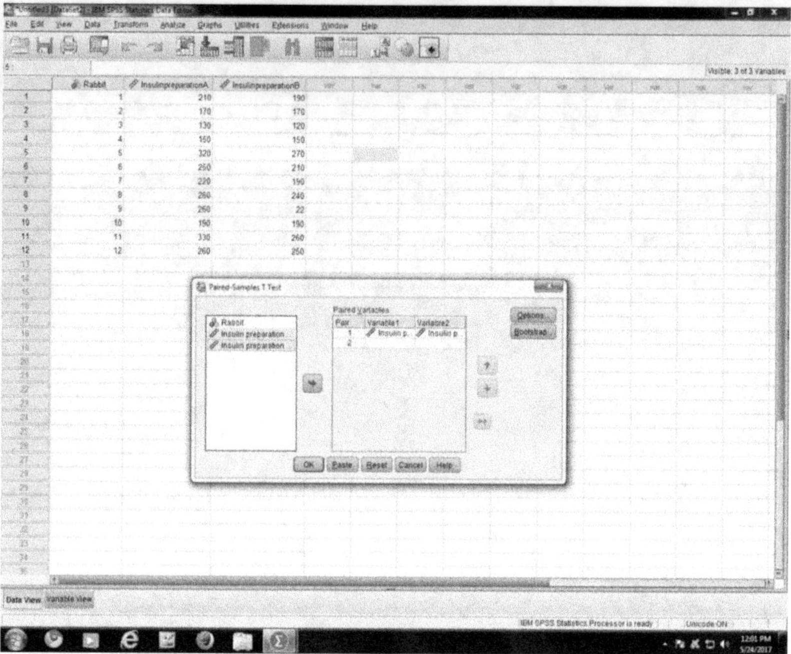

FIGURE 24.14 SPSS Software Application Paired 't' test Screen Shot 4

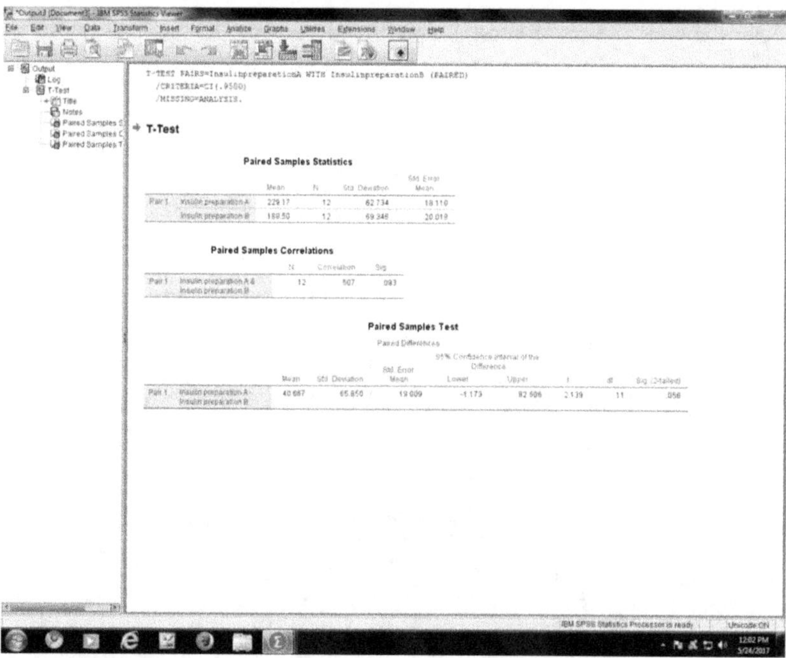

FIGURE 24.15 SPSS Software Application Paired 't' test Screen Shot 5 (Out put result)

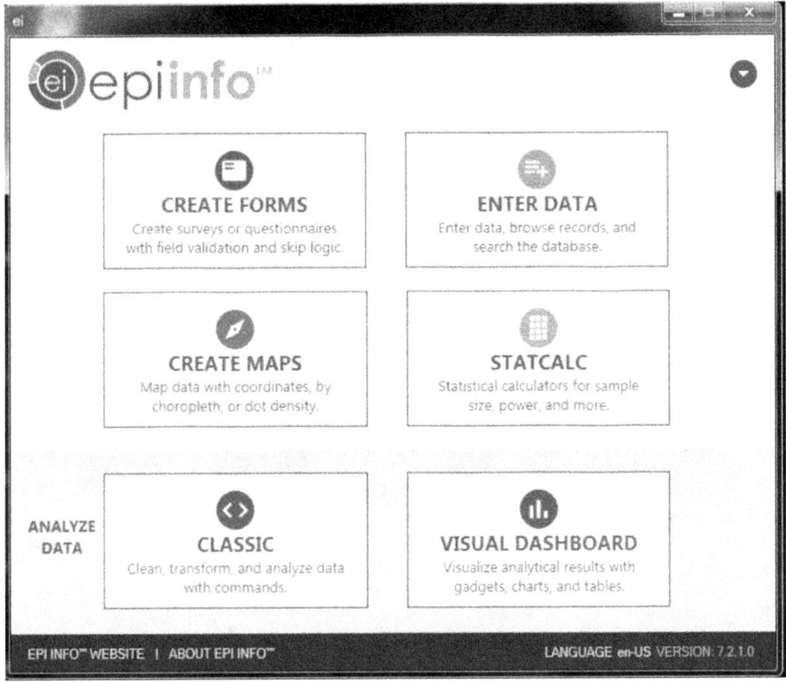

FIGURE 24.16 Epi Info Software Screen Shot 1

FIGURE 24.17 Epi Info Software Screen Shot 2 (Create Forms)

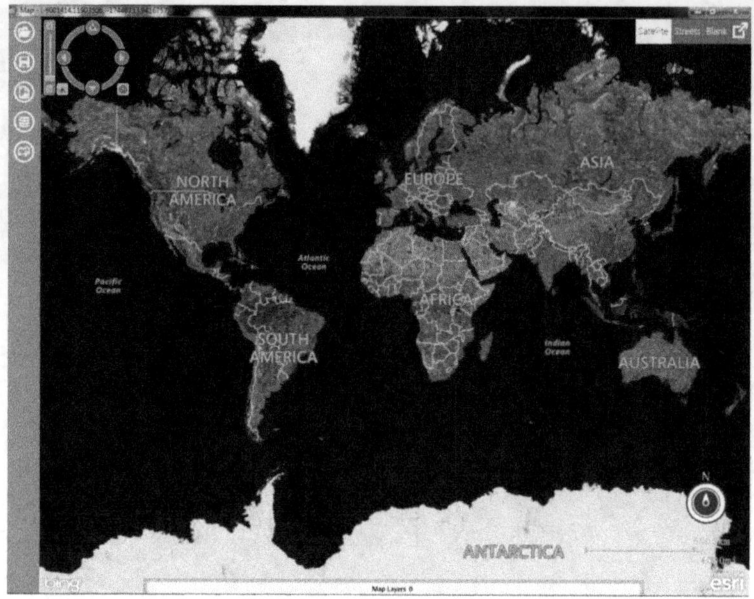

FIGURE 24.18 Epi Info Software Screen Shot 3 (Create Maps)

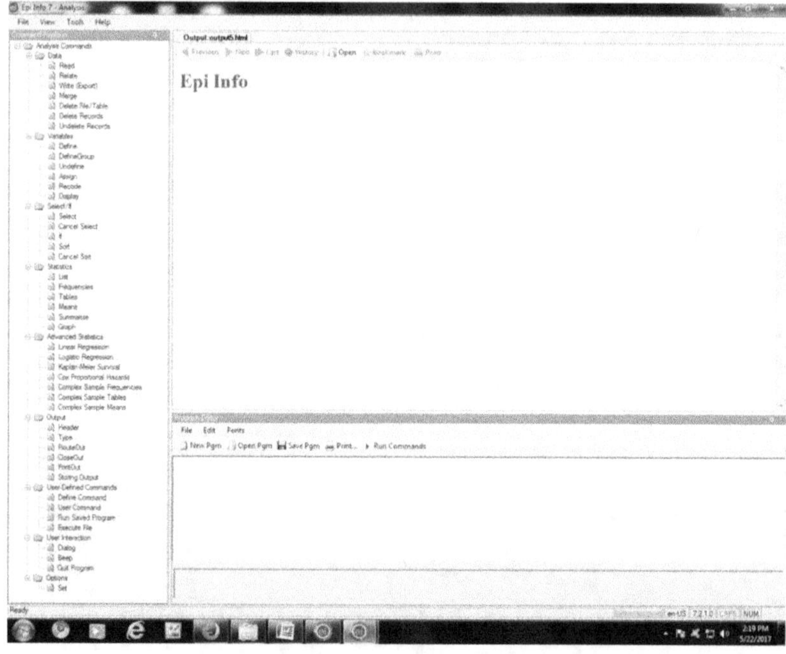

FIGURE 24.19 Epi Info Software Screen Shot 4 (Classic)

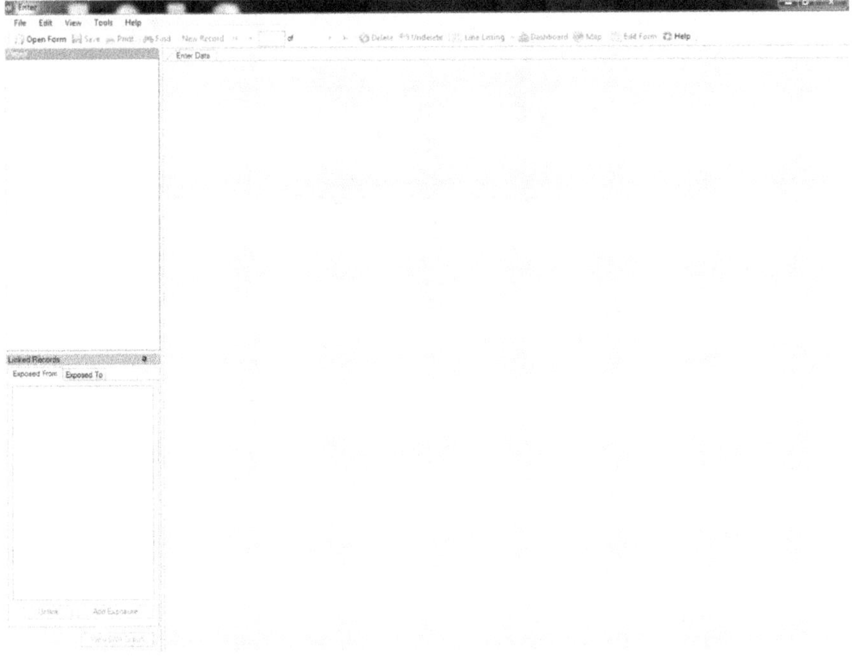

FIGURE 24.20 Epi Info Software Screen Shot 5 (Enter Data)

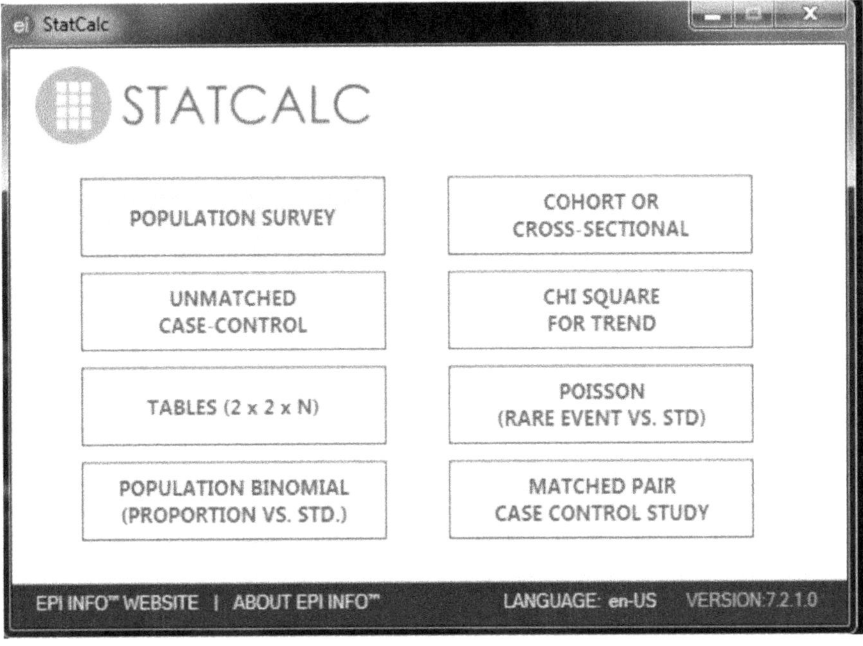

FIGURE 24.21 Epi Info Software Screen Shot 6 (Stat Calc)

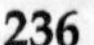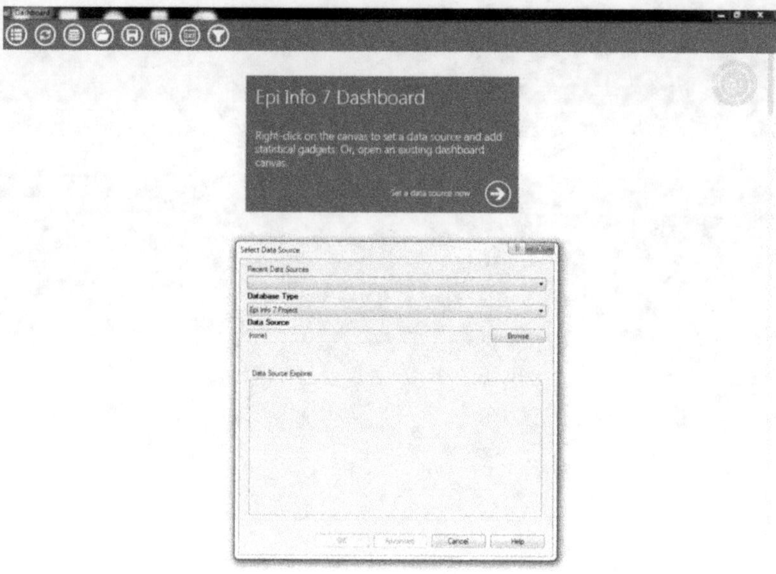

FIGURE 24.22 Epi Info Software Screen Shot 7 (Visual Dashboard)

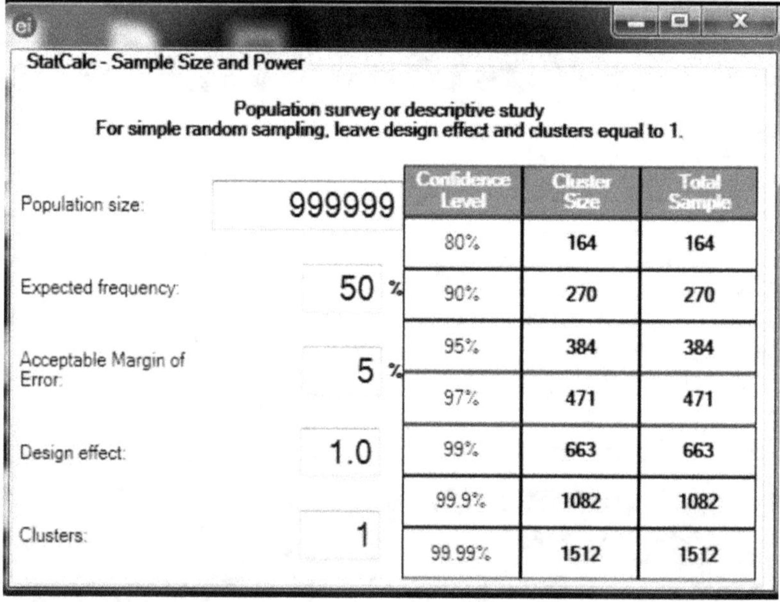

FIGURE 24.23 Epi Info Software Screen Shot 8-Stat Calc-Population Survey

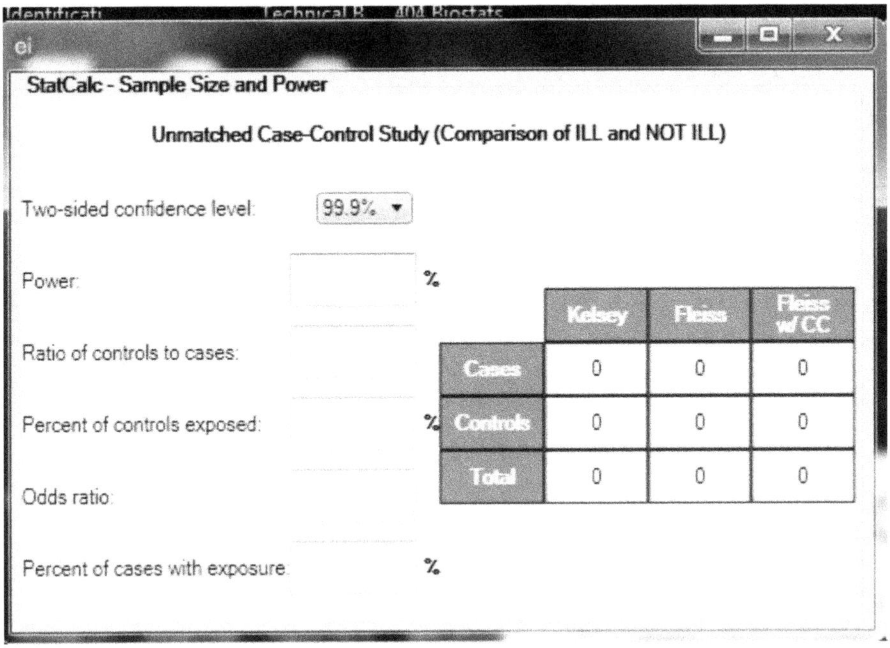

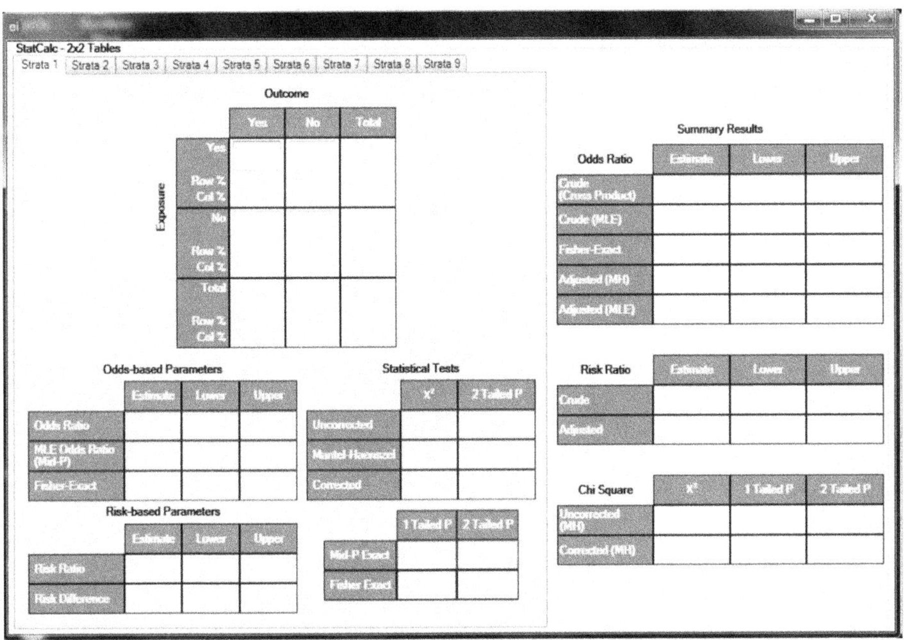

FIGURE 24.24 Epi Info Software Screen Shot 9-Stat Calc- Unmatched Case-Control Study

FIGURE 24.25 Epi Info Software Screen Shot 10 – Stat Calc – 2 x 2x N Table

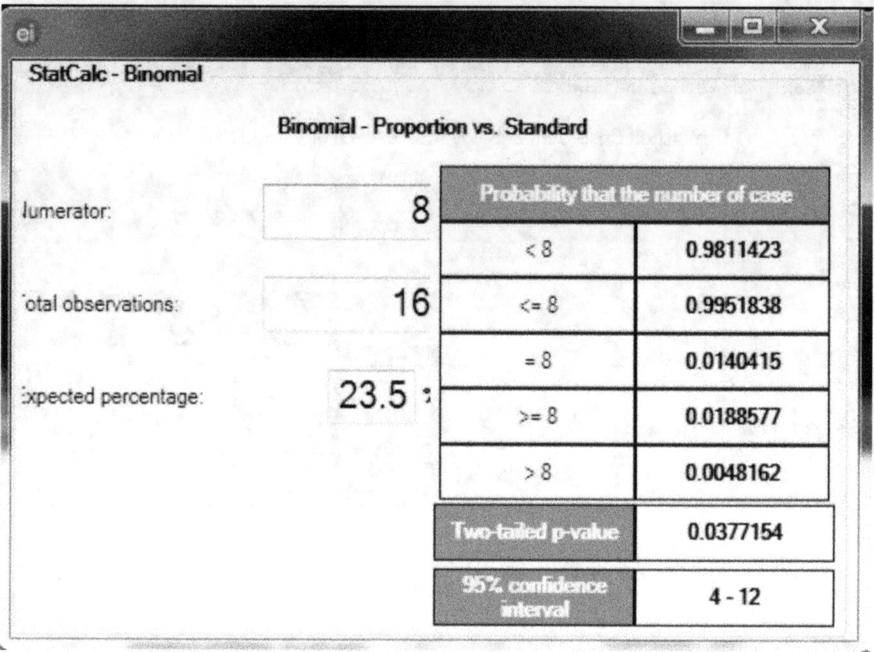

FIGURE 24.26 Epi Info Software Screen Shot 11 – Stat Calc – Population Binomial (Proportion vs. Standard)

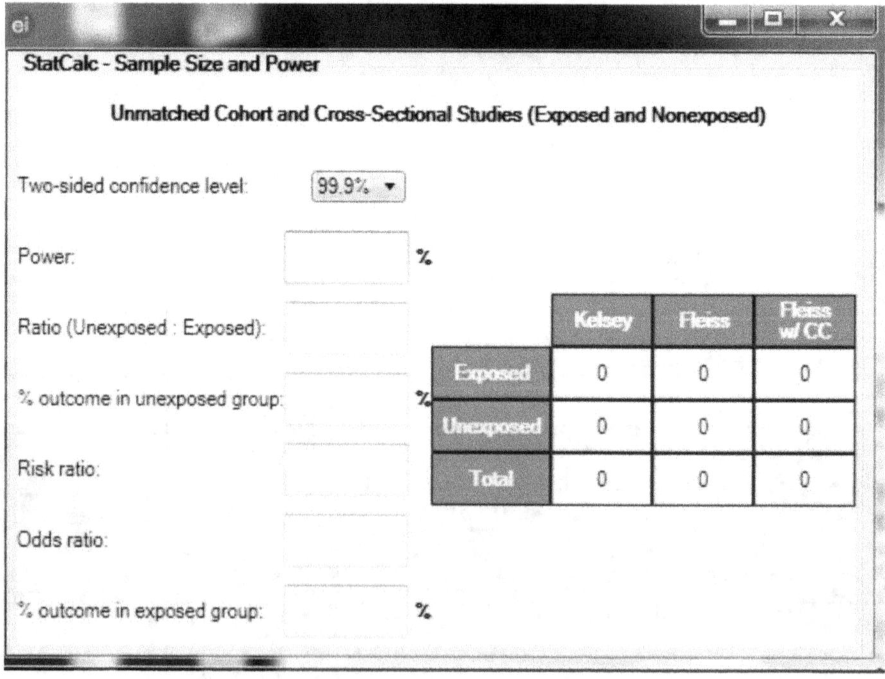

FIGURE 24.27 Epi Info Software Screen Shot 12 – Stat Calc – (Cohort or Cross-Sectional)

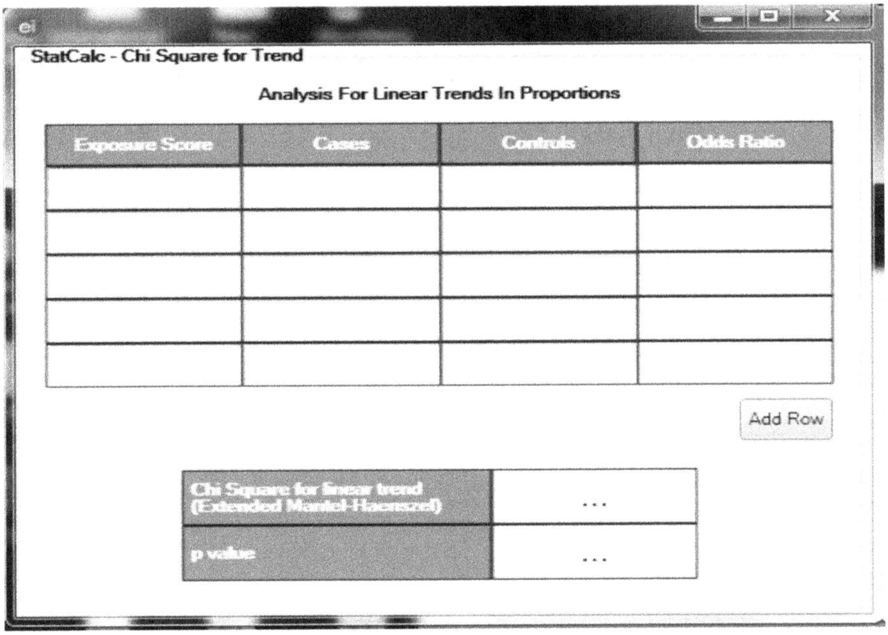

StatCalc - Chi Square for Trend

Analysis For Linear Trends In Proportions

Exposure Score	Cases	Controls	Odds Ratio

Add Row

Chi Square for linear trend (Extended Mantel-Haenszel)	...
p value	...

FIGURE 24.28 Epi Info Software Screen Shot – 13 – Stat Calc
(Chi-Square for Trend)

StatCalc - Poisson

Poisson - Rare Event vs. Standard

Observed # of events: 6

Expected # of events: 1.16

Probability that the number of events found is	
< 6	0.9987342
<= 6	0.9997950
= 6	0.0010608
>= 6	0.0012658
> 6	0.0002050

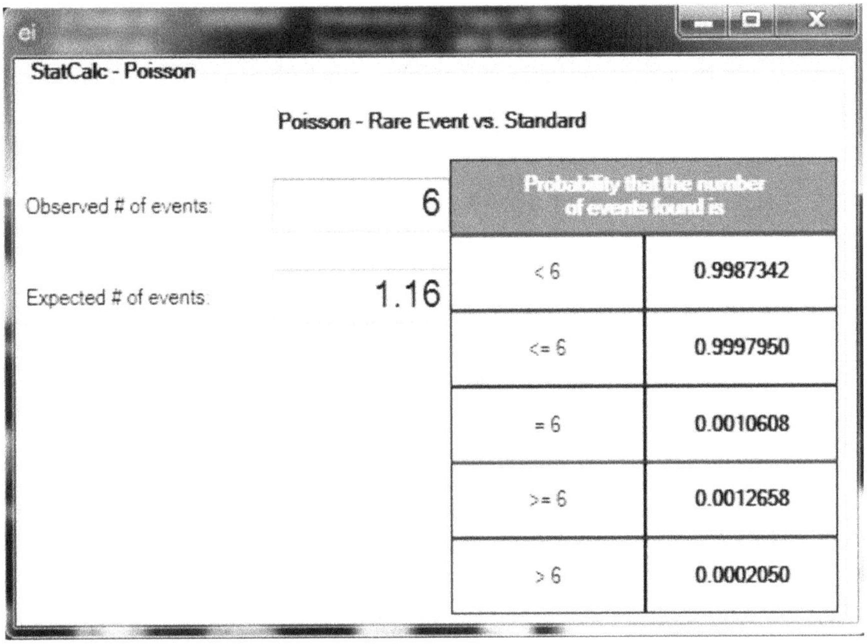

FIGURE 24.29 Epi Info Software Screen Shot – 14 – Stat Calc
(Poisson Rare Event vs. Std)

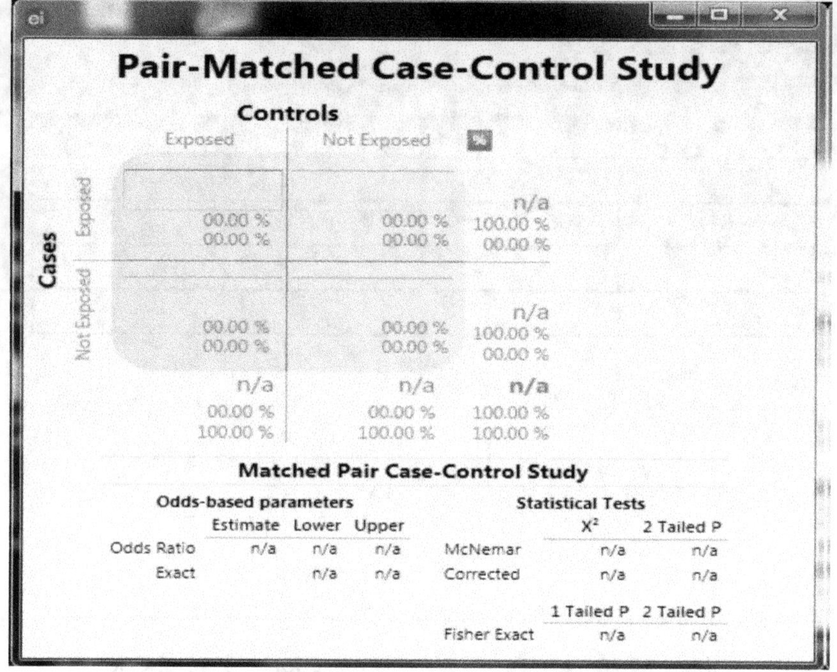

FIGURE 24.30 Epi Info Software Screen Shot – 15 – Stat Calc
(Matched Pair Case-Control)

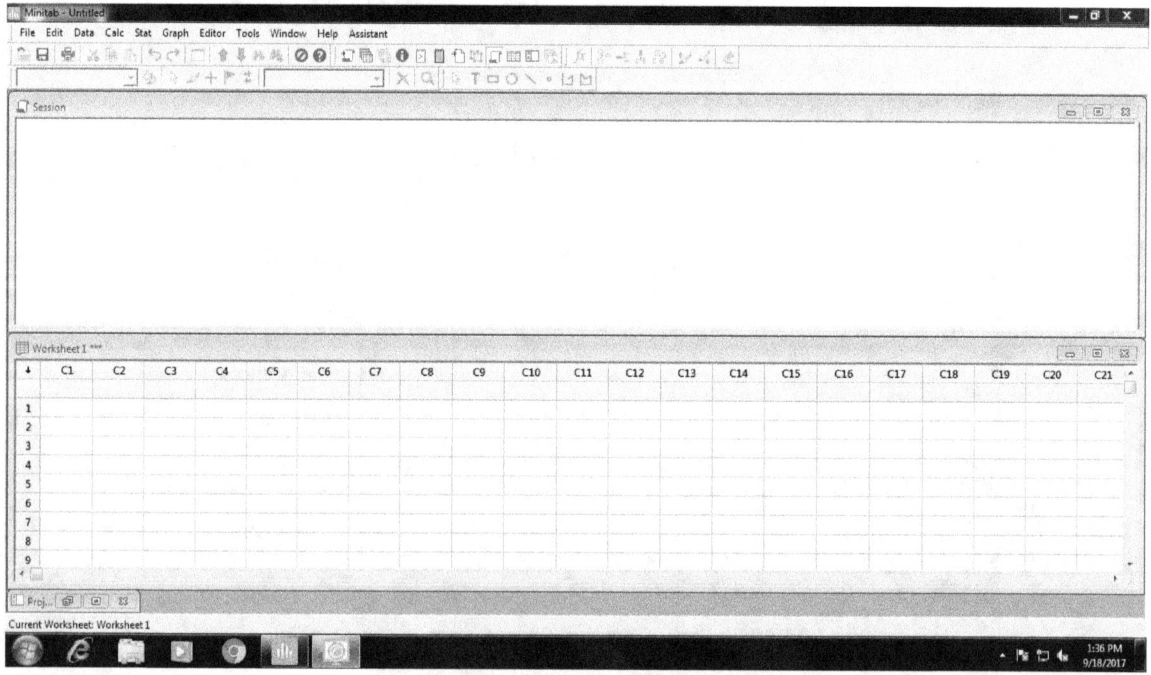

FIGURE 24.31 Minitab Screen Shot 1

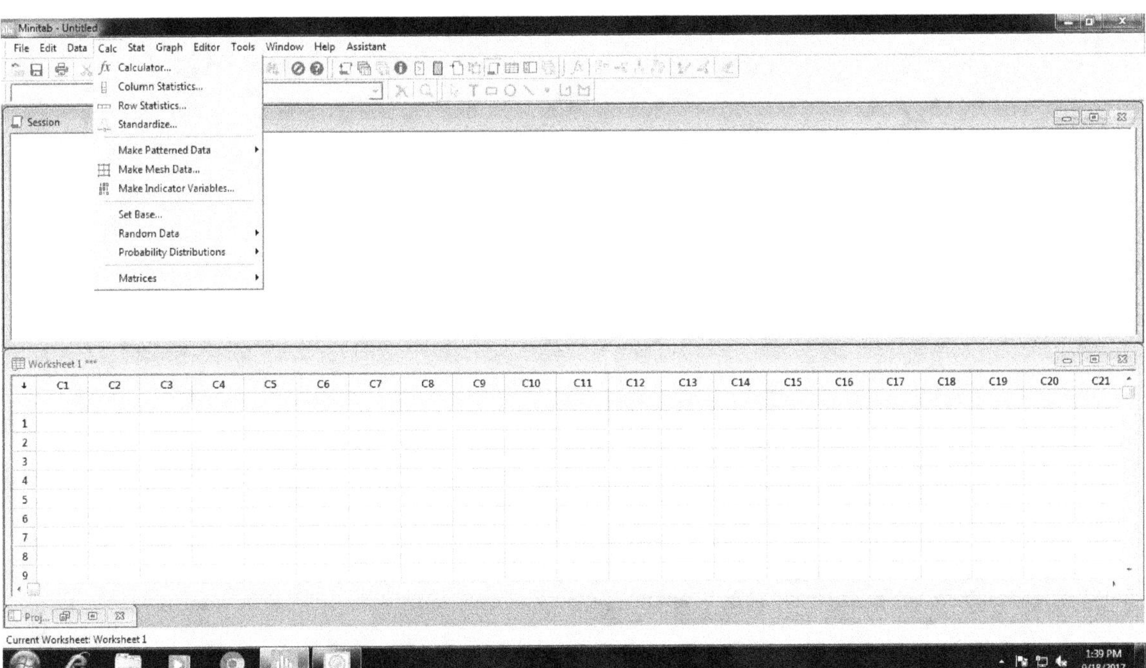

FIGURE 24.32 Minitab Screen Shot 2

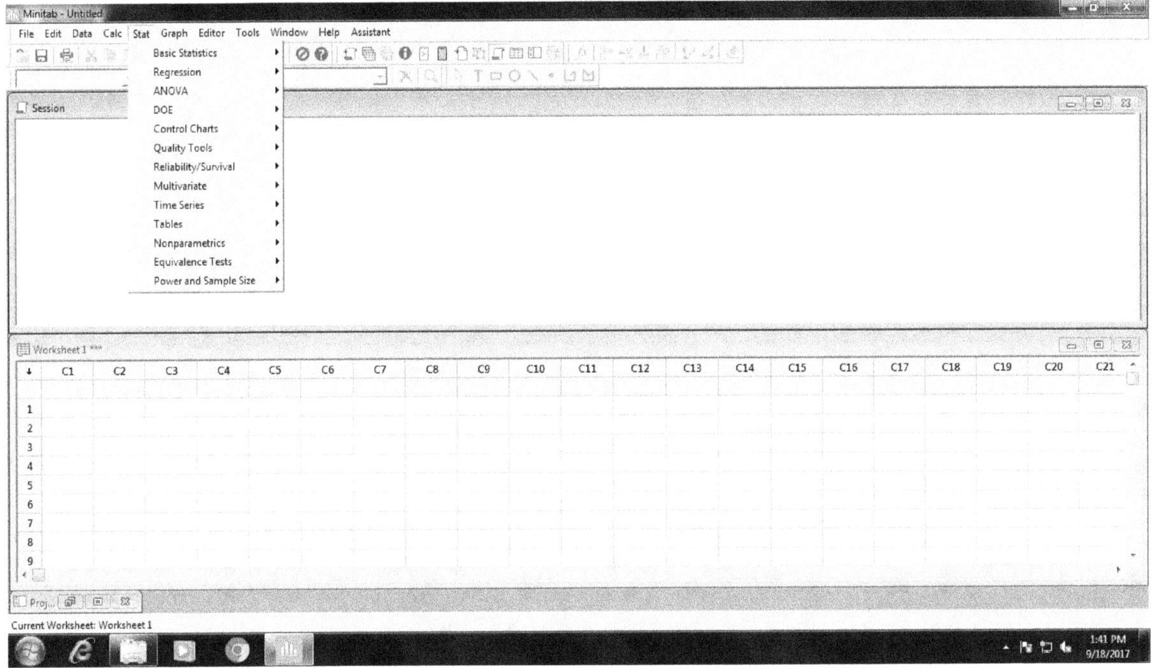

FIGURE 24.33 Minitab Screen Shot 3

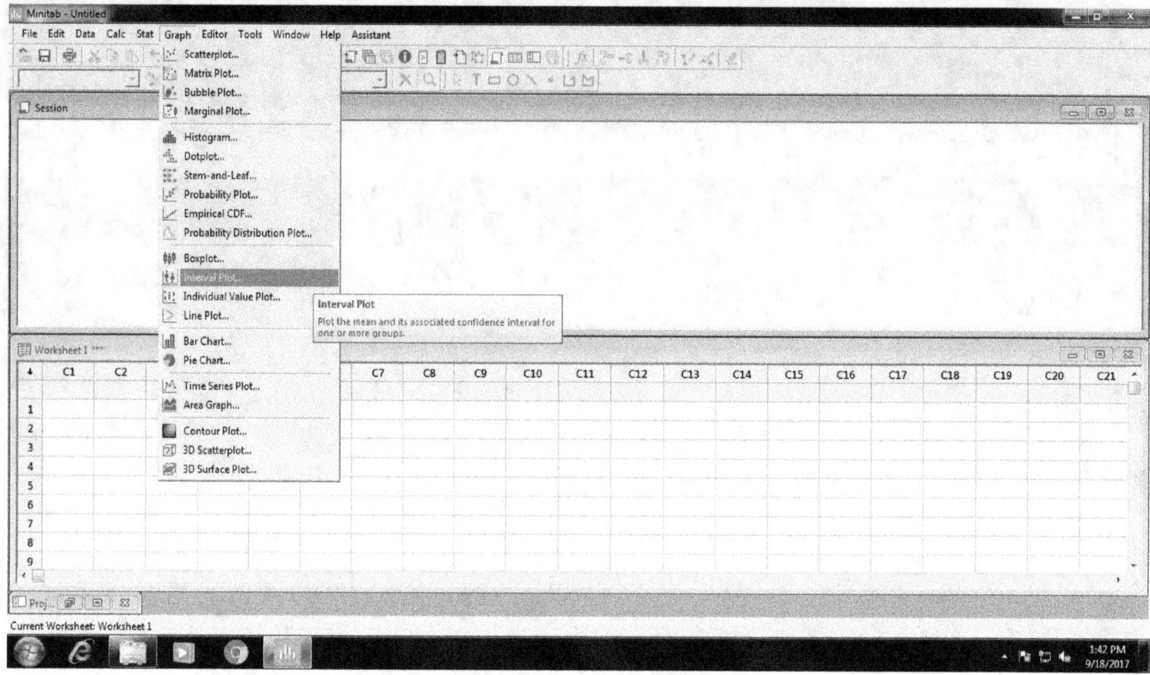

FIGURE 24.34 Minitab Screen Shot 4

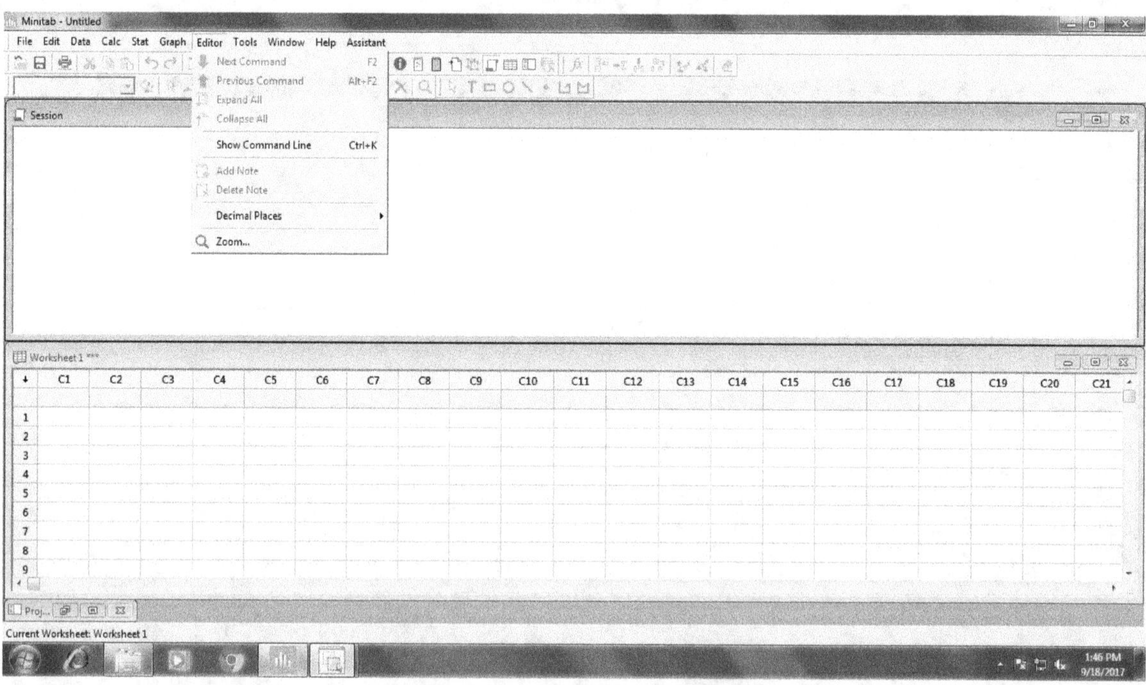

FIGURE 24.35 Minitab Screen Shot 5

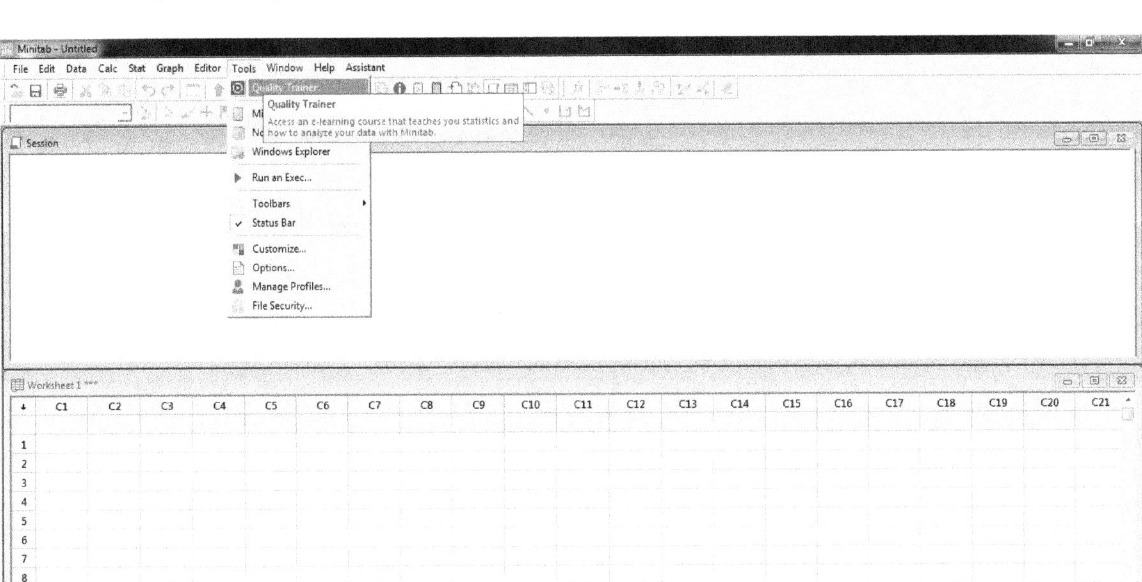

FIGURE 24.36 Minitab Screen Shot 6

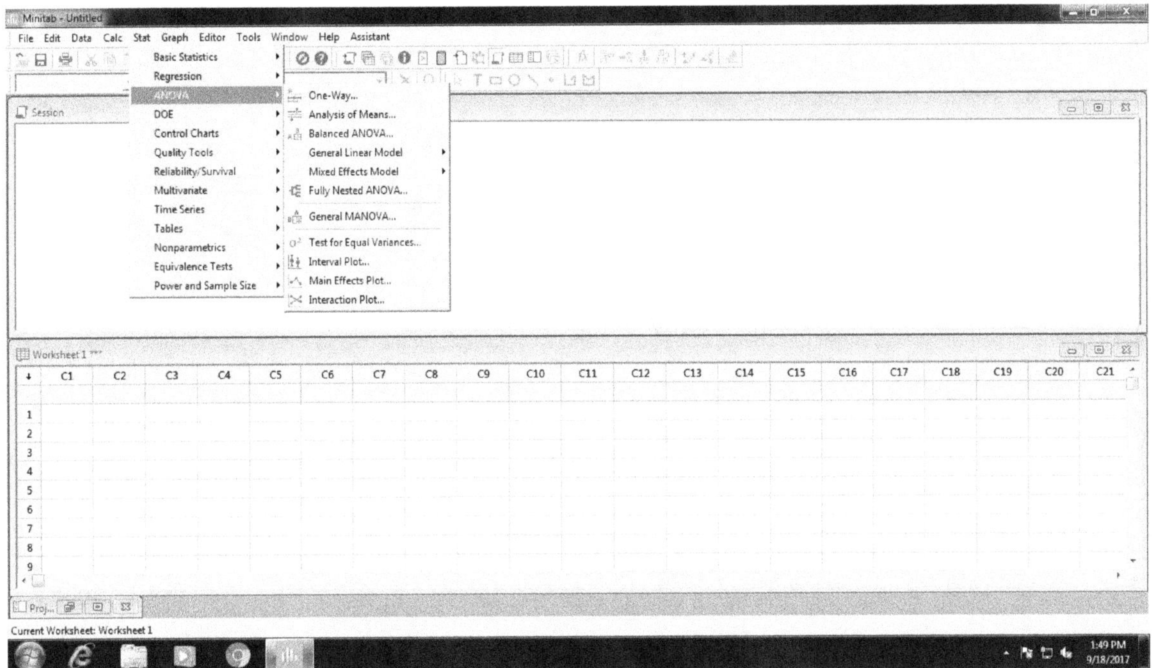

FIGURE 24.37 Minitab Screen Shot 7

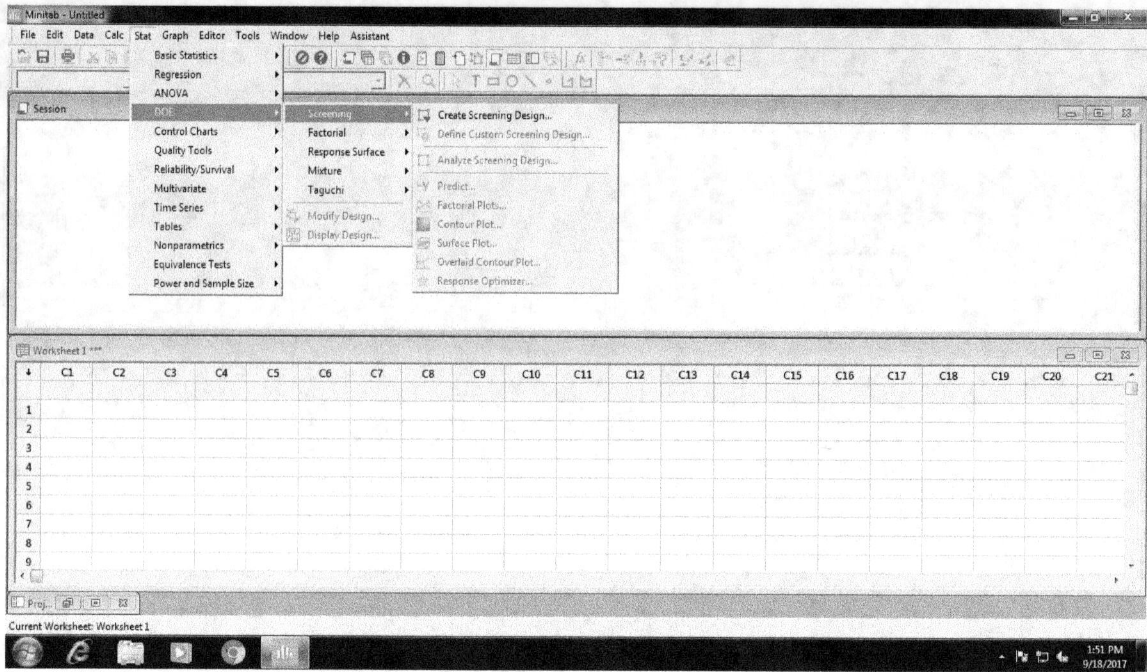

FIGURE 24.38 Minitab Screen Shot 8

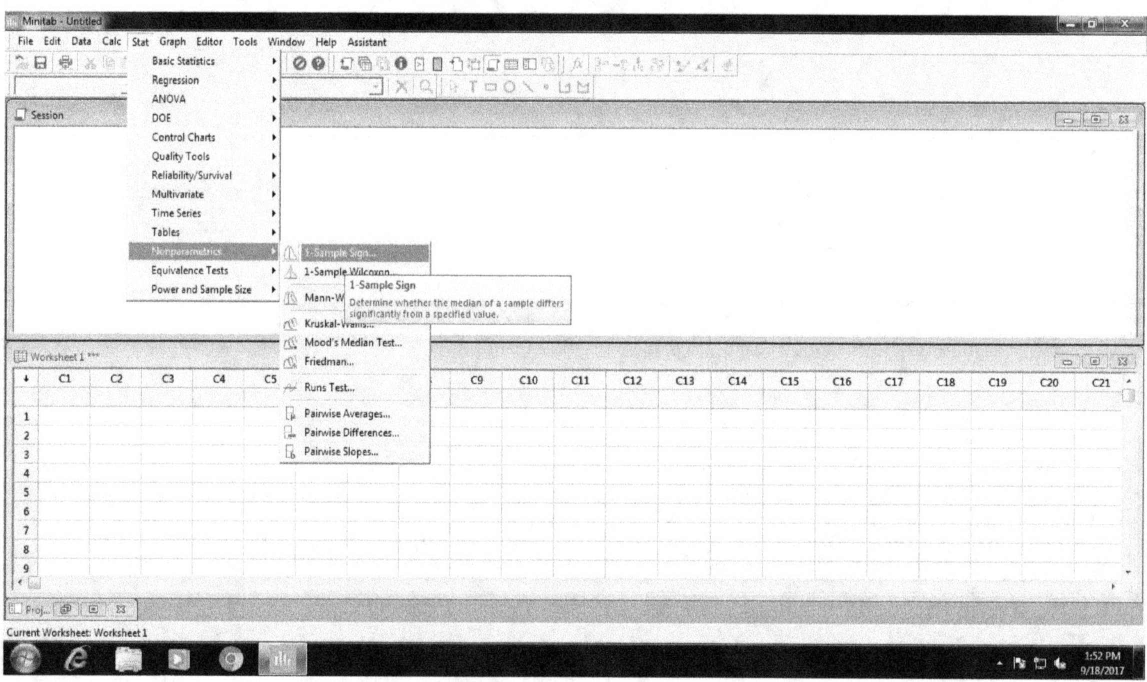

FIGURE 24.39 Minitab Screen Shot 9

25 Linear Regression, Correlation and Correlation Coefficient

25.0 Introduction

In pharmaceuticals, the relation between an independent and dependent variable is well understood when a plot of dependent variable (ordinate) vs. independent (abscissa) variable is made. The relation is either linear or non-linear. Such plots are quite commonly observed as absorbance vs. drug concentration for standard plots, drug concentration vs. time for kinetic studies to understand the drug release profile of a formulation or to understand the shelf life of a formulation or the degradation profile of drug with time with respect to stability studies of drug, drug product. Beers-Lambert's law defines that absorbance increases with concentration as well as with path length and is directly proportional in either the cases. In certain circumstances, upon crossing the Beers-Lambert's law limit, a linear relation among the variables tend towards a quench. In certain circumstances, in pharmaceuticals, a log form of a variable is used to achieve linearity.

25.1 Linear Regression

Let us imagine an experimental evaluation of absorbance vs. concentration of a drug. The pure drug is accurately weighed, accurately diluted and the diluted solution is subjected to UV spectroscopy (say) for absorbance. Let us imagine that, various concentrations of the drug solution are measured for its absorbance. When the values are subjected to a plot i.e., absorbance vs. concentration, theoretically a linear plot is expected. But, due to practical errors, all the plots with respect to concentration and corresponding absorbance whole together does not fall on a straight line. Thus theoretically expected straight line leads to a practically non-linear line. As linearity is required due to various reasons, the best fit line (sum of least squares line) has to be drawn or determined that is statistically significant. Hence, drawing a best fit line implies for statistical significance.

The advantage with a straight line relation is that, it not only helps in interpolation but also helps in extrapolations (i.e., helps in predicting the future conditions (i.e., determination of shelf life of formulation)). The quite commonly observed linear relations are for zero order kinetics, for first order kinetics and for log dose response curves. At the student level, during experimental plots, the best fit line is empirically drawn in such a way that the straight line passes through the maximum number of points leaving evenly those points not passing equally on either side of the line. But when the same plot is made in statistical software, the line is drawn by taking into consideration the statistical significant best fit line (sum of least squares).

Mathematically, a straight line is represented by y = mx + c, where y is the dependent variable, x is the independent variable, m is the slope of the straight line and c is the intercept of the straight line on the y-axis. If the straight line is passing from origin, the straight line is represented by y = mx, since c=0. If a straight line is ascending, the slope is positive and if the straight line is descending, the slope is negative and the straight line is represented as y = (-m)x + c. The negative sign in the latter case has no mathematical value but implies a descending slope of the straight line. In general, slope of the straight line is given by $(y_2 - y_1)/(x_2 - x_1)$, where (x_1, y_1), (x_2, y_2) are two points on the line.

For 'N' pairs of variables x, y, one can define the best straight line (or best fit line) by determining the line that minimizes the sum of squares of the vertical distances of each point from the fitted line. The sum of squares of the vertical distances of each point from the fitted line is determined mathematically by $\sum(y - y')$, where y is the experimental point and y' is the corresponding point on the fitted line. The line constructed is called the least squares line.

Using calculus, the slope (m) and intercept (c) are mathematically represented as follows:

$$slope = m = \frac{\sum(x - \bar{x})(y - \bar{y})}{\sum(x - \bar{x})^2}$$

Where x = independent variable, $\bar{x}$ bar = mean of independent variables, y = dependent variable, $\bar{y}$ bar = mean of corresponding dependent variables.

For ease of calculations, the equation for determination of slope is given by

$$slope = m = \frac{N \sum xy - (\sum x)(\sum y)}{N \sum x^2 - (\sum x)^2}$$

and the intercept is given by

$$c = \frac{\sum y - m(\sum x)}{N}$$

where N is number of observations   or

$$intercept = c = \bar{y} - m\bar{x}$$

Problem 25.1, on determination of slope and intercept: The drug potency (independent variable) and the corresponding assay (dependent variable) are as mentioned below:

Drug potency (x)	Assay (y)	xy
60	63	3780
80	75	6000
100	99	9900
120	116	13920
$\sum x = 360$	$\sum y = 353$	$\sum xy = 33,600$
$\sum x^2 = 34,400$	$\sum y^2 = 32,851$	

Solution: For the best fitted line or the least squares line,

$$slope = m = \frac{N \sum xy - (\sum x)(\sum y)}{N \sum x^2 - (\sum x)^2} = \frac{4\,(33600)(360)(353)}{4\,(34400) - (360)^2} = 0.915$$

and

$$intercept = c = \frac{353}{4} - (0.915)(90) = 5.9$$

An ideal slope is unity, which is theoretical and in majority of the practical conditions, the slope is observed near to unity and not unity.

When a straight line passes through origin, the slope of the straight line is given by

$$m = \frac{\sum xy}{\sum x^2}$$

For a linear regression, several test hypothesis are assumed i.e.,

i.   The 'x' variable is measured without error or with relatively little error. Usually, in pharmaceuticals, 'x' is the concentration of the drug in a solution form obtained by weighing and doing serial dilutions.

ii. For each 'x', y value is independent and normally distributed and 'y' value is a function of 'x'.

iii. The variance of 'y' is assumed to be the same at each 'x'.

iv. A linear relationship exists between 'x' and 'y' as $y = mx + c$.

Except for location (mean), the distribution of 'y' is the same at every value of 'x', that is, 'y' has the same variance at every value of 'x'.

In practice, when a standard plot is being established, six individual weightings for every concentration planned are made and serial individual dilutions are made and the respective six dilution absorbances are recorded. Hence, if we plan for five concentrations, then 5 X 6 weightings = 30 weightings leading to 30 absorbances (after dilutions) corresponding to 5 concentrations (average of six) are being made.

If average of every concentration for six weightings is considered as " $\bar{x}$ i.e., x bar" and average of six absorbances with respect to one concentration is considered as "$\bar{y}$ i.e., y bar", there are five " x bars" and five "y bars". A plot of "y bar" vs. "x bar" can be considered as best fit line (or line with least sum of squares). The six absorbances for a specific individual concentration (of six) is found to exhibit normal distribution.

The variances of the theoretical estimates, for slope 'm' and intercept 'c' are given by

$$\text{Variance for intercept} = \sigma_c^2 = \sigma_{y.x}^2 \left[\frac{1}{N} + \frac{\bar{x}^2}{\Sigma(x - \bar{x})^2}\right],$$

where y.x is y value is function of x

$$\text{Variance for slope} = \sigma_m^2 = \frac{\sigma_{y.x}^2}{\Sigma(x - \bar{x})^2}$$

For calculation of variance with respect to observed points, it is obtained from the sum of squares of deviations of the observed points from the fitted line by

$$s_{y.x}^2 = \frac{\Sigma(y - y')^2}{N - 2} = \frac{\Sigma(y - \bar{y})^2 - b^2[\Sigma(x - \bar{x})^2}{N - 2}$$

$$= \frac{[\Sigma y^2 - \frac{(\Sigma y)^2}{N}] - [b^2[\Sigma(x - \bar{x})^2]]}{N - 2}$$

Where, degrees of freedom = N-2, instead N-1. This is because two parameters are being estimated i.e., slope and intercept.

$$\text{Variance for intercept} = s_c^2 = s_{y.x}^2 \left[\frac{1}{N} + \frac{\bar{x}^2}{\Sigma(x - \bar{x})^2}\right],$$

where y.x is y value is function of x

$$\text{Variance for slope} = s_m^2 = \frac{s_{y.x}^2}{\Sigma(x - \bar{x})^2}$$

Statistically, for a linear regression, a null hypothesis is defined (say), H_0: c=0 i.e., there is no intercept. As an alternate hypothesis, H_A: c $\neq$ 0 implying there is intercept for the straight line. Here, the test is two sided indicating the intercept could be either positive or negative. For a slope, H_0: m=0 and H_A: m $\neq$ 0.

In order to find out whether there is any difference between theoretical and practical slopes as well as similarly for intercepts, a student 't' test is the one which gives conclusions. The equations that are suitable to the circumstances are as follows: for intercept:

$$t_{d.f} = \frac{|c - c'|}{\sqrt{s_c^2}}$$

where, c= practical intercept and c' = theoretical intercept
and for slope,

$$t_{d.f} = \frac{|m - m'|}{\sqrt{s_m^2}}$$

where, m = practical slope and m' = theoretical slope
For the calculations of student 't' tests, the corresponding variances can be calculated and substituted as per the earlier mentioned equations.

Likewise, for a linear regression, a confidence interval helps is making better conclusions, for instance, when determining shelf life of a drug (i.e., the time taken for drug content in a formulation reducing to final drug content of 90 percent) the equation is given by:

$$Confidence\ interval\ (C.I, 5\%\ probability, 95\ \%\ confidence\ level) =$$

$$y \pm t\,(s_{y.x}) \sqrt{[\frac{1}{N} + \frac{(x - \bar{x})^2}{\Sigma(x - \bar{x})^2}]}$$

The above confidence interval indicates for 'y' at a given value of 'x'. Usually, the lowest confidence interval is used for shelf life (expiry date) rather than the upper sided in a two sided test.

A confidence interval for 'x' at a given value of 'y' can be calculated by the following equation:

$$C.I = \frac{(x - g\bar{x}) \pm \left[\frac{t(s_{y.x})}{m}\right] [\sqrt{\frac{1-g}{N} + \frac{(x-\bar{x})^2}{\Sigma(x-\bar{x})^2}}]}{1 - g}$$

$$Where,\ g = \frac{t^2(s_{y.x}^2)}{m^2\,\Sigma(x-\bar{x})^2}$$

For instance, in research, standard plots (or calibration curves) are usually necessary and several international guidelines insist for statistical analysis. This can be illustrated as follows, Table 25.1, Figure 25.1.

TABLE 25.1 Weight of Drug Vs. Absorbance after Dilutions

Weight of Drug (g)	Average Weight (g)	Absorbance	Average of Absorbance
a1, a2, a3, a4, a5, a6	$\bar{a}$	A1, A2, A3, A4, A5, A6	$\bar{A}$
b1, b2, b3, b4, b5, b6	$\bar{b}$	B1, B2, B3, B4, B5, B6	$\bar{B}$
c1, c2, c3, c4, c5, c6	$\bar{c}$	C1, C2, C3, C4, C5, C6	$\bar{C}$
d1, d2, d3, d4, d5, d6	$\bar{d}$	D1, D2, D3, D4, D5, D6	$\bar{D}$
e1, e2, e3, e4, e5, e6	$\bar{e}$	E1, E2, E3, E4, E5, E6	$\bar{E}$
f1, f2, f3, f4, f5, f6	$\bar{f}$	F1, F2, F3, F4, F5, F6	$\bar{F}$

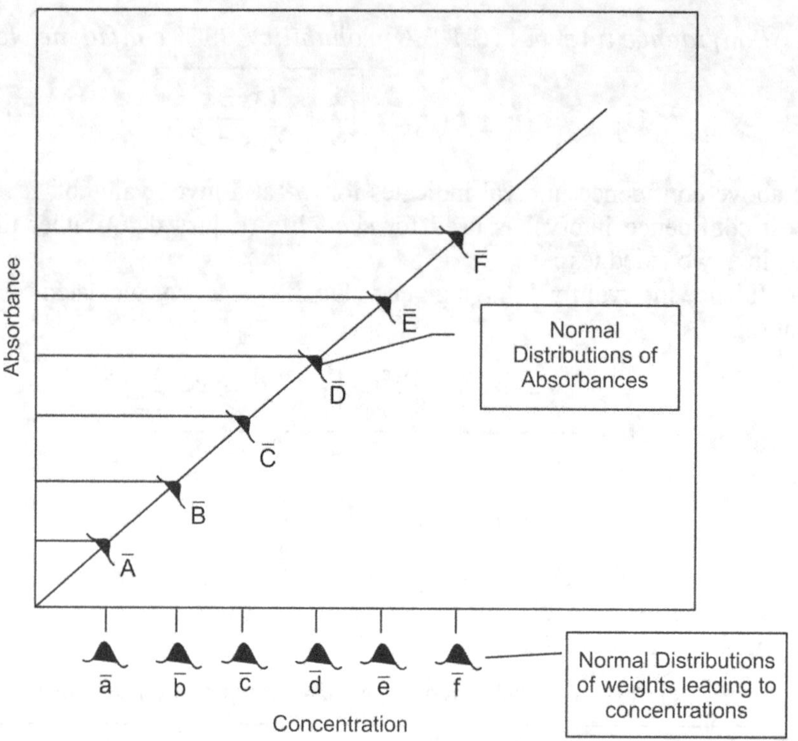

FIGURE 25.1 Absorbance vs. Concentration w.r.t to Six Individual Weights for One Concentration (Standard Curve-Theoretical)

Problem 25.2 on linear regression, shelf life of formulation

A tablet formulation is subjected to stability study at ambient temperature. Three randomly chosen tablets at every time period were assayed at 0, 3, 6, 9, 12 and 18 months. The assay values are as mentioned in the below Table 25.2. Calculate the shelf life of the formulation dosage form, statistically. The higher values in the assay are due to 4% overage, even though FDA discourages overages to compensate for poor stability.

Table 25.2 Assay Value of Tablet Formulation for Shelf Life Determination

Time, X (Months)	Assay 1 (mg)	Assay 2 (mg)	Assay 3 (mg)	Average
0	51	51	53	51.7
3	51	50	52	51
6	50	52	48	50
9	49	51	51	50.3
12	49	48	47	48
18	47	45	49	47

Solution: Shelf life is defined as that time when a tablet formulation contains 90% of the labeled drug potency.

When a plot of Assay (mg) vs. Time is plotted, Figure 25.2, illustrates that the order of decrease in concentration of the drug from the formulation is zero-order

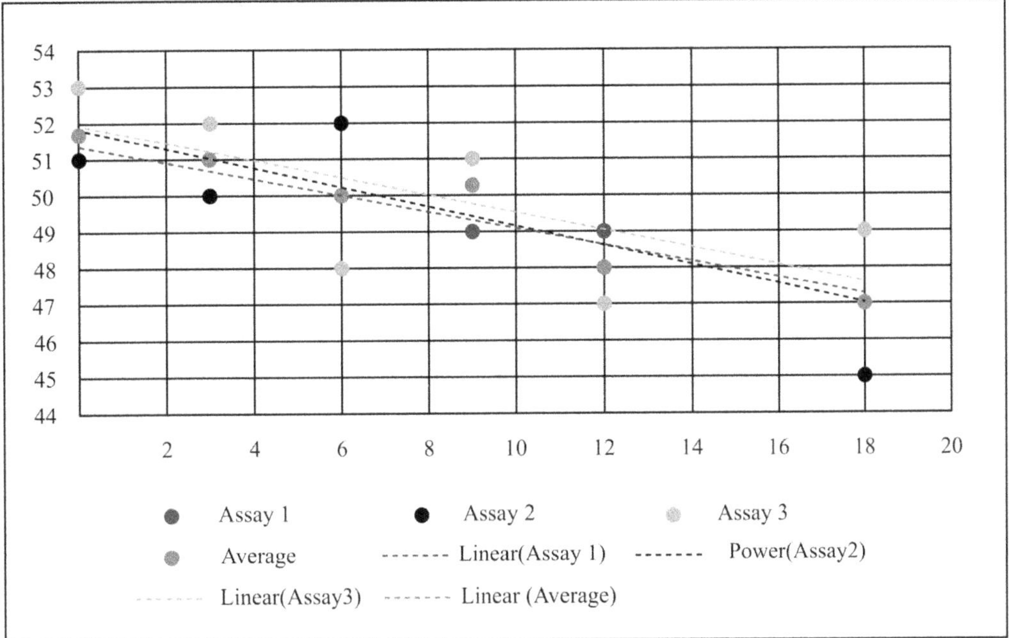

FIGURE 25.2 Trend in Assay Values for Tablet Formulation for Shelf Life Determination

and the equation of the linear equation can be given by

$$C = C_0 - kt$$

Where, C = concentration at time 't', C_0 = concentration at time 0 (y-intercept, c), k the rate constant (slope, -m) and 't' the time (storage time).

The equations to determine the intercept (c) and slope (m) are

$$\text{slope} = m = \frac{N \sum xy - (\sum x)(\sum y)}{N \sum x^2 - (\sum x)^2}$$

$$\text{intercept} = c = \bar{y} - m\bar{x}$$

Here,

$\sum x = (0 + 3 + 6 + 9 + 12 + 18) + (0 + 3 + 6 + 9 + 12 + 18) + (0 + 3 + 6 + 9 + 12 + 18) = 144$

$\sum x^2 = (0^2 + 3^2 + 6^2 + 9^2 + 12^2 + 18^2) + (0^2 + 3^2 + 6^2 + 9^2 + 12^2 + 18^2) + (0^2 + 3^2 + 6^2 + 9^2 + 12^2 + 18^2) = 1782$

$\sum y = (51 + 51 + 53) + (51 + 50 + 52) + (50 + 52 + 48) + (49 + 51 + 51) + (49 + 48 + 47) + (47 + 45 + 49) = 894$

$\sum y^2 = (51^2 + 51^2 + 53^2) + (51^2 + 50^2 + 52^2) + (50^2 + 52^2 + 48^2) + (49^2 + 51^2 + 51^2) + (49^2 + 48^2 + 47^2) + (47^2 + 45^2 + 49^2) = 44,476$

and N = total no. of observations = 18

Therefore,

$$\text{slope} = m = \frac{N \sum xy - (\sum x)(\sum y)}{N \sum x^2 - (\sum x)^2} = \frac{18\,(6984) - 144\,(894)}{18\,(1782) - (144)^2}$$

$$= \frac{125712 - 128736}{32076 - 20736} = \frac{-3024}{11340} = -0.267 \; mg/month$$

$$\text{intercept} = c = \bar{y} - m\bar{x} = \left[\frac{894}{18} - (-0.267)\frac{144}{18}\right] = [49.67 - (-2.136)] = 51.80$$

Therefore, the best fit line is given by

$$C = C_0 - kt$$

and when compared with y=mx + c, y = C, m = -k, C = C_0 and x=t.

Hence, $C = C_0 - kt = 51.80 - (0.267)t$

At a fixed time, the variance estimate is given by

$$s_{y.x}^2 = \frac{\left[\sum y^2 - \frac{(\sum y)^2}{N}\right] - [\, b^2[\sum(x - \bar{x})^2]\,]}{N - 2} = \frac{\left[44476 - \frac{(894)^2}{18}\right] - [(-0.267)^2(630)]}{18 - 2}$$

$$= \frac{74 - 44.91}{16} = 1.82$$

Since the initial concentration with overage is 51.80 mg and the variance estimate is 1.82, then the final initial concentration can be considered as 50 mg.

At shelf life, only 90 % of initial concentration is observed i.e., 50 X 90/100 = 45 mg.

Hence, $45 = C_0 - k\,t = 51.80 - (0.267)t$

Therefore, t = [51.80 – 45]/0.267 = 25.46 months.

All the above calculations are based on average of 18 tablets and the final value varies when each tablet is taken into consideration.

At 95 percent confidence interval for potency at fixed point of time is calculated by,

$$Confidence\ interval\ (C.I, 5\%\ probability, 95\ \%\ confidence\ level) =$$

$$y \pm t\,(s_{y.x}) \sqrt{\left[\frac{1}{N} + \frac{(x - \bar{x})^2}{\sum(x - \bar{x})^2}\right]} = 45 \pm 2.12\,(1.35) \sqrt{\frac{1}{18} + \frac{(25.5 - 8)^2}{630}}$$

$$= 45 \pm 2.1 \; mg$$

At 95 percent confidence interval for time at fixed value of potency is calculated by,

When x = 25.5, $\bar{x}$ (x bar) = 8, N =18

$$C.I = \frac{(x - g\bar{x}) \pm \left[\frac{t(s_{y.x})}{m}\right]\left[\sqrt{\frac{1-g}{N} + \frac{(x - \bar{x})^2}{\sum(x - \bar{x})^2}}\right]}{1 - g}$$

$$\text{Where, } g = \frac{t^2(s_{y.x}^2)}{m^2 \sum(x - \bar{x})^2} = \frac{(2.12)^2(1.825)}{(-0.267)^2(630)} = 0.183$$

Therefore,

$$C.I = \frac{(x - g\bar{x}) \pm \left[\frac{t(s_{y.x})}{m}\right] \left[\sqrt{\frac{1-g}{N} + \frac{(x-\bar{x})^2}{\Sigma(x-\bar{x})^2}}\right]}{1 - g}$$

$$= \frac{(25.5 - (0.183)8) \pm \left[\frac{2.12(1.35)}{-0.267}\right] \left[\sqrt{\frac{1-0.183}{18} + \frac{(17.5)^2}{630}}\right]}{0.817}$$

$$= \frac{(25.5 - 1.464) \pm (-10.72)\sqrt{0.0454 + 0.486}}{0.817}$$

$$= \frac{24.036 \pm (-7.815)}{0.817} = 19.8 \; to \; 39.0 \; months$$

But, USFDA suggest for one side (one tailed) rather than two sided for shelf-life (expiry date) study. That is only the lower limit is computed for 5% probability, d.f of 16 and with t = 1.75 and g = 0.1244, then CI

$$= \frac{(25.5 - (0.1244)8) \pm \left[\frac{1.75(1.35)}{-0.267}\right] \left[\sqrt{\frac{0.8756}{18} + \frac{(17.5)^2}{630}}\right]}{0.8756} = 20.6 \; months$$

Prediction interval is the determination of the confidence interval for a future determination. In the above calculations, confidence interval was calculated for 'y' for fixed value of 'x' or vice-versa. The new value of 'y' obtained from best fitted line leads to establishment of new concentration at the newly observed value of 'y', which is called as 'inverse prediction'. The calculation of prediction level, has similar equations but with one modification i.e.,

Prediction interval (C. I, 5% probability, 95 % confidence level) for $'x'$ at specified $'y'$

$$= y \pm t\,(s_{y.x}) \sqrt{[1 + \frac{1}{N} + \frac{(x - \bar{x})^2}{\Sigma(x - \bar{x})^2}]}$$

Prediction interval (C. I, 5% probability, 95 % confidence level) for $'y'$ at specified $'x'$

$$= \frac{(x - g\bar{x}) \pm \left[\frac{t(s_{y.x})}{m}\right] \left[\sqrt{\frac{(N+1)(1-g)}{N} + \frac{(x-\bar{x})^2}{\Sigma(x-\bar{x})^2}}\right]}{1 - g}$$

Likewise confidence interval for slope (m) and intercept (c) can be calculated as follows:

$$C.I \; for \; slope \; (m) = m \pm \frac{t\,(s_{y.x})}{\sqrt{\Sigma(x - \bar{x})^2}}$$

$$C.I \; for \; intercept \; (c) = c \pm t\,(s_{y.x}) \sqrt{\frac{1}{N} + \frac{(\bar{x})^2}{\Sigma(x - \bar{x})^2}}$$

25.2 Correlation

Correlation is a measure of association among two or more variables. Correlation helps in predicting one variable from the other variable. Correlation assumes a linear or straight line relationship between the two variables and it is applied for continuous variable. Scatter plots such as assay (potency) vs. tablet weight, absorbance vs. concentration are some of the representations for correlations. For instance, dissolution of a tablet based on tablet hardness is expected to exhibit correlation. It is believed that homogeneous granules tend towards larger weight in the tablet and with lower dissolution leading to a negative correlation.

25.3 Correlation Coefficient

Correlation Coefficient is a measure of degree of correlation and is a quantitative measure of the relationship between the two variables. Correlation Coefficient is not a measure of linearity. A strong correlation is sometimes interpreted as meaning that the relationship between variables is a straight line.

$$\textit{Correlation Coefficient} = r = \frac{\Sigma(x - \bar{x})(y - \bar{y})}{\sqrt{\Sigma(x - \bar{x})^2\, \Sigma(y - \bar{y})^2}}$$

Or

$$r = \frac{N\Sigma xy - \Sigma x \Sigma y}{\sqrt{\left[N\Sigma x^2 - (\Sigma x)^2\right]\left[N\Sigma y^2 - (\Sigma y)^2\right]}}$$

It is necessary to understand correlation coefficient is a test of correlation or independence among variables and with this one can estimate the degree of closeness of linear relationship between the two variables. The maximum value of correlation coefficient 'r' is equal to one. Due to practical errors, the value should be the nearest possible to unity (above 0.9).

Problem 25.3, on linear regression and correlation coefficient

A researcher wishes to establish blending operation parameters for a hand operated double cone blender. A 1 kg batch was planned with 10g of $KMnO_4$ and 1000 g of Starch. To ensure the uniform distribution of $KMnO_4$ in the final mixture, the researcher has initially established a standard plot of Absorbance vs. Concentration (μg/ml). A triplicate weighing and corresponding dilutions were made and subjected the coloured solution at 540nm in a colourimeter. The corresponding observations are as follows, Table 25.3:

TABLE 25.3 Establishment of Absorbance vs. Concentration of KMnO₄ (at 540 nm)

Concentration (mcg/ml)	Absorbance 1	Absorbance 2	Absorbance 3	Mean	SD	Mean ± SD
10	0.12	0.12	0.12	0.12	0	0.12 ± 0
20	0.22	0.23	0.23	0.23	0.006	0.23 ± 0.006
30	0.33	0.34	0.33	0.33	0.006	0.33 ± 0.006
40	0.44	0.45	0.45	0.45	0.006	0.45 ± 0.006
50	0.53	0.55	0.53	0.54	0.012	0.54 ± 0.012
60	0.63	0.64	0.63	0.63	0.006	0.63 ± 0.006
70	0.71	0.73	0.72	0.72	0.01	0.72 ± 0.01
80	0.79	0.8	0.78	0.79	0.01	0.79 ± 0.01
90	0.86	0.88	0.86	0.87	0.012	0.87 ± 0.012
100	0.92	0.94	0.92	0.93	0.012	0.93 ± 0.012

Using MS Office excel calculate the linear regression and correlation coefficient.

Solution:

Using MS Office Excel:

Step 1: The concentration and corresponding absorbances (triplicate values) were fed to the excel sheet.

Step 2: Mean of absorbances and standard deviation was concluded using excel functions.

Step 3: A plot of Absorbance (Mean) vs. Concentration (µg/ml) along with standard deviation, linear regression (slope, intercept) and correlation coefficient (R^2 or r) were obtained directly using the excel tools, Figure 25.3.

Step 4: A linear regression with respect to the best fitted line passing through origin is $y = 0.099x$ and a linear regression with respect to the best fitted having the intercept is $y = 0.090x + 0.062$.

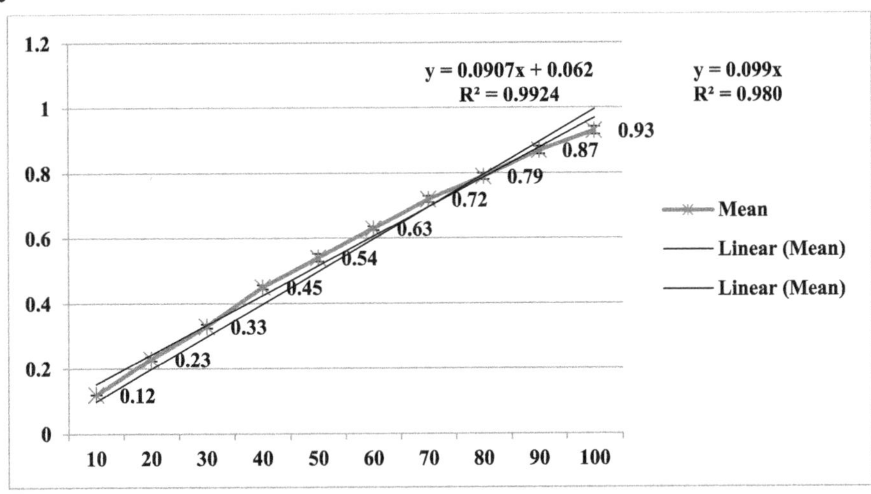

FIGURE 25.3 Standard Plot of KMnO4 (at 540 nm)

-Triplicate Study (Absorbance vs. Concentration - µg/ml)

25.4 Establishing a Multiple Regression Analysis

For a single dependent variable, there may exist with single or multiple independent variables for a relation. A single dependent and independent variable and their relation are usually given by y= mx + c (provided it is a linear relationship).

A multiple regression equation involves with a dependant variable and its relation with several independent variables in one single equation. Establishing a multiple regression equation involves with conducting several experiments. For instance, inducing anesthesia involves with administration of anesthetic gas (nitrous oxide) and a drug (thiopentone) to the patient. The fixation of dose for inducing anesthesia varies from individual to individual.   This implies that a dose given to one patient may induce anesthesia, but the same dose may not induce anesthesia to another patient. This is because of several factors such as height, weight, age, gender, body type, individual's regular habits etc.

Now, let us consider thiopentone dose induction study. This involves establishing a multiple regression equation that suits for any kind of patient and upon calculation that helps in fixing the dose. Thus, a compact multiple regression equation is built up in a series of steps. Firstly, each independent variable is separately regressed on the dependent variable. The independent variable that explains largest proportion of the outcome variation is selected as the first variable to enter the multiple regression equation.   Secondly, each remaining independent variable is regressed on the dependent variable jointly with the first variable.   The one which has largest proportion of outcome variation is selected as the second variable to the multiple regression equation. The remaining each independent variable is individually regressed with the combined first two independent variables that are considered and the process of establishing the multiple regression equation continues until required.

The final multiple regression equation is represented by

$$y = a + b_1 x_1 + b_2 x_2$$

Experimentally, the thiopentone induction dose study with ten possible independent variables is a follows:

Independent Variable	Additional Variation Explained After Step (%)					
	0	1	2	3	4	5
Gender	6.5	0.4	0.4	0.1	0.2	0.1
Age	0.1	2.2	3.3	2.9	---	---
Weight	22.3	4.5	---	---	---	---
Height	23.2	---	---	---	---	---
Body type	7.2	3.6	0.4	0.4	0.3	0.2
Cigarette consumption	3.0	1.0	1.1	0	0	0.1
Alcohol consumption	10.7	4.0	4.0	---	---	---
Degree of anxiety	2.3	1.3	1.5	1.2	1.0	0.8
Systolic BP	1.7	0.1	0	0	0.7	0.6
Heart rate	0.1	2.1	2.4	2.7	2.2	---

The multiple regression model is given by

Step	Variable added	Additional variation explained (%)	Influence
1	Height	23.2	Body mass
2	Weight	4.5	Body shape
3	Alcohol consumption	4.0	Drug tolerance
4	Age	2.9	Aging
5	Heart rate	2.2	Anxiety
	Total	36.8	

y = -239.77 + 1.78 x₁ + 1.83 x₂ + 20.49 x₃ -0.71 x₄ + 0.86 x₅

$$y = -239.77 + 1.78\,x_1 + 1.83\,x_2 + 20.49\,x_3 - 0.71\,x_4 + 0.86\,x_5$$

The five other independent variables and their influence has no further significant gain, and their not inclusion in the final equation is explained by proxy.   Gender differences are explained by height and weight differences, anxiety levels are reflected by heart rates and so the other.

25.4.1 Multi-linear Regression Analysis (Mathematical and Excel Calculations)

When one dependent variable is related to more than one independent variable, and if the relation is linear, then the equation or model generated is called multi-linear regression equation.   When the relation is non-linear, then it leads to polynomial equations of varying degrees i.e., second, third degree etc.   In case of two dependent variables having relation to several independent variables, then the equation or model generated is a multi-variant equation.

Now to the current context, as an example, let us take two independent variables and one dependent variable. The equation is given by

$$Y = b_0 + b_1 X_1 + b_2 X_2$$

$$b_1 = \frac{[(\sum x_2^2)(\sum x_1 y)] - [(\sum x_1 x_2)(\sum x_2 y)]}{[(\sum x_1^2)(\sum x_2^2) - ((\sum x_1 x_2)^2)]} \quad or \quad \frac{S_{xy}}{S_{xx}} = \frac{\sum xy - \frac{(\sum x)(\sum y)}{n}}{\sum x^2 - \frac{(\sum x)^2}{n}}$$

$$b_2 = \frac{[(\sum x_1^2)(\sum x_2 y)] - [(\sum x_1 x_2)(\sum x_1 y)]}{[(\sum x_1^2)(\sum x_2^2) - ((\sum x_1 x_2)^2)]}$$

$$b_0 = \bar{Y} - b_1 \overline{X_1} - b_2 \overline{X_2}$$

Where,

$$\sum x_i^2 = \sum X_i^2 - \frac{(X_i)^2}{N}$$

$$\sum x_i y = \sum X_i Y - \frac{(\sum X_i)(\sum Y)}{N}$$

$$\sum x_1 x_2 = \sum X_1 X_2 - \frac{(\sum X_1)(\sum X_2)}{N}$$

Now let us see how these equations are derived. Let us take five students with their marks in various pharmacy subjects, say instrumental methods of analysis (X_1), industrial pharmacy (X_2), pharmacy practice (X_3), novel drug delivery systems (X_4), instrumental methods of analysis practical (X_5), practice school (X_6). Let us take into consideration Percentage marks (Y) as dependent variable. Hence, for every student the dependent variable (y) is the sum of all the marks (x) of all the subjects. A question may arise whether to take mid 1 and mid 2 marks for every subject as two independent variables. The mid marks of the same subject may have same correlation with dependent variable and there may not be effect. Hence, either we have to selectively avoid one of the mid marks or take into consideration the average of mid marks as one independent variable. In order to understand whether there is any correlation between two independent variables, we can plot a scatter plot or calculate coefficient of correlation (or multi-colinearity) and if two independent variables have high correlation, it is better to consider one among them and definitely not both. It is necessary to understand that whatever independent variables available can be developed with a multi-linear regression equation, the resultant linear equation may give significance but there is no rationality and this may give incorrect interpretations at a later stage and hence to be avoided. The marks in the Table format are as follows:

Student No	Percentage Marks (Y)	Instrumental methods of analysis (X_1) Max. Marks: 100	Industrial pharmacy (X_2) Max. Marks: 100	Pharmacy practice (X_3) Max. Marks: 100	Novel drug delivery systems (X_4) Max. Marks: 100	Instrumental methods of analysis Practical (X_5) Max. Marks: 50	Practice school (X_6) Max. Marks: 150
1	y_1	X_{11}	X_{21}	X_{31}	X_{41}	X_{51}	X_{61}
2	y_2	X_{12}	X_{22}	X_{32}	X_{42}	X_{52}	X_{62}
3	y_3	X_{13}	X_{23}	X_{33}	X_{43}	X_{53}	X_{63}
4	y_4	X_{14}	X_{24}	X_{34}	X_{44}	X_{54}	X_{64}
5	y_5	X_{15}	X_{25}	X_{35}	X_{45}	X_{55}	X_{65}

In order to derive the multi-linear regression, we usually use least square method which in turn means smallest sum of square of residuals which in turn meaning difference between the data points and the predicted line.

Hence, the final one equation is as follows:

$$Y = B_0 + B_1 X_1 + B_2 X_2 + B_3 X_3 + B_4 X_4 + B_5 X_5 + B_6 X_6$$

Where, Y is over all dependent variable, X_1, X_2, X_3, X_4, X_5, X_6 are overall independent variables for the corresponding pharmacy subjects, B_0 is the overall intercept and B_1, B_2, B_3, B_4, B_5, and B_6 are the overall regression coefficients (overall individual pharmacy subject slopes) for the corresponding pharmacy subjects (independent variables).

Now let us take the observed regression equation for each student, then

$y_1 = b_{01} + b_{11}x_{11} + b_{21}x_{21} + b_{31}x_{31} + b_{41}x_{41} + b_{51}x_{51} + b_{61}x_{61} + \varepsilon_1$

$y_2 = b_{02} + b_{12}x_{12} + b_{22}x_{22} + b_{32}x_{32} + b_{42}x_{42} + b_{52}x_{52} + b_{62}x_{62} + \varepsilon_2$

$y_3 = b_{03} + b_{13}x_{13} + b_{23}x_{23} + b_{33}x_{33} + b_{43}x_{43} + b_{53}x_{53} + b_{63}x_{63} + \varepsilon_3$

$y_4 = b_{04} + b_{14}x_{14} + b_{24}x_{24} + b_{34}x_{34} + b_{44}x_{44} + b_{54}x_{54} + b_{64}x_{64} + \varepsilon_4$

$y_5 = b_{05} + b_{15}x_{15} + b_{25}x_{25} + b_{35}x_{35} + b_{45}x_{45} + b_{55}x_{55} + b_{65}x_{65} + \varepsilon_5$

$y_6 = b_{06} + b_{16}x_{16} + b_{26}x_{26} + b_{36}x_{36} + b_{46}x_{46} + b_{56}x_{56} + b_{66}x_{66} + \varepsilon_6$

Then the corresponding predicted regression equations are

$\hat{y}_1 = \hat{b}_{01} + \hat{b}_{11}x_{11} + \hat{b}_{21}x_{21} + \hat{b}_{31}x_{31} + \hat{b}_{41}x_{41} + \hat{b}_{51}x_{51} + \hat{b}_{61}x_{61}$

$\hat{y}_2 = \hat{b}_{02} + \hat{b}_{12}x_{12} + \hat{b}_{22}x_{22} + \hat{b}_{32}x_{32} + \hat{b}_{42}x_{42} + \hat{b}_{52}x_{52} + \hat{b}_{62}x_{62}$

$\hat{y}_3 = \hat{b}_{03} + \hat{b}_{13}x_{13} + \hat{b}_{23}x_{23} + \hat{b}_{33}x_{33} + \hat{b}_{43}x_{43} + \hat{b}_{53}x_{53} + \hat{b}_{63}x_{63}$

$\hat{y}_4 = \hat{b}_{04} + \hat{b}_{14}x_{14} + \hat{b}_{24}x_{24} + \hat{b}_{34}x_{34} + \hat{b}_{44}x_{44} + \hat{b}_{54}x_{54} + \hat{b}_{64}x_{64}$

$\hat{y}_5 = \hat{b}_{05} + \hat{b}_{15}x_{15} + \hat{b}_{25}x_{25} + \hat{b}_{35}x_{35} + \hat{b}_{45}x_{45} + \hat{b}_{55}x_{55} + \hat{b}_{65}x_{65}$

$\hat{y}_6 = \hat{b}_{06} + \hat{b}_{16}x_{16} + \hat{b}_{26}x_{26} + \hat{b}_{36}x_{36} + \hat{b}_{46}x_{46} + \hat{b}_{56}x_{56} + \hat{b}_{66}x_{66}$

In the matrix form, the multi-linear regression equation is in the form of

$$
\begin{bmatrix} y_1 \\ y_2 \\ y_3 \\ y_4 \\ y_5 \\ y_6 \end{bmatrix}_{6 \times 1}
=
\begin{bmatrix}
1 & x_{11} & x_{21} & x_{31} & x_{41} & x_{51} & x_{61} \\
1 & x_{12} & x_{22} & x_{32} & x_{42} & x_{52} & x_{62} \\
1 & x_{13} & x_{23} & x_{33} & x_{43} & x_{53} & x_{63} \\
1 & x_{14} & x_{24} & x_{34} & x_{44} & x_{54} & x_{64} \\
1 & x_{15} & x_{25} & x_{35} & x_{45} & x_{55} & x_{65} \\
1 & x_{16} & x_{26} & x_{36} & x_{46} & x_{56} & x_{66}
\end{bmatrix}_{6 \times 7}
X
\begin{bmatrix} b_0 \\ b_1 \\ b_2 \\ b_3 \\ b_4 \\ b_5 \\ b_6 \end{bmatrix}_{7 \times 1}
+
\begin{bmatrix} \varepsilon_1 \\ \varepsilon_2 \\ \varepsilon_3 \\ \varepsilon_4 \\ \varepsilon_5 \\ \varepsilon_6 \end{bmatrix}_{6 \times 1}
$$

Here, the distribution of Y is described as multivariate normal distribution and is represented by

$Y = [\text{mean (ie., xbar), variance (i.e., } \sigma^2)]$

The difference between the observed and predicted regression is given by residual error (e), which is equal to $(y - \hat{y})$, i.e., $e = y - \hat{y}$, where 'ε' is called as irreducible error.

In order to derive the overall multi-linear regression equation, it is necessary to reduce the error that is by reducing the Error Sum of Squares (SSE) $= \sum_{n=1}^{n=6} e^2 = \sum_{n=1}^{n=6}(y - \hat{y})^2$ or $= e^T e = (y - \hat{y})^T (y - \hat{y}) = (y - X\hat{B})^T (y - X\hat{B}) = (y^T - X^T\hat{B}^T)(y - X\hat{B})$

Now, let us take into consideration simple equation i.e., $Y = \hat{B}X$

Multiply both sides by X^T, then the equation is $X^TY = \hat{B}(X^TX)$

Rearranging the equation, then $[X^TY]/[X^TX] = \hat{B}$ and this can be written as $[X^TY][X^TX]^{-1} = \hat{B}$. Here, the left hand side represents least squares.

Therefore,

$$
\begin{bmatrix}
1 & 1 & 1 & 1 & 1 & 1 \\
x_{11} & x_{12} & x_{13} & x_{14} & x_{15} & x_{16} \\
x_{21} & x_{22} & x_{23} & x_{24} & x_{25} & x_{26} \\
x_{31} & x_{32} & x_{33} & x_{34} & x_{35} & x_{36} \\
x_{41} & x_{42} & x_{43} & x_{44} & x_{45} & x_{46} \\
x_{51} & x_{52} & x_{53} & x_{54} & x_{55} & x_{56} \\
x_{61} & x_{62} & x_{63} & x_{64} & x_{65} & x_{66}
\end{bmatrix}_{7 \times 6}
\begin{bmatrix}
y_1 \\ y_2 \\ y_3 \\ y_4 \\ y_5 \\ y_6
\end{bmatrix}_{6 \times 1}
* \left\{
\begin{bmatrix}
1 & 1 & 1 & 1 & 1 & 1 \\
x_{11} & x_{12} & x_{13} & x_{14} & x_{15} & x_{16} \\
x_{21} & x_{22} & x_{23} & x_{24} & x_{25} & x_{26} \\
x_{31} & x_{32} & x_{33} & x_{34} & x_{35} & x_{36} \\
x_{41} & x_{42} & x_{43} & x_{44} & x_{45} & x_{46} \\
x_{51} & x_{52} & x_{53} & x_{54} & x_{55} & x_{56} \\
x_{61} & x_{62} & x_{63} & x_{64} & x_{65} & x_{66}
\end{bmatrix}_{7 \times 6}
\begin{bmatrix}
1 & x_{11} & x_{21} & x_{31} & x_{41} & x_{51} & x_{61} \\
1 & x_{12} & x_{22} & x_{32} & x_{42} & x_{52} & x_{62} \\
1 & x_{13} & x_{23} & x_{33} & x_{43} & x_{53} & x_{63} \\
1 & x_{14} & x_{24} & x_{34} & x_{44} & x_{54} & x_{64} \\
1 & x_{15} & x_{25} & x_{35} & x_{45} & x_{55} & x_{65} \\
1 & x_{16} & x_{26} & x_{36} & x_{46} & x_{56} & x_{66}
\end{bmatrix}_{6 \times 7}
\right\}^{-1} = \hat{B}
$$

$$
\begin{bmatrix}
(1 * y_1 + 1 * y_2 + 1 * y_3 + 1 * y_4 + 1 * y_5 + 1 * y_6) \\
(x_{11} * y_1 + x_{12} * y_2 + x_{13} * y_3 + x_{14} * y_4 + x_{15} * y_5 + x_{16} + y_6) \\
(x_{21} * y_1 + x_{22} * y_2 + x_{23} * y_3 + x_{24} * y_4 + x_{25} * y_5 + x_{26} + y_6) \\
(x_{31} * y_1 + x_{32} * y_2 + x_{33} * y_3 + x_{34} * y_4 + x_{35} * y_5 + x_{36} + y_6) \\
(x_{41} * y_1 + x_{42} * y_2 + x_{43} * y_3 + x_{44} * y_4 + x_{45} * y_5 + x_{46} + y_6) \\
(x_{51} * y_1 + x_{52} * y_2 + x_{53} * y_3 + x_{54} * y_4 + x_{55} * y_5 + x_{56} + y_6) \\
(x_{61} * y_1 + x_{62} * y_2 + x_{63} * y_3 + x_{64} * y_4 + x_{65} * y_5 + x_{66} + y_6)
\end{bmatrix}_{7 \times 1}
$$

$$
* \left\{ \begin{bmatrix}
(1 * 1 + 1 * 1 + 1 * 1 + 1 * 1 + 1 * 1 + 1 * 1) \\
\vdots \\
(x_{31} * 1 + x_{32} * 1 + x_{33} * 1 + x_{34} * 1 + x_{35} * 1 + x_{36} * 1) \\
(x_{51} * 1 + x_{52} * 1 + x_{53} * 1 + x_{54} * 1 + x_{55} * 1 + x_{56} * 1) \\
(x_{61} * 1 + x_{62} * 1 + x_{63} * 1 + x_{64} * 1 + x_{65} * 1 + x_{66} * 1)
\end{bmatrix} \right.
$$

$$
(1 * x_{11} + 1 * x_{12} + 1 * x_{13} + 1 * x_{14} + 1 * x_{15} + 1 * x_{16})
$$

$$
(x_{31} * x_{11} + x_{32} * x_{12} + x_{33} * x_{13} + x_{34} * x_{14} + x_{35} * x_{15} + x_{36} * x_{16})
$$

$$
(x_{51} * x_{11} + x_{52} * x_{12} + x_{53} * x_{13} + x_{54} * x_{14} + x_{55} * x_{15} + x_{56} * x_{16})
$$

$$
(x_{61} * x_{11} + x_{62} * x_{12} + x_{63} * x_{13} + x_{64} * x_{14} + x_{65} * x_{15} + x_{66} * x_{16})
$$

$$
(1 * x_{61} + 1 * x_{62} + 1 * x_{63} + 1 * x_{64} + 1 * x_{65} + 1 * x_{66})
$$

$$
(x_{31} * x_{61} + x_{32} * x_{62} + x_{33} * x_{63} + x_{34} * x_{64} + x_{35} * x_{65} + x_{36} * x_{66})
$$

$$
(x_{51} * x_{61} + x_{52} * x_{62} + x_{53} * x_{63} + x_{54} * x_{64} + x_{55} * x_{65} + x_{56} * x_{66})
$$

$$
\left. (x_{51} * x_{61} + x_{52} * x_{62} + x_{53} * x_{63} + x_{54} * x_{64} + x_{55} * x_{65} + x_{56} * x_{66}) \right\}^{-1}_{7 \times 7} = \hat{B}
$$

$$
\begin{bmatrix}
(1 * y_1 + 1 * y_2 + 1 * y_3 + 1 * y_4 + 1 * y_5 + 1 * y_6) \\
(x_{11} * y_1 + x_{12} * y_2 + x_{13} * y_3 + x_{14} * y_4 + x_{15} * y_5 + x_{16} * y_6) \\
(x_{21} * y_1 + x_{22} * y_2 + x_{23} * y_3 + x_{24} * y_4 + x_{25} * y_5 + x_{26} * y_6) \\
(x_{31} * y_1 + x_{32} * y_2 + x_{33} * y_3 + x_{34} * y_4 + x_{35} * y_5 + x_{36} * y_6) \\
(x_{41} * y_1 + x_{42} * y_2 + x_{43} * y_3 + x_{44} * y_4 + x_{45} * y_5 + x_{46} * y_6) \\
(x_{51} * y_1 + x_{52} * y_2 + x_{53} * y_3 + x_{54} * y_4 + x_{55} * y_5 + x_{56} * y_6) \\
(x_{61} * y_1 + x_{62} * y_2 + x_{63} * y_3 + x_{64} * y_4 + x_{65} * y_5 + x_{66} * y_6)
\end{bmatrix}_{7 \times 1}
*
\begin{bmatrix}
6 & \left(\sum_{i=1}^{i=6} x_{1i}\right) & \left(\sum_{i=1}^{i=6} x_{2i}\right) & \left(\sum_{i=1}^{i=6} x_{3i}\right) & \left(\sum_{i=1}^{i=6} x_{4i}\right) & \left(\sum_{i=1}^{i=6} x_{5i}\right) & \left(\sum_{i=1}^{i=6} x_{6i}\right) \\
\sum_{i=1}^{i=6} x_{1i} & \sum_{i=1}^{i=6} x_{1i}x_{1i} & \sum_{i=1}^{i=6} x_{1i}x_{2i} & \sum_{i=1}^{i=6} x_{1i}x_{3i} & \sum_{i=1}^{i=6} x_{1i}x_{4i} & \sum_{i=1}^{i=6} x_{1i}x_{5i} & \sum_{i=1}^{i=6} x_{1i}x_{6i} \\
\sum_{i=1}^{i=6} x_{2i} & \sum_{i=1}^{i=6} x_{2i}x_{1i} & \sum_{i=1}^{i=6} x_{2i}x_{2i} & \sum_{i=1}^{i=6} x_{2i}x_{3i} & \sum_{i=1}^{i=6} x_{2i}x_{4i} & \sum_{i=1}^{i=6} x_{2i}x_{5i} & \sum_{i=1}^{i=6} x_{2i}x_{6i} \\
\sum_{i=1}^{i=6} x_{3i} & \sum_{i=1}^{i=6} x_{3i}x_{1i} & \sum_{i=1}^{i=6} x_{3i}x_{2i} & \sum_{i=1}^{i=6} x_{3i}x_{3i} & \sum_{i=1}^{i=6} x_{3i}x_{4i} & \sum_{i=1}^{i=6} x_{3i}x_{5i} & \sum_{i=1}^{i=6} x_{3i}x_{6i} \\
\sum_{i=1}^{i=6} x_{4i} & \sum_{i=1}^{i=6} x_{4i}x_{1i} & \sum_{i=1}^{i=6} x_{4i}x_{2i} & \sum_{i=1}^{i=6} x_{4i}x_{3i} & \sum_{i=1}^{i=6} x_{4i}x_{4i} & \sum_{i=1}^{i=6} x_{4i}x_{5i} & \sum_{i=1}^{i=6} x_{4i}x_{6i} \\
\sum_{i=1}^{i=6} x_{5i} & \sum_{i=1}^{i=6} x_{5i}x_{1i} & \sum_{i=1}^{i=6} x_{5i}x_{2i} & \sum_{i=1}^{i=6} x_{5i}x_{3i} & \sum_{i=1}^{i=6} x_{5i}x_{4i} & \sum_{i=1}^{i=6} x_{5i}x_{5i} & \sum_{i=1}^{i=6} x_{5i}x_{6i} \\
\sum_{i=1}^{i=6} x_{6i} & \sum_{i=1}^{i=6} x_{6i}x_{1i} & \sum_{i=1}^{i=6} x_{6i}x_{2i} & \sum_{i=1}^{i=6} x_{6i}x_{3i} & \sum_{i=1}^{i=6} x_{6i}x_{4i} & \sum_{i=1}^{i=6} x_{6i}x_{5i} & \sum_{i=1}^{i=6} x_{6i}x_{6i}
\end{bmatrix}^{-1}_{7 \times 7} = B
$$

$$
\begin{bmatrix}
\left(\sum_{i=1}^{i=6} y_i\right) \\
\left(\sum_{i=1}^{i=6} x_{1i}y_i\right) \\
\left(\sum_{i=1}^{i=6} x_{2i}y_i\right) \\
\left(\sum_{i=1}^{i=6} x_{3i}y_i\right) \\
\left(\sum_{i=1}^{i=6} x_{4i}y_i\right) \\
\left(\sum_{i=1}^{i=6} x_{5i}y_i\right) \\
\left(\sum_{i=1}^{i=6} x_{6i}y_i\right)
\end{bmatrix}_{7\times1}
*
\begin{bmatrix}
6 & \left(\sum x_{1i}\right) & \left(\sum x_{2i}\right) & \left(\sum x_{3i}\right) & \left(\sum x_{4i}\right) & \left(\sum x_{5i}\right) & \left(\sum x_{6i}\right) \\
\left(\sum x_{1i}\right) & \left(\sum x_{1i}^2\right) & \left(\sum x_{1i}x_{2i}\right) & \left(\sum x_{1i}x_{3i}\right) & \left(\sum x_{1i}x_{4i}\right) & \left(\sum x_{1i}x_{5i}\right) & \left(\sum x_{1i}x_{6i}\right) \\
\left(\sum x_{2i}\right) & \left(\sum x_{2i}x_{1i}\right) & \left(\sum x_{2i}^2\right) & \left(\sum x_{2i}x_{3i}\right) & \left(\sum x_{2i}x_{4i}\right) & \left(\sum x_{2i}x_{5i}\right) & \left(\sum x_{2i}x_{6i}\right) \\
\left(\sum x_{3i}\right) & \left(\sum x_{3i}x_{1i}\right) & \left(\sum x_{3i}x_{2i}\right) & \left(\sum x_{3i}^2\right) & \left(\sum x_{3i}x_{4i}\right) & \left(\sum x_{3i}x_{5i}\right) & \left(\sum x_{3i}x_{6i}\right) \\
\left(\sum x_{4i}\right) & \left(\sum x_{4i}x_{1i}\right) & \left(\sum x_{4i}x_{2i}\right) & \left(\sum x_{4i}x_{3i}\right) & \left(\sum x_{4i}^2\right) & \left(\sum x_{4i}x_{5i}\right) & \left(\sum x_{4i}x_{6i}\right) \\
\left(\sum x_{5i}\right) & \left(\sum x_{5i}x_{1i}\right) & \left(\sum x_{5i}x_{2i}\right) & \left(\sum x_{5i}x_{3i}\right) & \left(\sum x_{5i}x_{4i}\right) & \left(\sum x_{5i}^2\right) & \left(\sum x_{5i}x_{6i}\right) \\
\left(\sum x_{6i}\right) & \left(\sum x_{6i}x_{1i}\right) & \left(\sum x_{6i}x_{2i}\right) & \left(\sum x_{6i}x_{3i}\right) & \left(\sum x_{6i}x_{4i}\right) & \left(\sum x_{6i}x_{5i}\right) & \left(\sum x_{6i}^2\right)
\end{bmatrix}_{7\times7}^{-1}
= \hat{B}
$$

$$
\begin{bmatrix}
(n\,y) \\
\left(\sum x_{1i}y_i\right) \\
\left(\sum x_{2i}y_i\right) \\
\left(\sum x_{3i}y_i\right) \\
\left(\sum x_{4i}y_i\right) \\
\left(\sum x_{5i}y_i\right) \\
\left(\sum x_{6i}y_i\right)
\end{bmatrix}_{7\times1}
*
\begin{bmatrix}
6 & (n\,x_1) & (n\,x_2) & (n\,x_3) & (n\,x_4) & (n\,x_5) & (n\,x_6) \\
(n\,x_1) & \left(\sum x_{1i}^2\right) & \left(\sum x_{1i}x_{2i}\right) & \left(\sum x_{1i}x_{3i}\right) & \left(\sum x_{1i}x_{4i}\right) & \left(\sum x_{1i}x_{5i}\right) & \left(\sum x_{1i}x_{6i}\right) \\
(n\,x_2) & \left(\sum x_{2i}x_{1i}\right) & \left(\sum x_{2i}^2\right) & \left(\sum x_{2i}x_{3i}\right) & \left(\sum x_{2i}x_{4i}\right) & \left(\sum x_{2i}x_{5i}\right) & \left(\sum x_{2i}x_{6i}\right) \\
(n\,x_3) & \left(\sum x_{3i}x_{1i}\right) & \left(\sum x_{3i}x_{2i}\right) & \left(\sum x_{3i}^2\right) & \left(\sum x_{3i}x_{4i}\right) & \left(\sum x_{3i}x_{5i}\right) & \left(\sum x_{3i}x_{6i}\right) \\
(n\,x_4) & \left(\sum x_{4i}x_{1i}\right) & \left(\sum x_{4i}x_{2i}\right) & \left(\sum x_{4i}x_{3i}\right) & \left(\sum x_{4i}^2\right) & \left(\sum x_{4i}x_{5i}\right) & \left(\sum x_{4i}x_{6i}\right) \\
(n\,x_5) & \left(\sum x_{5i}x_{1i}\right) & \left(\sum x_{5i}x_{2i}\right) & \left(\sum x_{5i}x_{3i}\right) & \left(\sum x_{5i}x_{4i}\right) & \left(\sum x_{5i}^2\right) & \left(\sum x_{5i}x_{6i}\right) \\
(n\,x_6) & \left(\sum x_{6i}x_{1i}\right) & \left(\sum x_{6i}x_{2i}\right) & \left(\sum x_{6i}x_{3i}\right) & \left(\sum x_{6i}x_{4i}\right) & \left(\sum x_{6i}x_{5i}\right) & \left(\sum x_{6i}^2\right)
\end{bmatrix}_{7\times7}^{-1}
= B
$$

Upon calculating the above matrices, we are going to get out regression coefficients.

Problem 25.4 on Multi-Linear Regression:

The marks of ten pharmacy students who were successful in their examinations in the end semester are as follows. Construct a multi-linear regression using Excel and report the equation.

Student No	Percentage Marks (Y)	(X₁)	(X₂)	(X₃)	(X₄)	(X₅)	(X₆)
1	73	75	80	50	80	40	110
2	73	60	92	55	66	45	120
3	66	50	65	60	50	30	140
4	71	88	78	51	77	30	100
5	63	90	50	65	50	35	90
6	81	77	88	51	88	48	134
7	74	80	50	78	55	35	145
8	63	40	53	58	56	47	123
9	60	65	43	51	70	30	99
10	60	70	50	78	45	35	79

Solution:

When correlation operation was conducted on MS Office Excel relating to independent variables (i.e., subjects marks), the following matrix is observed.

	(X1)	(X2)	(X3)	(X4)	(X5)	(X6)
(X1)	1					
(X2)	0.0838248	1				
(X3)	0.1018281	-0.570630904	1			
(X4)	0.2737306	0.67222642	-0.784452	1		
(X5)	-0.289992	0.474531812	-0.209235	0.31945438	1	
(X6)	-0.33736	0.283692815	-0.055571	0.151496644	0.300719648	1

When a linear regression operation was conducted on MS Office Excel relating to one dependent variable and six independent variables, the output was found to be

SUMMARY OUTPUT

Regression Statistics	
Multiple R	1
R Square	1
Adjusted R Square	1
Standard Error	1.505E-15
Observations	10

ANOVA

	df	SS	MS	F	Significance F
Regression	6	449.7805556	74.963426	3.3108E+31	8.11958E-48
Residual	3	6.79262E-30	2.264E-30		
Total	9	449.7805556			

	Coefficients	Standard Error	t Stat	P-value	Lower 95%	Upper 95%	Lower 95.0%	Upper 95.0%
Intercept	-1.42E-14	8.05321E-15	-1.764619	0.175815912	-3.98398E-14	1.14181E-14	-3.98398E-14	1.14181E-14
(X1)	0.1666667	5.3476E-17	3.117E+15	**7.28453E-47**	0.166666667	0.166666667	0.166666667	0.166666667
(X2)	0.1666667	4.25484E-17	3.917E+15	**3.66923E-47**	0.166666667	0.166666667	0.166666667	0.166666667
(X3)	0.1666667	1.07889E-16	1.545E+15	**5.98218E-46**	0.166666667	0.166666667	0.166666667	0.166666667
(X4)	0.1666667	8.77808E-17	1.899E+15	**3.22198E-46**	0.166666667	0.166666667	0.166666667	0.166666667
(X5)	0.1666667	9.69896E-17	1.718E+15	**4.34611E-46**	0.166666667	0.166666667	0.166666667	0.166666667
(X6)	0.1666667	2.85078E-17	5.846E+15	**1.10361E-47**	0.166666667	0.166666667	0.166666667	0.166666667

Hence, the equation can be written as

$Y = -1.42 * 10^{-14} + 0.17 * X1 + 0.17 * X2 + 0.17 * X3 + 0.17 * X4 + 0.17 * X5 + 0.17 * X6$

Here, the p-value for all the independent variables is less than 0.05 and hence significant enough.

In MS Office Excel, it is necessary to add at every step one independent variable and conduct regression and check for p value for significance and up on adding at each step one independent variable, we can expect six linear regression equations. Of which we have to ensure for best fit regression line.

When the same operation was conducted using an online regression calculator (say statistics kingdom), the equation generated is as follows:

$Y = -0.93 + 0.15 X_1 + 0.17 X_2 + 0.20 X_3 + 0.20 X_4 + 0.14 X_5 + 0.16 X_6$

26 Inventory Control

26.0 Introduction

Inventory can be defined as a statistical numerical compilation of stock position in a drug store at a defined time. Especially in terms of monetary value, inventory value is a better term for knowing the stock position. For a drug store, it is believed that about 30 percent of the working capital is invested on purchasing and maintaining the stock.

26.1 Objectives

The three objectives of an inventory control system in a drug store or in a hospital are as follows:

1. For providing better customer service i.e., when a customer reaches with the prescription, the drug store should be in a position to provide the drug product immediately.

2. To reduce the cost of inventory itself so that, the working capital may be used for other requirements in a drug store or the hospital.

3. To reduce the manufacturing cost. This can be considered with manufacturing pharmacy in a hospital or in a pharmaceutical manufacturing company. In either the case, a poor inventory system may lead short fall of the drug product or the raw materials and this lead to delay in the manufacturing process leading to extra expenditures.

26.2 Methods of Establishing Inventory Control

In order to maintain proper inventory, the following are some of the methods that can be used.

i. Always Better Control (ABC) Analysis

In this method, the items are categorized into A, B and C items. The classification of the items is made using cost as well as volume as parameters. In case of 'A' items, they have a volume of 10 % (say) and cost of 70% (say). In case of 'B' items, they have a volume of 20 % and cost of 20 %. In case of 'C' items, they have a volume of 70 % and cost of 10 % of the entire stock in the pharmacy store.

While reviewing the inventory and for new purchase, the pharmacist have to be cautious and stringent for A items, bit liberal to B items and completely liberal for C items.

ii. Economic Order Quantity (EOQ)

For this method, order cost and inventory carrying cost are the two parameters to be taken into consideration. Order cost is the expenditure relating to paper, typing, posting, filing for preparing the purchase order. In case of inventory carrying cost, the expenditure incurred for transport, insurance, taxes, storage and breakage or damaged products.

a. Tabular method:

This method helps in understanding how many purchase order for a better inventory can be planned. The method helps in establishing the number of purchase orders per year that are suitable for the organization.

Let us assume annual purchase orders as 12, 6, 4, 3, 2, 1 for monthly, bi-monthly, quarterly, every four months, half yearly, and yearly respectively. Among these which is the best inventory for the organization has to be established. For this, preliminary establishment of order cost and inventory carrying cost is necessary. Let us imagine the order cost is Rs. 10/- and inventory carrying cost is 10% of the rupee value of annual usage. Let us image the purchase order is planned for Rs. 1000/-

Number of Orders per Year (a)	Annual Ordering Cost (b) = a X Rs. 10/-	Annual Inventory Carrying Cost (c) = Inventory Carrying Cost X Investment Rupee Value/No. of Months	Total Annual Cost (b + c)
12	120	8.33	128.33
6	60	16.66	76.66
4	40	25.00	65.00
3	30	33.33	63.33
2	20	50.00	70.00
1	10	100.00	110.00

Among above computations, the best inventory plan is for three purchase order per year (purchase order for every four months) corresponding to the lowest annual cost of 63.33.

b. Graphical method:

In this case a plot of order quantity (on x-axis) and cost to order and carry (on y-axis) is plotted, Figure 26.1. Two curves are established as annual ordering cost and as total annual cost to order and carry. The sum of the annual ordering cost and total annual cost to order and carry lead to another line in the plot which is a straight line from origin. The best 'Economic Order Quantity' is the lowest coinciding value for both the annual ordering cost and the total annual cost to order and carry which coincides on the straight line of ordering cost. This coinciding value on the straight line is taken as best Economic Order

Quantity.

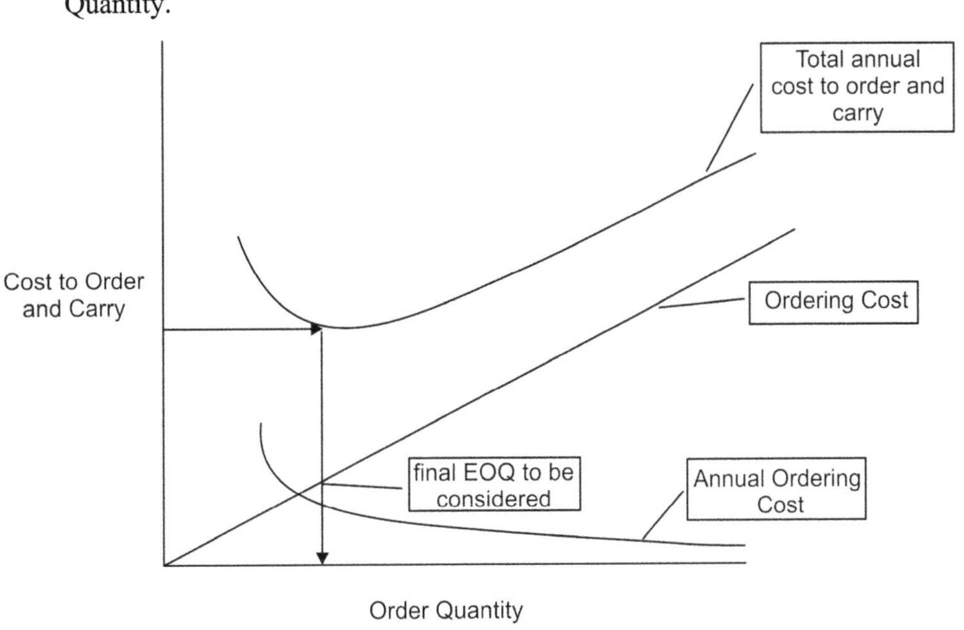

FIGURE 26.1 Graphical Representation for EOQ

c. Arithmetic method:

In this method, a simple mathematical equation is used for determining the Economic Order Quantity (EOQ).

$$EOQ = \sqrt{\frac{2\,a\,b}{c\,s}}$$

Where, a = annual consumption, b = buying cost per order, c = cost per unit of material, s = storage and other inventory carrying cost.

Problem 26.1, to calculate EOQ using arithmetic method: Annual usage of a material is 1200 units and its cost is Rs. 10/- to handle an order for this material. The price is Rs. 1/- per unit regardless of the quantity purchased and carrying cost of inventory is 24% per year.

Solution: The equation for calculating EOQ is

$$EOQ = \sqrt{\frac{2\,a\,b}{c\,s}}$$

Here a = 1200 units, b= Rs. 10/- per order, c= Rs. 1/- per unit and s= 24/100

Therefore,

$$EOQ = \sqrt{\frac{2\,(1200)(10)}{(1)(\frac{24}{100})}} = 316 \text{ units}$$

iii. Perpetual Inventory System

a. Bin card method

In this method, a bin card is used every time when the stock entered into the pharmacy during purchase and stock sold to customer by making an entry in the card. Using of such a card method updates every time the stock position of the drug product.

Hence, bin card method helps in monitoring the product when received, issued and the stock position. This card can be compared with the card system used in a library for a book. Hence, in a pharmacy, several times picking up the card may be alphabetical or item code etc. Figure 26.2, illustrates a model bin card used in a pharmacy store.

BIN CARD					
Description of Material:			Bin No:		
Code No:			Normal Quantity to Order:		
Stores Ledger Folio No:			Maximum Stock Level:		
			Re-order stock Level		
Date	Receipt		Issue		Balance Quantity
	G. R. No.	Quantity	S. R. No:	Quantity	

FIGURE 26.2 M/s. ABC Pharmacy, Hyderabad - Bin Card

b. Store ledger method

In this method, the leaf lets of each product and its stock status is maintained at the accounting department. The stock position in the main stores, issued to main pharmacy etc is recorded. Figure 26.3 illustrates the leaflet.

Stores Ledger Account													
Description of Material:			Bin No:										
Code No:			Maximum Stock Level:										
Stores Ledger Folio No:			Minimum Stock Level:										
Location:			Re-order Level:										
Unit:			Ordering Quantity:										
Date	Receipt				Issue				Balance Quantity			Stock Verified	
	G. R. No.	Qty	Rate	Amt	S. R. No.	Qty	Rate	Amt	Qty	Rate	Amt	Date	Initial	Remarks

FIGURE 26.3 M/s. ABC Pharmacy, Hyderabad – Store Ledger Account Leaflet

c. Continuous stock monitoring method

In this method, every item in the pharmacy store is checked for stock position at fixed number of times but not all at once but at fixed intervals. For instance, if a drug store has 1000 products, every product is checked six times in a year for stock position out of a total of say 12 reviews for stock in a year.

The advantage with perpetual inventory system is that the product status is reviewed at periodically defined and any discrepancies can be identified at the next stage of stock verification.

iv. Review of Slow and Non-moving Items

As discussed earlier, cost of the inventory is about 30 percent of the working capital. Under such circumstances it is necessary to identify slow and not-moving drug products so that such products are not planned for purchase in future or purchased on just in time basis. In order to identify slow and non-moving items, the pharmacist may have to follow one or more of the following methods:

a. Periodic report

In this method, the pharmacist reviews the stock position of the items periodically i.e., monthly, quarterly and such review indicates how much purchased, how much consumed and how much balance left.

b. Obsolete items

In this method, during the regular review process of stock position, the pharmacist identifies those drug products that are becoming useless. The reason behind the product becoming useless may be due to no relevant cases etc.

c. Moving ratios

In this method, ratios are developed to identify stock that is slow moving, dormant (seasonal products) and dead stock. Once identified, a further review is made whether to purchase the product or not.

v. Input-Output Ratio Analysis Method

This method can best be illustrated with tablet manufacturing. For instance, in an organisation Paracetamol bulk drug is being used to manufacture Paracetamol tablets. Under such circumstances, let us imagine that 2 kg of bulk drug is needed and when the final product obtained as tablets was re-checked for practical yield, it was identified that only 1.6 kg of the Paracetamol was consumed for the tablets. Thus, the input was 2 kg and the output was 1.6 kg. When a ratio of input/output is calculated, then it is found to be $2/1.6 \times 100 = 125\%$.

Such method helps in careful monitoring of the inventory both in terms of purchase as well as better management to minimize wastage.

Problem 26.2, on input-ouput ratio analysis: A pharmaceutical company uses 'A' as raw material @ Rs. 10/- per kg. The input-output ratio is 125%. Due to non availability of the raw material, the company wishes to use a supplement. The company has identified two supplements i.e., A1, A2 and using input-output ratio method, identify the supplement which is economical to purchase. The rate and input-output ratio values of the supplements are as follows:

Material	Rate per Kg	Input-Output Ratio
A1	Rs. 15/-	110%
A2	Rs. 12/-	140%

Solution:

The first step is to find out the cost of each substitute in the finished product per unit. Using the following formula one can determine the cost i.e.,

$$\textit{The Cost of the raw material} = \frac{\textit{Input}}{\textit{Output}} \times \textit{Rate per unit in the finished product}$$

Hence,

$$\textit{The Cost of the raw material (A1)} = \frac{110}{100} \times 15 = Rs.\,16.50\ per\ kg$$

$$\textit{The Cost of the raw material (A2)} = \frac{140}{100} \times 12 = Rs.\,16.80\ per\ kg$$

Among the two substitutes, it is found that substitute A1 is economical than A2.

vi. Setting up of Various Levels

In this method, upon preliminary study of various drug products used in an hospital, every product is established for its maximum stock level, minimum stock level, re-order level and danger level.

a. Maximum stock level

This is the total number of units of a drug product that can be maximum purchased for use in the hospital. A purchase crossing this value at any stage indicates a bad inventory system and unnecessary blockage of working capital on such products. The equation used to calculate maximum stock level is as follows:

$$\textit{Maximum Stock Level} = Re - order\ level + Re - order\ quantity - Minimum\ Consumption$$

$$\textit{Minimum Consumption} = Minimum\ consumption\ per\ week \times Minimum\ re - order\ period$$

b. Minimum stock level (buffer stock level or safety stock level)

In this, the pharmacist sets a drug product that go up to a minimum stock level in the pharmacy. This level indicates a preliminary warning that the drug product stock position is reaching for fresh purchase. The method of calculation of this level takes into consideration two factors i.e., average rate of consumption, lead time (the time consumed to recognize the need of the item till the time it is received into the pharmacy store).

Minimum stock Level

$$= Re - order\ level$$
$$- [Normal\ Consumption\ per\ week \times Average\ delivery\ time]$$

c. Re-Order level

This is the stage where the inventory for the drug product indicates the pharmacist has to place a fresh order for the drug product. This level is slightly more than the minimum stock level to guard against abnormal use, abnormal delay in supply of the item.

Re − order Level = Minimum Consumption during the period × Maximum

reorder period

d. Danger level

If the drug product inventory reaches this stage it indicates the inventory system has a flaw and a pharmacist should not achieve this level at any stage and ensures always the products are maintained at the safe levels to prevent lack of stock.

vii. Material Budgeting

In this method, every drug product is established for inventory, inventory value and budget with simultaneous monitoring of the budget for entire drug products in the pharmacy. This system helps in understanding what is the current stock position for a drug product, how much was purchased and consumed in previous month and how much was purchased and consumed in the previous year for the same month. Such system helps in monitoring and prevent from over buying and under buying of the product.

It is necessary in several cases; every purchase made is subtracted from the balance of the purchase budget maintained in a separate purchase journal. This prevents from over and under buying of the product.

viii. Establishing Effective Purchase Procedures

In this system, the pharmacist upon maintaining the basic inventory parameters, he/she systematically maintains procedures such as identifying vendors, release of purchase order, receiving and verification of stock, maintaining the invoice and release of payment etc.

ix. Scrap and Surplus Disposal

Anything that is useless is a scrap and this scrap has very less economical value. In several circumstances, a scarp is re-processed and product is manufactured. Where scarp that is not re-usable it is completely destroyed, incinerated etc. For instance, during a tablet manufacture, certain amount of loose powder is witnessed and such scarp is re-processed to get again tablets. In case of a reactor in a pharmaceutical manufacturing industry, after ware and tare of the reactor certain weak spots are developed and further use may lead defective products. In such circumstance, the reactor is completely a scrap.

Scarp can be classified into legitimate, administrative and defective types. In case of legitimate scrap, the wastage occurring is anticipated beforehand (for instance loose powder during tablet manufacture), in case of administrative scrap, the wastage is generated due to change in administrative policy (for instance due to change in tablet strip design) and in case of defective scrap, the waste is generated during the process of manufacture (for instance chipping of tablet during manufacture).

In case of the concept of surplus, a week and improper inventory system may lead to production of the product in surplus. Such surplus may have to be forcibly released into the market or has to be completely destroyed in certain circumstances.

x. **VED Analysis (Vital, Essential, Desirable analysis)**

Let us imagine only Paracetamol containing tablets. Based on the number of prescriptions dispensed, the various brands of the Paracetamol tablets are sorted into Vital, Essential and Desirable items. If 70% of the total prescriptions suggest for brand 'A', then this item brand is vital. If 20% of the total prescriptions suggest for brand 'B', then this item brand is essential. If 10% of the total prescriptions suggest for brand 'C', then this item brand is desirable.

Hence, different brands of the same drug and strength are sorted under VED analysis and inventory is planned.

27 Accountancy and Book Keeping

27.0 Introduction

In an organisation every single transaction relating to either cash or good movement is recorded and this procedure is called as book keeping. Hence, a book keeping helps in monitoring a transaction and its influence on assets and liabilities of a business.

A book keeping involves with entry of transactions in a journal along with the basic supporting documents (such as cash vouchers, receipts, bills, invoice etc.). A book keeping entries are usually made by a sub-ordinate personnel and such entries helps in developing ledger entries to know the balance. A book keeping is accessed only for the individual company and from the information compiled; one may not assess the profits and loss of a company.

In contrast to book keeping, accountancy is a process of ensuring correct and quality entries of transactions were made. This helps in better interpreting of the profit and loss of a company and is usually helpful for the authority that is inspecting the entries and assessing the financial status of a company. Maintenance of accountancy involves with generation of balance sheet, trial balance and such activity is made by responsible higher authority. The true financial position of the company can be understood by accountancy.

Book keeping is usually of double entry system. This means that a transaction made between two parties is entered in the book with respect to both the parties. For instance, Company A has sold its products to Company B. The number of goods sold and cash received by company A is maintained in Goods A/c and Cash A/c of company 'A' as well as in Goods received and cash given by Company B. This is an indication of maintenance of book-keeping with respect to Company A only.

The demarcation point between book-keeping and accountancy is that book-keeping is the responsibility of junior staff where as accounting working is the responsibility of the higher authority of the department or organisation. In addition to this, book-keeping does not reveal the profit and loss of the organisation, where as in the accountancy books it provide the details.

It is also necessary to understand that maintenance of various books such as journal, various cash books, purchase books/registers, sales books/registers, purchase return book/register, sales return book/register etc depends on the size of business and the number of transactions. However, in any type of business one can expect the fundamental book such as journal, cash book, day book, and ledger.

When an accounts audit is made for the company, a third party or government or inspector scrutinizes the main books such as ledger and if necessary the other reference books are referred.

For maintaining a book keeping, various kinds of books are being used and they are as follows:

1. **Journal**
2. **Cash book**
    i.   Simple cash book
    ii. Double column cash book
    iii. Petty cash book
3. **Other day books/registers**
    i.   Purchase book/register
    ii. Sales book/register
    iii. Purchase returns book/register
    iv. Sales return book/register

A journal is usually of all kinds of transactions and such transactions are based on supporting documents. Cash books usually handle entries relating all cash transactions of the day. In case of day book, all the transactions that were made without cash are usually entered and such transactions receive the cash payment at a later day. For instance, a company has sold its products to another company on credit basis and immediate cash payment was not made.

27.1 Types of Accounts

There are two types of accounts i.e., personal and non-personal accounts. In non-personal accounts again there are two types of accounts i.e., real and nominal accounts.

This can be illustrated as below Figure 27.1.

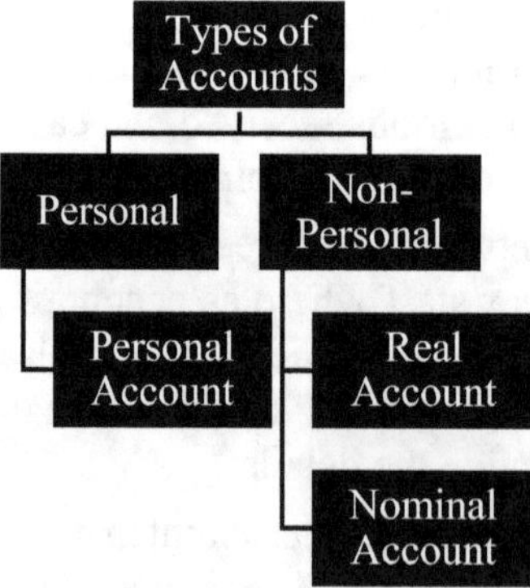

FIGURE 27.1 Types of Accounts

Personal Account: An individual account is opened in the name of person, company or institute, creditors (vendor accounts), debtors (customer accounts), advances. For instance, accounts are opened in the book in the name of Mr. ABC, M/s. Hyderabad Pharmacy, XYZ Educational Trust, capital A/c. All debtor accounts are relating to amounts receivable from customers/others. All creditor accounts are relating to amounts payable to vendors/others.

Real Account: In this case accounts are opened in the name of building, cash, furniture, stock (i.e., purchase, sales), land, machinery, bank etc.

Nominal Account: In this case accounts are opened in the book in the name of discount, insurance, rent, wages, salaries, cost of stationery items, interest, commission, goodwill, etc. Hence, nominal accounts are fictitious.

27.2 Types of Entry

In any account related book, transactions are entered as debit or credit. The receiver of a benefit is called as debtor and transaction is debited on the left hand side (debit side). Whereas, the giver of a benefit is called as creditor and transaction is credited on the right hand side (credit side).

Based on the type of account, the entry is decided whether it is debit or credit.

The fundamental definitions for debit and credit with respect to account type are as follows:

1. **Personal Account:** In case of personal account, debit the receiver and credit the giver.

2. **Real Account:** In case of real account, debit what comes in and credit what goes out.

3. **Nominal Account:** In case of nominal account, debit all expenses, loss and credit all income, profits.

This is better illustrated by the below given table:

Name of Account	Debit	Credit
Personal Account	Debit the Receiver	Credit the Giver
Real Account	Debit what comes in	Credit what goes out
Nominal Account	Debit all expenses and losses	Credit all incomes and profits

Hence, it is necessary to understand a transaction on what type of account it falls and later to determine the debit and credit transactions with respect to the account and make entries in the journal, cash book, day book etc.

While making an entry in journal, cash book, day book, ledger for a transaction, it is habitual to prefix the transaction narration with 'by' or 'Dr' for debit and with 'To' or 'Cr' for credit, for a transaction.

27.3 Anatomy of a Journal

It is usual that every organisation maintains a journal and a typical work sheet of a journal is as follows:

Date	Narration	Ledger Folio Page No	Debit (Rs.)	Credit (Rs.)

In a journal, every transaction is made in a chronological order by entering date in the first column. In the second column, based on the type of account and transaction, a debit or credit is prefixed to the narration (a small briefing of transaction made) and the corresponding money value is entered either on debit or credit side. The usage of column of ledger folio comes into picture only when the journal entry transaction is posted into the ledger. During ledger positing, details of ledger page no, and date of entry are mentioned in the ledger folio column for the corresponding transaction. Simultaneously, while making entries in the journal, the page number of journal and date of entry in the journal are made on the supporting documents of the transactions (such as bills, vouchers etc.,)

27.4 Rules for Journal Entries

In addition to type of accounts (personal, real and nominal) and corresponding debiting and crediting, several other accounts and their debiting and crediting have to be acquainted with.

a. **Goods Account:** The goods accounts are divided into purchase account, sales account, purchase return account and sales returns account. The corresponding debit and credit transactions are made in a chronological order.

b. **Capital Account:** When a businessman starts his business, some money is invested and such money is credited in the Capital Account of journal. Simultaneously in cash account the same amount is debited.

c. **Drawing Account:** It is usual that a businessman withdraws some amount of money for his personal usage and in such circumstances, in the 'drawings account' the amount is debited and in 'cash account' the same amount is credited.

d. **Trade Discount:** During a trade transaction certain amount of discount is given for the product. Such discount is mentioned along with reduced price, which in turn is mentioned in the bill. Such transactions while entering in the journal should be mentioned with the final discounted price.

e. **Cash Discount:** In several cases, during a trade transaction the business man provides an offer of cash discount, if entire cash is paid for the product within the stipulated time. In such circumstances, the discounted price reflects in a separate account called as 'Discount Account' in addition to other accounts. At the time of payment to the creditor net of discount relating to purchase amount is credited to cash or bank account and balance amount is credited to discount account and liability account of vendor is debited for full purchase amount.

Based on the various books on accounts maintained, a ledger is the final record and from this a trial balance is developed which is the summary of all the accounts recorded. A trial balance gives all debits, credit balances relating to all accounts including carry forward balances.

In case of balance sheet, it is a statement that gives the exact financial statement of affairs of the business on a particular date (normally year end and period end). It is prepared from trial balance sheet. A balance sheet indicates all the assets and liabilities that are possessed and owed respectively of a business. If assets are over liabilities, it indicates surplus/accumulated reserves of the entry. If liabilities are more than assets, the difference indicate deficit/accumulated losses of that entity.

A trial balance comprises of all account balances relating to incomes, expenses, assets, liabilities and capital. A trial balance is re-classified into balance sheet and profit & loss account. A balance sheet comprises individual account balances relating to assets, liabilities and capital. All the accounts relating to incomes, expenditures are reflected in profit and loss account.

27.5 Procedure for Making Entries in the Account Books (Journal)

For every transaction, while making an entry, the individual has to enter date of transaction and then has to provide brief narration of the transaction made. In order to judge whether on debit side or credit side the entry has to be made, by judging whether the account name comes under personal or real or nominal account and later has to keep in mind the various rules for debit and credit depending on type of account (i.e., personal or real or nominal) and then finally make an entry on the appropriate side (debit or credit). It is necessary to follow a double entry system so that at the end of every day or month or year, the transaction is well understood. Hence, in a double entry system it is not only making the entries on the company side which is maintaining the books, but also making entries from whom the transaction is made (of the other party). Finally at the end of the day, month or year both the debit and credit transactions are to be balanced (equated), else it is an indication of wrong entries or duplicate entries. It is quite commonly observed b/d (for brought down) and c/d (for carried down). The former is used for fresh entry made for adopting previous year/page account balance in the new page and the latter is used for end of the page with respect to net balance either on debit or credit side made. In certain circumstances, one cash payment receipt is provided for two transactions i.e., purchase of good as well as transport of the good to the premises. Under such circumstances, a compound entry is made for one single debit with two corresponding credits or the vice-versa. As the entries are made based on bills, while making entry of the transaction in the account book, it is necessary to make an entry on the bill indicating the page number of the account book where the entry is made as well as the date of entry in the account book (cross-reference). It is a regular practice that every day accountants working in the organisation make cash book entries, day book entries and transfer all the entries from both the books into ledger and finally ensures the total debit and total credit are equal. In other words the difference between total debit and total credit should be zero, which is called as balance.

In case of very big organisations, as the transactions are very high in number, minor and repetitive transactions in a day relating to cash are maintained separately by using petty cash book. The accounts department releases a certain amount of money as advance (or imprest account). This money is released to the concerned authority in the department in such a way that at every end of month, the detailed transactions along with petty cash entries made are submitted. Immediately, the accounts department releases petty cash for subsequent month and makes necessary entry as one transaction w.r.t petty cash transactions in the main accounts book of the previous month. This process is a cycle process so as to reduce the work load of the accounts department.

Problem 27.1, on Journal Entries: Enter the following transactions in the general journal of M/s. ABC Pharmacy for the month of May 2017:

Date	Transaction Details	Amount in Rs.
May 1	Mr. Raj Kumar started his business with a capital	Rs. 1, 00, 000=00
May 1	Bought furniture for cash from M/s. Modern Furniture	Rs. 15, 000=00
May 2	Purchased goods for cash	Rs. 25, 000=00
May 3	Purchased goods from Ram Gopal on Credit	Rs. 30, 000=00
May 5	Sold goods to Harish Kumar on Credit	Rs. 8, 000=00
May 14	Paid advertisement expenses	Rs. 2, 400=00
May 15	Received interest from Nand Lal	Rs. 150=00
May 18	Deposited Cash into bank	Rs. 1, 000=00

Solution: Journal register of M/s. ABC Pharmacy

Date		Narration	Ledger Folio	Debit (Rs.)	Credit (Rs.)
May 1, 2017	i.	Cash Account Cash for starting business by Mr. Raj Kumar Capital A/c (Cash account is real account and cash comes in)	Entry will be made here when the transaction is posted in the ledger.	Rs. 1, 00, 000 = 00	-----
	ii.	To Capital Account (implies Mr. Raj Kumar's Capital Account). To Capital Account (Capital account is personal account and here credit the giver)	Entry will be made here when the transaction is posted in the ledger.	-----	Rs. 1, 00, 000=00
May 1, 2017	i.	Furniture A/c (Furniture comes under the category of real account) for purchase of furniture from M/s. Modern Furniture. Debit what comes in	Entry will be made here when the transaction is posted in the ledger.	Rs. 15, 000 = 00	-----
	ii.	To Cash A/c (Comes under the category of real account) Credit what goes out. Here cash is going out and hence the entry is made on the credit side	Entry will be made here when the transaction is posted in the ledger.	-----	Rs. 15, 000 = 00

Contd...

Date	Narration	Ledger Folio	Debit (Rs.)	Credit (Rs.)
May 2, 2017	Purchase A/c (Goods were purchased and falls under the category of real account). Here goods are coming in and hence to be debited	Entry will be made here when the transaction is posted in the ledger.	Rs. 25, 000 = 00	-----
	To Cash A/c (Comes under the category of real account). Here, cash goes out. Hence, to be credited with brief narration saying cash given to M/s xyz for purchase of goods.	Entry will be made here when the transaction is posted in the ledger.	-----	Rs. 25, 000 = 00
May 3, 2017	Purchase A/c (Real Account). Here goods are purchased from Ram Gopal and goods come in.	Entry will be made here when the transaction is posted in the ledger.	Rs. 30, 000 = 00	-----
	To Ram Gopal A/c (Personal Account). Here cash has to be paid to Ram Gopal but transaction was made on credit. Here, goods are given by Ram Gopal and w.r.t to Ram Gopal personal account, credit the giver. This is because; Ram Gopal has given the goods.	Entry will be made here when the transaction is posted in the ledger.	-----	Rs. 30, 000 = 00
May 5, 2017	Harish Kumar A/c (Personal Account). Here goods were sold on credit to Harish Kumar and for Harish Kumar account, debit the receiver of goods.	Entry will be made here when the transaction is posted in the ledger.	Rs. 8, 000 = 00	-----
	To Sales A/c (Real Account). Here goods were sold to Harish Kumar on credit by M/s. ABC Pharmacy. Hence in the book of ABC Pharmacy, goods goes out and hence credited.	Entry will be made here when the transaction is posted in the ledger.	-----	Rs. 8, 000 = 00
May 14, 2017	Advertisement A/c (Nominal Account since it is expenditure). As advertisement is an expenditure and under nominal account, debit all expenses.	Entry will be made here when the transaction is posted in the ledger.	Rs. 2,400 = 00	-----
	To Cash A/c (Real Account) Here cash has been paid for advertisement. Under real account, credit what goes out and here cash is going out. Hence credit to Cash A/c.	Entry will be made here when the transaction is posted in the ledger.	-----	Rs. 2, 400 = 00

Contd...

Date	Narration	Ledger Folio	Debit (Rs.)	Credit (Rs.)
May 15, 2017	Cash A/c (Real Account). Here interest is received from Nand Lal. Hence, debit what comes in. As cash is coming into the business, the transaction is debited w.r.t Cash A/c.	Entry will be made here when the transaction is posted in the ledger.	Rs. 150 = 00	-----
	To Interest A/c (Nominal Account). Here, credit all incomes. As cash is coming into M/s. ABC Pharmacy as income, hence credited.	Entry will be made here when the transaction is posted in the ledger.	-----	Rs. 150 = 00
May 18, 2017	By Bank A/c (Real Account). Debit what comes in. As cash is coming into bank A/c, hence debited. Here in the book of M/s. ABC Pharmacy, under Bank Account, the transaction is debited.	Entry will be made here when the transaction is posted in the ledger.	Rs. 1, 000 = 00	-----
	To Cash A/c. (Real Account). Here, M/s. ABC Pharmacy has deposited cash into the bank. Credit what goes out. Here cash is going out and hence credited	Entry will be made here when the transaction is posted in the ledger.	-----	Rs. 1, 000 = 00
Total			**Rs. 1, 81, 550 =00**	**Rs. 1, 81, 550 = 00**

Layout formats of various types of account books:

Layout of accounts books are usually available in two formats i.e., 'T' form and the vertical forms. Usually Cash accounts are practiced in 'T' form layout format and only either cash account or bank account in single column registers/books. A two column book is a combined account of cash and bank transactions. Cash book is classified into different columns basing on nature of expenditure.

1. Single Column Cash book (T-form layout format):

Dr		Single Column Cash Book (T-layout format)					Cr
Date	Particulars	L. F	Amount (Rs.)	Date	Particulars	L. F	Amount (Rs.)
	Opening balance		xyz		Payments		abc
	Receipts		zzz		Closing balance		
	Total				Total		

Or

Single Column Cash Book (Vertical Layout format)					
Date	**Particulars**	**L. F**	**Receipts (Debit-Dr)**	**Payments (Credit-Cr)**	**Balance Amount (Rs.)**
Date	Opening balance		abc		
Date	Receipts		xyz		
Date	Payments			lmn	Net balance

2. Two Column Cash/Bank book (Vertical layout format):

Dr	Two Column Cash Book										Cr
Date	Particulars	L. F	Bank Rs.	Cash Rs.	Amount (Rs.)	Date	Particulars	L. F	Bank Rs.	Cash Rs.	Amount (Rs.)

3. Petty Cash book (or columnar cash book):

Dr													Cr
Date	Particulars	Total Amount (Rs.)	Date	Particulars	Voucher No	Total Amount (Rs.)	Conveyance (Rs.)	Stationery (Rs.)	Postage & Courier (Rs.)	Cartage (Rs.)	Misc. (Rs.)	Remarks	
1st Jun	To Cash Received	2000=00	2nd Jun	By Taxi Fare	1	120=00	120=00	---	---	---	---	---	
			5th Jun	By wages	2	500=00					500=00		

4. Purchases Register:

Date	Invoice No	Name of the supplier	L. F	Amount (Rs.)

5. Sales Register:

Date	Invoice No	Name of the customer	L. F	Amount (Rs.)

6. Purchases Returns Register:

Date	Debit Note No	Name of the supplier	L. F	Amount (Rs.)

7. Sales Return Register:

Date	Credit Note No	Name of the customer	L. F	Amount (Rs.)

8. Ledger:

Dr	Ledger Book						Cr
Date	Particulars	J.F	Amount (Rs.)	Date	Particulars	J. F	Amount (Rs.)

27.6 Posting of Ledger

Every transaction which was entered in various books is finally posted in the ledger book. In a ledger book, a separate page is used for every account such as bank account, salaries account, cash account, capital account, machinery account, purchase account, building account, individual's name account, sales account, and interest account etc. A transaction which is debited in a journal entry is posted on the credit side of the ledger and a transaction credited in a journal entry is posted to the debit side of ledger. This is because the postings are made in the particular account. Hence the rules are to be framed basing on the nature of transaction relating to that account.

Problem 27.2, on postings in Ledger:

M/s. ABC Pharmacy journal entries are as given below. Illustrate the Ledger book entries for the same.

Date	Narration	Ledger Folio	Debit (Rs.)	Credit (Rs.)
May 1, 2017	i. Cash Account Cash for starting business by Mr. Raj Kumar Capital A/c (Cash account is real account and cash comes in)	Entry will be made here when the transaction is posted in the ledger.	Rs. 1, 00, 000 = 00	-----
	ii. To Capital Account (implies Mr. Raj Kumar's Capital Account). To Capital Account (Capital account is personal account and here credit the giver)	Entry will be made here when the transaction is posted in the ledger.	-----	Rs. 1, 00, 000=00
May 1, 2017	i. Furniture A/c (Furniture comes under the category of real account) for purchase of furniture from M/s. Modern Furniture. Debit what comes in	Entry will be made here when the transaction is posted in the ledger.	Rs. 15, 000 = 00	-----
	ii. To Cash A/c (Comes under the category of real account) Credit what goes out. Here cash is going out and hence the entry is made on the credit side	Entry will be made here when the transaction is posted in the ledger.	-----	Rs. 15, 000 = 00
May 2, 2017	Purchase A/c (Goods were purchased and falls under the category of real account). Here goods are coming in and hence to be debited	Entry will be made here when the transaction is posted in the ledger.	Rs. 25, 000 = 00	-----
	To Cash A/c (Comes under the category of real account). Here, cash goes out. Hence, to be credited with brief narration saying cash given to M/s xyz for purchase of goods.	Entry will be made here when the transaction is posted in the ledger.	-----	Rs. 25, 000 = 00

Contd...

Date	Narration	Ledger Folio	Debit (Rs.)	Credit (Rs.)
May 3, 2017	Purchase A/c (Real Account). Here goods are purchased from Ram Gopal and goods come in.	Entry will be made here when the transaction is posted in the ledger.	Rs. 30, 000 = 00	-----
	To Ram Gopal A/c (Personal Account). Here cash has to be paid to Ram Gopal but transaction was made on credit. Here, goods are given by Ram gopal and w.r.t to Ram Gopal personal account, credit the giver. This is because; Ram Gopal has given the goods.	Entry will be made here when the transaction is posted in the ledger.	-----	Rs. 30, 000 = 00
May 5, 2017	Harish Kumar A/c (Personal Account). Here goods were sold on credit to Harish Kumar and for Harish kumar account, debit the receiver of goods.	Entry will be made here when the transaction is posted in the ledger.	Rs. 8, 000 = 00	-----
	To Sales A/c (Real Account). Here goods were sold to Harish Kumar on credit by M/s. ABC Pharmacy. Hence in the book of ABC Pharmacy, goods goes out and hence credited.	Entry will be made here when the transaction is posted in the ledger.	-----	Rs. 8, 000 = 00
May 14, 2017	Advertisement A/c (Nominal Account since it is expenditure). As advertisement is an expenditure and under nominal account, debit all expenses.	Entry will be made here when the transaction is posted in the ledger.	Rs. 2,400 = 00	-----
	To Cash A/c (Real Account) Here cash has been paid for advertisement. Under real account, credit what goes out and here cash is going out. Hence credit to Cash A/c.	Entry will be made here when the transaction is posted in the ledger.	-----	Rs. 2, 400 = 00
May 15, 2017	Cash A/c (Real Account). Here interest is received from Nand Lal. Hence, debit what comes in. As cash is coming into the business, the transaction is debited w.r.t Cash A/c.	Entry will be made here when the transaction is posted in the ledger.	Rs. 150 = 00	-----
	To Interest A/c (Nominal Account). Here, credit all incomes. As cash is coming into M/s. ABC Pharmacy as income, hence credited.	Entry will be made here when the transaction is posted in the ledger.	-----	Rs. 150 = 00

Contd...

Date	Narration	Ledger Folio	Debit (Rs.)	Credit (Rs.)
May 18, 2017	By Bank A/c (Real Account). Debit what comes in. As cash is coming into bank A/c, hence debited. Here in the book of M/s. ABC Pharmacy, under Bank Account, the transaction is debited.	Entry will be made here when the transaction is posted in the ledger.	Rs. 1, 000 = 00	-----
	To Cash A/c. (Real Account). Here, M/s. ABC Pharmacy has deposited cash into the bank. Credit what goes out. Here cash is going out and hence credited	Entry will be made here when the transaction is posted in the ledger.	-----	Rs. 1, 000 = 00
Total			**Rs. 1, 81, 550 =00**	**Rs. 1, 81, 550 = 00**

Solution w.r.t to M/s. ABC Pharmacy Ledger Postings:

Dr			Ledger Book Page No: 2 Cash A/c				Cr
Date	Particulars	J. F	Amount (Rs.)	Date	Particulars	J. F	Amount (Rs.)
1 May, 2017	To Capital A/c		Rs. 1, 00, 000=00	1 May, 2017	By Furniture A/c		Rs. 15, 000=00
15 May, 2017	To Interest A/c		Rs. 150=00	2 May 2017	By Purchase A/c		Rs. 25, 000=00
				14 May, 2017	By Advertisement A/c		Rs. 2, 400=00
				18 May, 2017	By Bank A/c		Rs. 1, 000=00

Dr			Ledger Book Page No: 3 Capital A/c				Cr
Date	Particulars	J. F	Amount (Rs.)	Date	Particulars	J. F	Amount (Rs.)
				1 May, 2017	By Cash A/c		Rs. 1, 00, 000=00

Dr			Ledger Book Page No: 4 Furniture A/c				Cr
Date	Particulars	J. F	Amount (Rs.)	Date	Particulars	J. F	Amount (Rs.)
1 May, 2017	To Cash A/c		Rs. 15, 000=00				

Dr			Ledger Book Page No: 5 Purchase A/c				Cr
Date	Particulars	J. F	Amount (Rs.)	Date	Particulars	J. F	Amount (Rs.)
2 May, 2017	To Cash A/c		Rs. 25, 000=00				
2 May, 2017	To Ram Gopal A/c		Rs. 30, 000=00				

Dr			Ledger Book Page No: 6 Ram Gopal A/c				Cr
Date	**Particulars**	**J. F**	**Amount (Rs.)**	**Date**	**Particulars**	**J. F**	**Amount (Rs.)**
				3 May, 2017	By Purchase A/c		Rs. 30, 000=00

Dr			Ledger Book Page No: 7 Harish Kumar A/c				Cr
Date	**Particulars**	**J. F**	**Amount (Rs.)**	**Date**	**Particulars**	**J. F**	**Amount (Rs.)**
5 May 2017	To Sales A/c		Rs. 8, 000=00				

Dr			Ledger Book Page No: 8 Sales A/c				Cr
Date	**Particulars**	**J. F**	**Amount (Rs.)**	**Date**	**Particulars**	**J. F**	**Amount (Rs.)**
				5 May 2017	By Harish Kumar A/c		Rs. 8, 000=00

Dr			Ledger Book Page No: 9 Advertisement A/c				Cr
Date	**Particulars**	**J. F**	**Amount (Rs.)**	**Date**	**Particulars**	**J. F**	**Amount (Rs.)**
14 May, 2017	To Cash A/c		Rs. 2, 400=00				

Dr			Ledger Book Page No: 10 Interest A/c				Cr
Date	**Particulars**	**J. F**	**Amount (Rs.)**	**Date**	**Particulars**	**J. F**	**Amount (Rs.)**
				15 May, 2017	By Cash A/c		Rs. 150=00

Dr			Ledger Book Page No: 11 Bank A/c				Cr
Date	**Particulars**	**J. F**	**Amount (Rs.)**	**Date**	**Particulars**	**J. F**	**Amount (Rs.)**
18 May, 2017	To Cash A/c		Rs. 1, 000=00				

28 Management Report

28.0 Introduction

Management report is defined as a system of communication, normally in the written form, of facts which should be brought to the attention of various levels of management who use them to take suitable action.

In a broad sense, management reporting can be categorized into reporting the status of work to the immediate authority and the other as a report of a company being submitted to the owner of the company so as to bring it to public, stake holders, investors, bank, financial institutions etc.,

28.1 Objectives

i.   To acquire the information and execute the managerial functions such as planning, organizing, controlling, directing, and decision making etc., efficiently and effectively.

ii. To assess the operational efficiency of an organisation.

iii. To provide better and maximum resources for use.

iv. To bring out an understanding of the various activities executed among the personnel.

v.   To improve discipline and moral principles.

vi. To help the management to come out with effective decision makings.

28.2 Essentials of a Good Management Reporting System

For a better management system, the responsible authority should be aware of all aspects of work taking place in his department or organisation. Such aspects are recorded and are suitable for taking decisions at any point of time. Hence, such records either of the past, present or to be drafted in the future should be uniform for comparison within a domain as well as a whole. To fulfill, uniformity (harmonization) in reporting system should be proposed for implementation. Hence, every individual who is reporting to immediate higher authority has to ensure his reporting document comprises of proper format, contents available in a logical sequence, maintain promptness, accurate in documenting by providing correct information, should be comparable with past reports documented, consistent in maintaining uniformity, relevant to the aspect being under discussion, simple such that every individual understand the contents by avoiding technical terms, conduct cost-benefit analysis with respect to reporting, involving managing authority on the principle of management by exception instead as a rule of the day, and has control over control and beyond the control parameters.

28.3 Classification of Management Reporting

The management reporting is of either of oral or written report forms. An oral reporting system may be in the form of intangible form but, such reporting can be made into tangible form by audio-video recording. In case of written report system, it can be further sub-classified that is,

I. **According to Objects:**

    A. External Reports

    B. Internal Reports

        i. Reports meant for top management

        ii. Reports meant for middle level management

        iii. Reports meant for junior level management

II. **According to Period:**

        i. Routine Reports: Such as daily, weekly, monthly reports

        ii. Special Reports: Specific cases where separate reports are required

III. **According to Functions:**

    A. Operating Reports

        i. Control Reports

        ii. Information Reports

        iii. Venture Measurement Reports

    B. Financial Reports

        i. Static Reports

        ii. Dynamic Reports

A. External Reports:

External Reports are reports assumed as authored by the head of the organisation and he/she is responsible as per law with the information provided. External reports are meant for Government, share holders, bankers, investors, financial institutions etc. Such reports are drafted as per international or national laws and guidelines. With respect to international, drafting of an external report is based on combined country efforts of drafting guidelines such as European Union (EU) directive 2006/46/EC. The directive indicates that the responsibility for the preparation and publication of the financial statements and the management reports, at separate and consolidated level, will be based on national law. With respect to India, Article VI of The Indian Companies Act, 1956 provides the guidelines for planning, drafting and implementing a management report. Such reports are widely observed from pharmaceutical industries as 'Annual Reports'.

B. Internal Reports:

The reports are meant for internal communication purpose and are not meant for outsiders. Internal reports can be classified into three levels:

i.   **Report meant for top management:** Here the sub-ordinate authority submits to either Board of Directors including Chairman, Managing Directors, General Manager or Chief Executive of the organisation. The aspects usually covered in the report are reports on budgeted and actual profit, sales and production, capital budget, master budget, periodical financials, plant utilization, machine and labour utilization, research and development activities, project evaluation, stock of raw materials, work in progress and finished goods, overhead cost absorption and efficiency, selling and distribution overhead.

ii. **Report meant for middle level management:** The middle level management are the department heads such as production, marketing etc managers. Such managers develop reports with respect to the department with the help of their subordinates. Some of the specific reports concerned to the various departments are as follows:

   a.   **Purchase department report:** The report includes individual reports of material and price and usage variance, material carrying cost, loss of material in the storage, trends in the pertaining of various items of materials.

   b.   **Materials department report:** The report includes individual reports of stock of raw materials, work in progress and finished goods, material wastage and losses, stock of materials planning and control, level of materials at the stores, surplus and deficiency status.

   c.   **Production department report:** The report includes budgeted and actual production, overtime work and ideal time, labour utilization statement, machine utilization statement, scrap production cost, accidents causing dislocation of activity.

   d.   **Sales department report:** The report includes budgeted and actual sales, sales efficiency, orders received and orders executed, cash and credit sales, stock of finished goods, market share and potential, sales promotion efficiency.

iii. **Report meant for junior level management:** The junior level management comprises of foremen, supervisors, sectional in-charges. Such authority develop reports on labour efficiency variance, ideal time, overtime and machine utilization, materials usage variance, credit collections and outstanding.

   For instance, in case of routine reports, in a pharmaceutical industry, project status are submitted on day to day work basis, entire work status and progress of the week and finally by the end of the month the review of the work status of the previous months and how current month work has overcome the set targets. Such reviews are expected to know the status of work and also help in making firm decisions whether to continue the projects. Hence, a report depends on the nature of work such as research, administrative, financial or market status of the products etc.

In case of special reports, a long term project that is in progress, upon circumstances a higher authority wishes to review the entire status and seeks for. A special report may arise in emergency circumstances or a project has un-expected outcomes.

Control reports are developed in order to maintain quality standards for a product. Such control reports include standard ranges of every attribute of unit operation in a pharmaceutical manufacturing industry. A control report includes installation, operational and quality validations so that a product standard set provides with reproducible results.

Information reports are developed in order to pass message from the giving end to the receiving end. This can be from one department to another department or to the stake holders in case of a company status. Information reports are quite commonly observed in news papers wherein a company declares the status of the company over the past years to the current and finally projecting to the future expected status.

Venture measurements reports are developed when a project is proposed and an estimate is developed so that the practicality of the project is assessed by funding organisations (Banks, Government approvals etc.,). Such reports also help in assessing when a breakeven is achieved.

In case of financial reports, a static may be considered as regular routine financial status reports where as dynamic may be one that is developed to assess the current situation.

28.4 Structure of External Management Report

As discussed earlier, external management report is drafted keeping in view of the eyes of the management. This is because a management report (or Annual Report) is presented to third parties.

International and national guidelines insists on pillar 1 for objective, pillar 2 for minimum content and pillar 3 for the principles and rule to be followed when preparing the management report.

Pillar 1: Objectives of the management report:

1.1 Provide a fair explanation of the situation of the entity and its business performance

1.2 Disclose the entity's risks, uncertainties and opportunities

1.3 Supplement the information contained in the financial statements

1.4 Present information that is relevant, reliable, understandable, verifiable, timely and useful for the user

Pillar 2: Content of the management report:

2.1 Situation of the entity:

2.1.1 Organizational structure: Includes company's organizational structure

       2.1.2   Modus oprandi: Includes entity's objectives, strategies for action, group it heads, environment in which it operates such as materials, energy, emissions, effluents and waste, water, biodiversity, transport, products and services, regulatory compliance.

2.2   Business performance and results:

       2.2.1   Key financial and non-financial indicators

       2.2.2   Issues relating to the environment and employees

2.3   Liquidity and capital resources:

       2.3.1   Liquidity

       2.3.2   Capital resources

       2.3.3   Analysis of contractual obligations and off balance sheet transactions

2.4   Main risks and uncertainities:

       2.4.1   Operational risks

           a.   Regulatory risks

           b.   Other operational risks

       2.4.2   Financial risks

           a.   Market risk

              i.   Interest rate risk

              ii.   Foreign currency risk

              iii.   Financial instrument price risk

              iv.   Commodity price risk

           b.   Credit risk

           c.   Liquidity risk

2.5   Significant events after the reporting period

2.6   Information on the outlook for the entity

2.7   Research and Development and Innovations

2.8   Acquisition and disposal of treasury shares

2.9   Other salient information

       2.9.1   Stock market information

       2.9.2   Other information: Past performance, current situation, making forecasts

Pillar 3: Principles and rules for the preparation of the management report

3.1   Discussion through the eyes of the management

3.2   Clear, concise and consistent wording

3.3   Objectiveness when explaining and analyzing events, plans, forecasts and their consequences.

3.4   Specifications of the sources, bases and assumptions contained in the forward-looking information

3.5   Consistency with prior reports

3.6   Avoid, to the extent possible, duplication with the financial statements and other information

3.7   Avoid immaterial information that renders the report scantly useful or unmanageable

3.8   Avoid the use of generic and standard disclosures

3.9   Identity information from external sources and that produced by the entity

3.10   Tailor the management report to the nature of the business, taking into account the size and complexity there of

As a whole, a good management report comprises of executive summary, introduction, analysis of data, findings and recommendations. An executive summary is included with summary of main findings, conclusions. A busy executive upon reading the executive summary decides whether to read further report. The report is included with useful but not essential appendices, tables and figures. It is necessary to understand that drafting a management report should be of simple English avoiding or minimizing technical vocabulary.

29 Role of Computers in Healthcare System

29.0 Introduction

During the decade of 1980s the concept of computers and machine languages started pouring into Indian territory. Transformation of alphabets and numerical into "0"s and "1"s and final conversion into bits and bytes made the scope of computers faster in data entering, data handling, data calculations, data analysis, data interpretations, data retrieving easier, which was earlier manual in documentations. As time has advanced, internet communications made even faster beyond one's territory.

Within a span of almost 30-40 years, the entire Indian work culture transformed with computerization. Several computer based languages and operating systems are helping to develop user friendly soft wares that are work specific. The scope of computers and their role is beyond the scope of the book; however an emphasis is made relating to health sector. Computer software comprises of user interface at the front end and with a back end programming languages developed by field experts. Such soft wares are developed in a logical and sequential work flow manner. Developing a program initiates with understanding the sequential work flow of events, leading to development of a flowchart that finally leads to development of programming as a software.

29.1 Role of Computers in Hospitals

Right from entry of a patient into a hospital to the final discharge of patients, the computers are programmed and are being accessible at various work stations by the concerned authority. A programming has to be developed right from entry of the patient details through directing him to the concerned department where he is expected with a doctor's counseling, entry of counseling information, leading to diagnosis protocols, finally leading to either medical, surgical type of treatments. Hence, an out –patient and in-patient details have be clearly sorted by the computer. The patient needs several medicines, medical devices during his visit and stay at the hospital. Under such situations, the patient is directed to the pharmacy where in the patient is being dispensed with the prescribed medicines, which the concerned pharmacist should access the prescription details by accessing the patient id number etc. Hence, there is a need of bills and accounting the expenditures incurred with respect to the patient. There is a need of computer based counseling to the patient and the counselor should have ample information as drug information system so as to pass the drug usage information to the patient. Upon discharge of an in-patient or out-patient, the entire case details of the patient should be stored at the hospital as well as a copy to be furnished to the patient. By the end of the day, computers should be well programmed in retrieving a report that provide entire demography of patients, age wise, gender wise, in-patient/out-patient, department wise, total money transactions, through health policies (non-money transactions), inventory levels so that where resources have to be procured on day to day basis can be fulfilled. In certain circumstances, an hospital administration structure is well framed in usage of controlled medicines, which need access and approval of dispensing through authorized authority. In addition to this, where an expert is not available for a diseased condition, the hospital should be in a position to access and communicate the expert across the globe so that diagnosis and treatment can be initiated. Inventory at the levels of stores, main hospital pharmacy, manufacturing pharmacy, satellite pharmacies and different out-patient and in-patient wards have to be monitored.

29.2   Role of Computers in Inventory Control

About 40 percent of the working capital is invested on inventory. Hence, keeping all the objectives, an inventory of every medicine, hospital equipment, medical devices etc., have to be monitored and procured. Hence, setting of inventory controls needs monitoring of stock on day to basis and the computer programming should be planned in such a way that it alerts the pharmacist or the hospital staff in preventing from scarcity levels. It is necessary to understand that various principles of inventory control are tuned through computer programming for their implementation.

29.3   Role of Computers in Pharmacy

At pharmacy, drugs are dispensed and if necessary to be constituted and dispensed. Hence, the pharmacist should be in a position to retrieve patient prescription data. The pharmacist and the computer should cross check whether for right aliment, right patient, right drug, right dosage form, right dosage calculations were made prior dispensing. Hence in a pharmacy that is either associated with hospital or with community, upon placing the order on the computer should give immediate response which drug product has to be dispensed on first come first serve basis (for a specific product). Where a drug product has to be constituted, the computer through the pharmacist should direct the order for manufacturing pharmacy to constituting and dispensing. The computer dispensing process should be well programmed that the drug products dispensed are valid with the expiry dates. In addition to this, if necessary, the computer should give access to various drug information sources so that the patient is provided with necessary counseling with regarding to usage of medicines.

29.4 Role of Computers for Diagnosis and Treatment

Several hospitals have limited facility and such hospitals also should have enough access to advanced and latest information. In certain circumstances, an expert scarcity for advice is observed. Under such circumstances, through computers and internet conferences, the expert can be contacted and with the aid of computers the diagnostic reports can be accessed for immediate start of treatment.

29.5 Role of Computers in Patient Record Database Management

Certain back end computer programs developed for an hospital retrieve all the patient data right from name of patient to the final discharge summary sheet that was recorded by authorized personnel in the hospital. Such data can be only retrieved if proper database management system is implemented in the hospital. Hence, hospital administration should ensure all the information of a patient is available in the computer database by ensuring appropriate entries are made at the work stations of the hospital. Development and maintenance of such databases need regular saving of hospital data in the final database. The purpose of databases is not only helpful in having the statistics but also helps in research and development of the hospital.

29.6 Role of Computers in Literature Retrieval

Computers with the aid of internet are currently helping to access various national and international databases and search engines. Such information is helping the health care providers with right diagnosis, appropriate treatment at right time. Literature retrieval is mainly from primary and secondary literature sources. Hence, an hospital should have access not only to internet but also subscribe and provide access to information sources such as journals, conferences, talks, pre-recorded treatment procedures, contraindications etc.

As a whole, digitization led to the usage and access of conventional information through computers.

30 Parenterals Admixture

It is believed that among the various formulations dosage forms, 40 percent of the dosage forms are relating to parenterals route of administration. A parenteral route of administration is preferred where the patient is un-conscious, patient not comfortable with conventional route of administration, for immediate electrolyte, fluids, energy balance. A parenteral can be dextrose solution, normal saline or of a drug. Especially for parenteral drug powder dosage form, a container with sterile water for injection is provided for re-constitution and administration. Several parenteral dosage forms are of multiple dose containers. Such containers are sealed with a rubber stopper that is heat resistant and convenient for pierce through of the injection needle several times keeping intact the drug product sterile.

Parenterals are usually administered as bolus or for a long duration of time. In the latter condition, it is necessary to ensure that the drug or the supplements are provided at a suitable rate preventing from hazard conditions. Specially designed drips apparatus with necessary tubing and needle system, the parenteral is usually administered to the patient. Such devices are more reliable and prevents from multiple punctures of the skin with several injections. The design of the drips apparatus is such that a "Y" junction is provided for multiple injections being given at several intervals for the same dextrose or saline solution being administered.

Administering several drugs at one time as parenteral admixture needs knowledge on incompatibilities. A parenteral admixture has to be ensured for physical, physiological, chemical, pharmacological (therapeutic) incompatibilities. Several admixtures lead to colour change, drug precipitation, synergic or antagonistic effects that may lead to fatal effects to the patient. Where a parental formulation is available in a multiple dosage container, under aseptic laminar air flow mechanisms, should be transferred into single dose containers and used. Labeling of parenteral containers needs extra precautions and cautions must be indicated to discard the formulation if any particulate matter is observed. An emphasis on storage conditions have to be made. An emphasis on which parenteral route of administration the formulation is meant for has to be indicated. In general, a label comprises of Generic name of drug, Brand name, Name and address of manufacturer, declaration of net contents, adequate direction for safe use, warning, caution and special directions required to be observed by the consumer, a distinctive batch number, manufacturing licence number, expiry date (shelf life), special symbols or coloured lines for prescription, narcotic, hazardous and poisonous drugs and finally with a trace and track barcode (2D or 3D) to safe guard from counterfeits.

Annexure - I
Standard Statistical Tables

Annexure 1

TABLE 1 Critical Values for Number of Runs at the 5% Level of Significance

Sample Size N	Two Sided Test		One-Sided Test
	Lower Number	Upper Number	Lower Number
10	2	9	3
12	3	10	3
14	3	12	4
16	4	13	5
18	5	14	6
20	6	15	6
22	7	16	7
24	7	18	8
26	8	19	9
28	9	20	10
30	10	21	11
32	11	22	11
34	11	24	12
36	12	25	13
38	13	26	14
40	14	27	15

Note: If number of runs is less than or equal to the lower number or greater than or equal to the upper value, the sequence is considered non-random at the 5% level of significance. The sample size (N) is the number of values above and below the median. For odd-size samples where one value is the median, use the next smaller sample size for the critical values.

TABLE 2 Individual Terms of the Binomial Distribution for N=2 to 10 and p = 0.5

| | N | | | | | | | | |
X	2	3	4	5	6	7	8	9	10
0	0.25	0.125	0.0625	0.031	0.016	0.008	0.004	0.002	0.001
1	0.5	0.375	0.25	0.156	0.094	0.055	0.031	0.018	0.01
2	0.25	0.375	0.375	0.313	0.234	0.164	0.109	0.07	0.044
3		0.125	0.25	0.313	0.313	0.273	0.219	0.164	0.117
4			0.0625	0.156	0.234	0.273	0.273	0.246	0.205
5				0.031	0.094	0.164	0.219	0.246	0.246
6					0.016	0.055	0.109	0.164	0.205
7						0.008	0.031	0.07	0.117
8							0.004	0.018	0.044
9								0.002	0.01
10									0.001

TABLE 3 Cumulative Normal Distribution: Cumulative Area under the Normal Distribution

Z	Area	Z	Area	Z	Area	Z	Area
-3.25	0.0006	-1.5	0.0668	0.25	0.5987	2	0.9772
-3.2	0.0007	-1.45	0.0735	0.3	0.6179	2.05	0.9798
-3.15	0.0008	-1.4	0.0808	0.35	0.6368	2.1	0.9821
-3.1	0.001	-1.35	0.0885	0.4	0.6554	2.15	0.9842
-3.05	0.0011	-1.3	0.0968	0.45	0.6736	2.2	0.9861
-3	0.0013	-1.25	0.1056	0.5	0.6915	2.25	0.9878
-2.95	0.0016	-1.2	0.1151	0.55	0.7088	2.3	0.9893
-2.9	0.0019	-1.15	0.1251	0.6	0.7257	2.35	0.9906
-2.85	0.0022	-1.1	0.1357	0.65	0.7422	2.4	0.9918
-2.8	0.0026	-1.05	0.1469	0.7	0.758	2.45	0.9929
-2.75	0.003	-1	0.1587	0.75	0.7732	2.5	0.9938
-2.7	0.0035	-0.95	0.1711	0.8	0.7881	2.55	0.9946
-2.65	0.004	-0.9	0.1841	0.85	0.8023	2.6	0.9953
-2.6	0.0047	-0.85	0.1977	0.9	0.8159	2.65	0.996
-2.55	0.0054	-0.8	0.2119	0.95	0.8289	2.7	0.9965
-2.5	0.0062	-0.75	0.2266	1	0.8413	2.75	0.997
-2.45	0.0071	-0.7	0.242	1.05	0.8531	2.8	0.9974
-2.4	0.0082	-0.65	0.2578	1.1	0.8643	2.85	0.9978
-2.35	0.0094	-0.6	0.2743	1.15	0.8749	2.9	0.9981

Table 3 *Contd...*

Z	Area	Z	Area	Z	Area	Z	Area
-2.3	0.0107	-0.55	0.2912	1.2	0.8849	2.95	0.9984
-2.25	0.0122	-0.5	0.3085	1.25	0.8944	3	0.9987
-2.2	0.0139	-0.45	0.3264	1.3	0.9032	3.25	0.9994
-2.15	0.0158	-0.4	0.3446	1.35	0.9115		
-2.1	0.0179	-0.35	0.3632	1.4	0.9192	**Z**	**Area**
-2.05	0.0202	-0.3	0.3821	1.45	0.9265	1.282	0.9
-2	0.0228	-0.25	0.4013	1.5	0.9332	1.645	0.95
-1.95	0.0256	-0.2	0.4207	1.55	0.9394	1.96	0.975
-1.9	0.0287	-0.15	0.4404	1.6	0.9452	2.326	0.99
-1.85	0.0322	-0.1	0.4602	1.65	0.9505	2.576	0.995
-1.8	0.0359	-0.05	0.4801	1.7	0.9554	3.09	0.999
-1.75	0.0401	0	0.5	1.75	0.9599		
-1.7	0.0446	0.05	0.5199	1.8	0.9641		
-1.65	0.0495	0.1	0.5398	1.85	0.9678		
-1.6	0.0548	0.15	0.5596	1.9	0.9713		
-1.55	0.0606	0.2	0.5793	1.95	0.9744		

TABLE 4 Chi-Square Distributions

Degrees of Freedom	Probability		Degrees of Freedom	Probability	
	0.01	0.05		0.01	0.05
1	6.634897	3.841459	32	53.48577	46.19426
2	9.21034	5.991465	33	54.77554	47.39988
3	11.34487	7.814728	34	56.06091	48.60237
4	13.2767	9.487729	35	57.34207	49.80185
5	15.08627	11.0705	36	58.61921	50.99846
6	16.81189	12.59159	37	59.8925	52.19232
7	18.47531	14.06714	38	61.16209	53.38354
8	20.09024	15.50731	39	62.42812	54.57223
9	21.66599	16.91898	40	63.69074	55.75848
10	23.20925	18.30704	41	64.95007	56.94239
11	24.72497	19.67514	42	66.20624	58.12404
12	26.21697	21.02607	43	67.45935	59.30351
13	27.68825	22.36203	44	68.70951	60.48089
14	29.14124	23.68479	45	187.5299	174.101
15	30.57791	24.99579	46	71.2014	62.82962
16	31.99993	26.29623	47	72.44331	64.00111

Table 4 *Contd...*

Degrees of Freedom	Probability		Degrees of Freedom	Probability	
	0.01	0.05		0.01	0.05
17	33.40866	27.58711	48	73.68264	65.17077
18	34.80531	28.8693	49	74.91947	66.33865
19	36.19087	30.14353	50	76.15389	67.50481
20	37.56623	31.41043	51	77.38596	68.66929
21	38.93217	32.67057	52	78.61576	69.83216
22	40.28936	33.92444	53	79.84334	70.99345
23	41.6384	35.17246	54	81.06877	72.15322
24	42.97982	36.41503	55	82.29212	73.31149
25	44.3141	37.65248	56	83.51343	74.46832
26	45.64168	38.88514	57	84.73277	75.62375
27	46.96294	40.11327	58	85.95018	76.7778
28	48.27824	41.33714	59	87.16571	77.93052
29	49.58788	42.55697	60	88.37942	79.08194
30	50.89218	43.77297	80	112.3288	101.8795
31	52.19139	44.98534	100	135.8067	124.3421
			500	576.4928	553.1268

TABLE 5 Student -t- distribution

Two-Sided:	10%	5%	1%	Two-Sided:	10%	5%	1%
One-sided:	5%	3%	0.50%	One-sided:	5%	3%	0.50%
d.f:	t (0.95)	t(0.975)	t(0.995)	d.f:	t (0.95)	t(0.975)	t(0.995)
1	6.313752	12.7062	63.65674	28	1.701131	2.048407	2.763262
2	2.919986	4.302653	9.924843	29	1.699127	2.04523	2.756386
3	2.353363	3.182446	5.840909	30	1.697261	2.042272	2.749996
4	2.131847	2.776445	4.604095	31	1.695519	2.039513	2.744042
5	2.015048	2.570582	4.032143	32	1.693889	2.036933	2.738484
6	1.94318	2.446912	3.707428	33	1.69236	2.034515	2.733277
7	1.894579	2.364624	3.499483	34	1.690924	2.032244	2.728394
8	1.859548	2.306004	3.355387	35	1.689572	2.030108	2.723806
9	1.833113	2.262157	3.249836	36	1.688298	2.028094	2.719485
10	1.812461	2.228139	3.169273	37	1.687094	2.026192	2.715409
11	1.795885	2.200985	3.105807	38	1.685954	2.024394	2.711558
12	1.782288	2.178813	3.05454	39	1.684875	2.022691	2.707913
13	1.770933	2.160369	3.012276	40	1.683851	2.021075	2.704459
14	1.76131	2.144787	2.976843	41	1.682878	2.019541	2.701181

Table 5 *Contd...*

Two-Sided:	10%	5%	1%	Two-Sided:	10%	5%	1%
One-sided:	5%	3%	0.50%	One-sided:	5%	3%	0.50%
d.f:	t (0.95)	t(0.975)	t(0.995)	d.f:	t (0.95)	t(0.975)	t(0.995)
15	1.75305	2.13145	2.946713	42	1.681952	2.018082	2.698066
16	1.745884	2.119905	2.920782	43	1.681071	2.016692	2.695102
17	1.739607	2.109816	2.898231	44	1.68023	2.015368	2.692278
18	1.734064	2.100922	2.87844	45	1.679427	2.014103	2.689585
19	1.729133	2.093024	2.860935	46	1.67866	2.012896	2.687013
20	1.724718	2.085963	2.84534	47	1.677927	2.01174	2.684556
21	1.720743	2.079614	2.83136	48	1.677224	2.010635	2.682204
22	1.717144	2.073873	2.818756	49	1.676551	2.009575	2.679952
23	1.713872	2.068658	2.807336	50	1.675905	2.008559	2.677793
24	1.710882	2.063899	2.796939	75	1.665425	1.992102	2.642983
25	1.708141	2.059539	2.787436	100	1.660234	1.983971	2.625891
26	1.705618	2.055529	2.778715	500	1.647907	1.96472	2.585998
27	1.703288	2.05183	2.770683	Infinity	1.644855	1.959966	2.575834

TABLE 6 Number of Positive or Negative Signs Needs for Significance for the Sign Test

Sample Size	Number of Positive or Negative signs for significance(@)	
	5% Level	1% Level
6	6	Nil
7	7	Nil
8	8	8
9	8	9
10	9	10
11	10	11
12	10	11
13	11	12
14	12	13
15	12	13
16	13	14
17	13	15
18	14	15
19	15	16
20	15	17

(@) This is a two-sided test. Choose positive or negative signs, which ever is larger

TABLE 7 Values Leading to Significance for the Wilcoxon Signed Rank Test (Two-Sided Test)

Sample Size, N	5 % Level (@)	1% Level
6	0	Nil
7	2	Nil
8	3	0
9	5	1
10	8	3
11	10	5
12	13	7
13	17	10
14	21	13
15	25	16
16	30	19
17	35	23
18	40	28
19	46	32
20	52	37

(@) If the smaller rank sum is less than or equal to the table value, the comparative groups are different at the indicated level of significance

TABLE 8 Critical Values for Wilcoxon Rank Sum Test (α=0.05)

Size of Larger Sample	Size of Smaller Sample (M)						
	M=3	M=4	M=5	M=6	M=7	M=8	M=9
M	5, 16	11, 25	18, 37	26, 52	37, 68	49, 87	63, 108
M+1	6, 18	12, 28	19, 41	28, 56	39,73	51, 93	66, 114
M+2	6, 21	12, 32	20, 45	29, 61	41, 78	54, 98	68, 121
M+3	7, 23	13, 35	21, 49	31, 65	43, 83	56, 104	71, 127
M+4	7, 26	14, 38	22, 53	32, 70	45, 88	58, 110	74, 133
M+5	8, 28	15, 41	24, 56	34, 74	46, 94	61, 115	77, 139
M+6	8, 31	16, 44	25, 60	36, 78	48, 99	63, 121	79, 146
M+7	9, 33	17, 47	26, 64	37, 83	50, 104	65, 127	82, 152
M+8	10, 35	17, 51	27, 68	39, 87	52, 109	68, 132	85, 158
M+9	10, 38	18, 54	29, 71	41, 91	54, 114	70, 138	88, 164
M+10	11, 40	19, 57	30, 75	42, 96	56,119	72, 144	90, 171
M+15	13, 53	24, 72	36, 94	50, 118	66, 144	84, 172	104, 202
M+20	16, 65	28, 88	42, 113	58, 140	76, 169	96, 200	118, 223
M+25	18, 78	32, 104	48, 132	66, 162	86, 194	108, 228	132, 264

Note: If rank sum of smaller sample is equal to or lower than smaller numbers in table or equal to or larger than larger number, groups are significantly different at 0.05 level

TABLE 9 Critical Difference for Significance (α=0.05) Comparing All Possible Pairs of Treatments for Non-parametric One-way ANOVA

N (for each treatment)	Number of Treatments				
	3	4	5	6	7
3	15	23	30	37	45
4	24	35	46	57	69
5	33	48	63	79	96
6	43	63	83	104	125
7	54	79	105	131	158
8	66	96	128	160	192
9	79	115	152	190	229
10	92	134	178	223	268
11	106	155	205	257	309
12	121	176	233	292	352
13	136	199	263	329	397
14	152	222	294	368	444
15	169	246	326	408	492
16	186	271	359	449	542
17	203	296	393	492	593
18	221	323	428	536	646
19	240	350	464	581	700
20	259	378	501	627	756
21	278	406	538	674	814
22	298	435	577	723	872
23	319	465	617	773	932
24	340	496	657	824	994
25	361	527	699	875	1056

TABLE 10 Critical Differences for Significance (α=0.05) Comparing All Possible Pairs of Treatments for Non-parametric Two-way ANOVA

N (for each treatment)	Number of Treatments				
	3	4	5	6	7
3	6	8	10	13	15
4	7	10	12	15	18
5	8	11	14	17	20
6	9	12	15	18	22
7	9	13	16	20	24
8	10	14	17	21	25

Table 10 *Contd...*

N (for each treatment)	Number of Treatments				
	3	4	5	6	7
10	11	15	19	24	28
11	11	16	20	25	30
12	12	16	21	26	31
13	12	17	22	27	32
14	13	18	23	28	34
15	13	18	24	29	35
16	13	19	24	30	36
17	14	19	25	31	37
18	14	20	26	32	38
19	14	20	27	33	39
20	15	21	27	34	40
21	15	21	28	35	41
22	16	22	29	35	42
23	16	22	29	36	43
24	16	23	30	37	44
25	17	23	31	38	45

TABLE 11 The Rank Sum Table

Values of T or T`, whichever is smaller, significant at the 10%, 5%, and 1% levels																	
		N1 (Smaller Sample)															
N2	p	4	5	6	7	8	9	10	11	12	13	14	15	16	17	18	19	20
8	0.01	15	23	31	41	51			When n1>20 and n2>20, significance values are given to a good approximation by n1(n1+n2+1)/2-z(sqrt(n1n2(n1+n2+1)/12)), where z is 1.64 for the 10% , 1.96 for the 5%, and 2.58 for the 1% levels. The probability figures given are for a two-tailed test. For a one-tailed test, p is halved.									
	0.05	14	21	29	38	49												
	0.01	11	17	25	34	43												
9	0.1	16	24	33	43	54	66											
	0.05	14	22	31	40	51	62											
	0.01	11	18	26	35	45	56											
10	0.1	17	26	35	45	56	69	82										
	0.05	15	23	32	42	53	65	78										
	0.01	12	19	27	37	47	58	71										
11	0.1	18	27	37	47	59	72	86	100									
	0.05	16	24	34	44	55	68	81	96									
	0.01	12	20	28	38	49	61	73	87									
12	0.1	19	28	38	49	62	75	89	104	120								
	0.05	17	26	35	46	58	71	84	99	115								
	0.01	13	21	30	40	51	63	76	90	105								
13	0.1	20	30	40	52	64	78	92	108	125	142							
	0.05	18	27	37	48	60	73	88	103	119	136							
	0.01	14	22	31	41	53	65	79	93	109	125							
14	0.1	21	31	42	54	67	81	96	112	129	147	166						
	0.05	19	28	38	50	62	76	91	106	123	141	160						
	0.01	14	22	32	43	54	67	81	96	112	129	147						
15	0.1	22	33	44	56	69	84	99	116	133	152	171	192					
	0.05	20	29	40	52	65	79	94	110	127	145	164	184					
	0.01	15	23	33	44	56	69	84	99	115	133	151	171					
16	0.1	24	34	46	58	72	87	103	120	138	156	176	197	219				
	0.05	21	30	42	54	67	82	97	113	131	150	169	190	211				
	0.01	15	24	34	46	58	72	86	102	119	136	155	175	196				
17	0.1	25	35	47	61	75	90	106	123	142	161	182	203	225	249			
	0.05	21	32	43	56	70	84	100	117	135	154	174	195	217	240			
	0.01	16	25	36	47	60	74	89	105	122	140	159	180	201	223			
18	0.1	26	37	49	63	77	93	110	127	146	166	187	208	231	255	280		
	0.05	22	33	45	58	72	87	103	121	139	158	179	200	222	246	270		
	0.01	16	26	37	49	62	76	92	108	125	144	163	184	206	228	252		
19	0.1	27	38	51	65	80	96	113	131	150	171	192	214	237	262	287	313	
	0.05	23	34	46	60	74	90	107	124	143	163	182	205	228	252	277	303	
	0.01	17	27	38	50	64	78	94	111	129	147	168	189	210	234	258	283	
20	0.1	28	40	53	67	83	99	117	135	155	175	197	220	243	268	294	320	348
	0.05	24	35	48	62	77	93	110	128	147	167	188	210	234	258	283	309	337
	0.01	18	28	39	52	66	81	97	114	132	151	172	193	215	239	263	289	315

TABLE 12 Upper 5% Values of the F Distribution

Degrees of freedom in denominator	Degrees of freedom in numerator																											
	1	2	3	4	5	6	7	8	9	10	11	12	13	14	15	16	17	18	19	20	25	30	40	50	60	80	100	Inf
1	161.448	199.5	215.707	224.583	230.162	233.986	236.768	244.69	240.543	241.882	242.983	243.906	244.69	245.364	245.95	244.69	246.918	247.323	247.686	248.013	249.26	250.095	251.143	251.774	252.196	252.724	253.041	254.314
2	18.513	19	19.164	19.247	19.296	19.33	19.353	19.371	19.385	19.396	19.405	19.413	19.419	19.424	19.429	19.433	19.437	19.44	19.443	19.446	19.456	19.462	19.471	19.476	19.479	19.483	19.486	19.496
3	10.128	9.552	9.277	9.117	9.013	8.941	8.887	8.845	8.812	8.786	8.763	8.745	8.729	8.715	8.703	8.692	8.683	8.675	8.667	8.66	8.634	8.617	8.594	8.581	8.572	8.561	8.554	8.526
4	7.709	6.944	6.591	6.388	6.256	6.163	6.094	6.041	5.999	5.964	5.936	5.912	5.891	5.873	5.858	5.844	5.832	5.821	5.811	5.803	5.769	5.746	5.717	5.699	5.688	5.673	5.664	5.628
5	6.608	5.786	5.409	5.192	5.05	4.95	4.876	4.818	4.772	4.735	4.704	4.678	4.655	4.636	4.619	4.604	4.59	4.579	4.568	4.558	4.521	4.496	4.464	4.444	4.431	4.415	4.405	4.365
6	5.987	5.143	4.757	4.534	4.387	4.284	4.207	4.147	4.099	4.06	4.027	4	3.976	3.956	3.938	3.922	3.908	3.896	3.884	3.874	3.835	3.808	3.774	3.754	3.74	3.722	3.712	3.669
7	5.591	4.737	4.347	4.12	3.972	3.866	3.787	3.726	3.677	3.637	3.603	3.575	3.55	3.529	3.511	3.494	3.48	3.467	3.455	3.445	3.404	3.376	3.34	3.319	3.304	3.286	3.275	3.23
8	5.318	5.318	4.066	3.838	3.687	3.581	3.5	3.438	3.388	3.347	3.313	3.284	3.259	3.237	3.218	3.202	3.187	3.173	3.161	3.15	3.108	3.079	3.043	3.02	3.005	2.986	2.975	2.928
9	5.117	4.256	3.863	3.633	3.482	3.374	3.293	3.23	3.179	3.137	3.102	3.073	3.048	3.025	3.006	2.989	2.974	2.96	2.948	2.936	2.893	2.864	2.826	2.803	2.787	2.768	2.756	2.707
10	4.965	4.103	3.708	3.478	3.326	3.217	3.135	3.072	3.02	2.978	2.943	2.913	2.887	2.865	2.845	2.828	2.812	2.798	2.785	2.774	2.73	2.7	2.661	2.637	2.621	2.601	2.588	2.538
11	4.844	3.982	3.587	3.357	3.204	3.095	3.012	2.948	2.896	2.854	2.818	2.788	2.761	2.739	2.719	2.701	2.685	2.671	2.658	2.646	2.601	2.57	2.531	2.507	2.49	2.469	2.457	2.404
12	4.747	3.885	3.49	3.259	3.106	2.996	2.913	2.849	2.796	2.753	2.717	2.687	2.66	2.637	2.617	2.599	2.583	2.568	2.555	2.544	2.498	2.466	2.426	2.401	2.384	2.363	2.35	2.296
13	4.667	3.806	3.411	3.179	3.025	2.915	2.832	2.767	2.714	2.671	2.635	2.604	2.577	2.554	2.533	2.515	2.499	2.484	2.471	2.459	2.412	2.38	2.339	2.314	2.297	2.275	2.261	2.206
14	4.6	3.739	3.344	3.112	2.958	2.848	2.764	2.699	2.646	2.602	2.565	2.534	2.507	2.484	2.463	2.445	2.428	2.413	2.4	2.388	2.341	2.308	2.266	2.241	2.223	2.201	2.187	2.131
15	4.543	3.682	3.287	3.056	2.901	2.79	2.707	2.641	2.588	2.544	2.507	2.475	2.448	2.424	2.403	2.385	2.368	2.353	2.34	2.328	2.28	2.247	2.204	2.178	2.16	2.137	2.123	2.066
16	4.494	3.634	3.239	3.007	2.852	2.741	2.657	2.591	2.538	2.494	2.456	2.425	2.397	2.373	2.352	2.333	2.317	2.302	2.288	2.276	2.227	2.194	2.151	2.124	2.106	2.083	2.068	2.01
17	4.451	3.592	3.197	2.965	2.81	2.699	2.614	2.548	2.494	2.45	2.413	2.381	2.353	2.329	2.308	2.289	2.272	2.257	2.243	2.23	2.181	2.148	2.104	2.077	2.058	2.035	2.02	1.96
18	4.414	3.555	3.16	2.928	2.773	2.661	2.577	2.51	2.456	2.412	2.374	2.342	2.314	2.29	2.269	2.25	2.233	2.217	2.203	2.191	2.141	2.107	2.063	2.035	2.017	1.993	1.978	1.917
19	4.381	3.522	3.127	2.895	2.74	2.628	2.544	2.477	2.423	2.378	2.34	2.308	2.28	2.256	2.234	2.215	2.198	2.182	2.168	2.155	2.106	2.071	2.026	1.999	1.98	1.955	1.94	1.878
20	4.351	3.493	3.098	2.866	2.711	2.599	2.514	2.447	2.393	2.348	2.31	2.278	2.25	2.225	2.203	2.184	2.167	2.151	2.137	2.124	2.074	2.089	1.994	1.966	1.946	1.922	1.907	1.843
21	4.325	3.467	3.072	2.84	2.685	2.573	2.488	2.42	2.366	2.321	2.283	2.25	2.222	2.197	2.176	2.156	2.139	2.123	2.109	2.096	2.045	2.01	1.965	1.936	1.916	1.891	1.876	1.812
22	4.301	3.443	3.049	2.817	2.661	2.549	2.464	2.397	2.342	2.297	2.259	2.226	2.198	2.173	2.151	2.131	2.114	2.098	2.084	2.071	2.02	1.984	1.938	1.909	1.889	1.864	1.849	1.783
23	4.279	3.422	3.028	2.796	2.64	2.528	2.442	2.375	2.32	2.275	2.236	2.204	2.175	2.15	2.128	2.109	2.091	2.075	2.061	2.048	1.996	1.961	1.914	1.885	1.865	1.839	1.823	1.757
24	4.26	3.403	3.009	2.776	2.621	2.508	2.423	2.355	2.3	2.255	2.216	2.183	2.155	2.13	2.108	2.088	2.07	2.054	2.04	2.027	1.975	1.939	1.892	1.863	1.842	1.816	1.8	1.733
25	4.242	3.385	2.991	2.759	2.603	2.49	2.405	2.337	2.282	2.236	2.198	2.165	2.136	2.111	2.089	2.069	2.051	2.035	2.021	2.007	1.955	1.919	1.872	1.842	1.822	1.796	1.779	1.711
26	4.225	3.369	2.975	2.743	2.587	2.474	2.388	2.321	2.265	2.22	2.181	2.148	2.119	2.094	2.072	2.052	2.034	2.018	2.003	1.99	1.938	1.901	1.853	1.823	1.803	1.776	1.76	1.691
27	4.21	3.354	2.96	2.728	2.572	2.459	2.373	2.305	2.25	2.204	2.166	2.132	2.103	2.078	2.056	2.036	2.018	2.002	1.987	1.974	1.921	1.884	1.836	1.806	1.785	1.758	1.742	1.672
28	4.196	3.34	2.947	2.714	2.558	2.445	2.359	2.291	2.236	2.19	2.151	2.118	2.089	2.064	2.041	2.021	2.003	1.987	1.972	1.959	1.906	1.869	1.82	1.79	1.769	1.742	1.725	1.654

TABLE 12 *Contd...*

Degrees of freedom in denominator	Degrees of freedom in numerator																											
	1	2	3	4	5	6	7	8	9	10	11	12	13	14	15	16	17	18	19	20	25	30	40	50	60	80	100	Inf
29	4.183	3.323	2.934	2.701	2.545	2.432	2.346	2.278	2.223	2.177	2.138	2.104	2.075	2.05	2.027	2.007	1.989	1.973	1.958	1.945	1.891	1.854	1.806	1.775	1.754	1.726	1.71	1.638
30	4.171	3.316	2.922	2.69	2.534	2.421	2.334	2.266	2.211	2.165	2.126	2.092	2.063	2.037	2.015	1.995	1.976	1.96	1.945	1.932	1.878	1.841	1.792	1.761	1.74	1.712	1.695	1.622
31	4.16	3.305	2.911	2.679	2.523	2.409	2.323	2.255	2.199	2.153	2.114	2.08	2.051	2.026	2.003	1.983	1.965	1.948	1.933	1.92	1.866	1.828	1.779	1.748	1.726	1.699	1.681	1.608
32	4.149	3.295	2.901	2.668	2.512	2.399	2.313	2.244	2.189	2.142	2.103	2.07	2.04	2.015	1.992	1.972	1.953	1.937	1.922	1.908	1.854	1.817	1.767	1.736	1.714	1.686	1.669	1.594
33	4.139	3.285	2.892	2.659	2.503	2.389	2.303	2.235	2.179	2.133	2.093	2.06	2.03	2.004	1.982	1.961	1.943	1.926	1.911	1.898	1.844	1.806	1.756	1.724	1.702	1.674	1.657	1.581
34	4.13	3.276	2.883	2.65	2.494	2.38	2.294	2.225	2.17	2.123	2.084	2.05	2.021	1.995	1.972	1.952	1.933	1.917	1.902	1.888	1.833	1.795	1.745	1.713	1.691	1.663	1.645	1.569
35	4.121	3.267	2.874	2.641	2.485	2.372	2.285	2.217	2.161	2.114	2.075	2.041	2.012	1.986	1.963	1.942	1.924	1.907	1.892	1.878	1.824	1.786	1.735	1.703	1.681	1.652	1.635	1.558
36	4.113	3.259	2.866	2.634	2.477	2.364	2.277	2.209	2.153	2.106	2.067	2.033	2.003	1.977	1.954	1.934	1.915	1.899	1.883	1.87	1.815	1.776	1.726	1.694	1.671	1.643	1.625	1.547
37	4.105	3.252	2.859	2.626	2.47	2.356	2.27	2.201	2.145	2.098	2.059	2.025	1.995	1.969	1.946	1.926	1.907	1.89	1.875	1.861	1.806	1.768	1.717	1.685	1.662	1.633	1.615	1.537
38	4.098	3.245	2.852	2.619	2.463	2.349	2.262	2.194	2.138	2.091	2.051	2.017	1.988	1.962	1.939	1.918	1.899	1.883	1.867	1.853	1.795	1.76	1.708	1.676	1.653	1.624	1.606	1.527
39	4.091	3.238	2.845	2.612	2.456	2.342	2.255	2.187	2.131	2.084	2.044	2.01	1.981	1.954	1.931	1.911	1.892	1.875	1.86	1.846	1.791	1.752	1.7	1.668	1.645	1.616	1.597	1.518
40	4.085	3.232	2.839	2.606	2.449	2.336	2.249	2.18	2.124	2.077	2.038	2.003	1.974	1.948	1.924	1.904	1.885	1.868	1.853	1.839	1.783	1.744	1.693	1.66	1.637	1.608	1.589	1.509
50	4.034	3.183	2.79	2.557	2.4	2.286	2.199	2.13	2.073	2.026	1.986	1.952	1.921	1.895	1.871	1.85	1.831	1.814	1.798	1.784	1.727	1.687	1.634	1.599	1.576	1.544	1.525	1.438
60	4.001	3.15	2.758	2.525	2.368	2.254	2.167	2.097	2.04	1.993	1.952	1.917	1.887	1.86	1.836	1.815	1.796	1.778	1.763	1.748	1.69	1.649	1.594	1.559	1.534	1.502	1.481	1.389
80	3.96	3.111	2.719	2.486	2.329	2.214	2.126	2.056	1.999	1.951	1.91	1.875	1.845	1.817	1.793	1.772	1.752	1.734	1.718	1.709	1.644	1.602	1.545	1.508	1.482	1.448	1.426	1.325
100	3.936	3.041	2.696	2.463	2.305	2.191	2.103	2.032	1.975	1.927	1.886	1.85	1.819	1.792	1.768	1.746	1.726	1.708	1.691	1.676	1.616	1.573	1.515	1.477	1.45	1.415	1.392	1.283
200	3.888	3.041	2.65	2.417	2.259	2.144	2.056	1.985	1.927	1.878	1.837	1.801	1.769	1.742	1.717	1.694	1.674	1.656	1.639	1.623	1.561	1.516	1.455	1.415	1.386	1.346	1.321	1.189
Infinity	3.842	3.912	2.605	2.372	2.214	2.099	2.01	1.939	1.88	1.831	1.789	1.752	1.72	1.692	1.666	1.644	1.623	1.604	1.587	1.571	1.506	1.459	1.394	1.35	1.318	1.274	1.244	1

TABLE 13 Upper 10 % Values of the F Distribution

Degrees of freedom in denominator	Degrees of freedom in numerator																											
	1	2	3	4	5	6	7	8	9	10	11	12	13	14	15	16	17	18	19	20	25	30	40	50	60	80	100	Inf
1	39.863	49.5	53.593	55.833	57.24	58.204	58.906	60.903	59.858	60.195	60.473	60.705	60.903	61.073	61.22	60.903	61.464	61.566	61.658	61.74	62.055	62.265	62.529	62.688	62.794	62.927	63.007	63.328
2	8.526	9	9.162	9.243	9.293	9.326	9.349	9.367	9.381	9.392	9.401	9.408	9.415	9.42	9.425	9.429	9.433	9.436	9.439	9.441	9.451	9.458	9.466	9.471	9.475	9.479	9.481	9.491
3	5.538	5.462	5.391	5.343	5.309	5.285	5.266	5.252	5.24	5.23	5.222	5.216	5.21	5.205	5.2	5.196	5.193	5.19	5.187	5.184	5.175	5.168	5.16	5.155	5.151	5.147	5.144	5.134
4	4.545	4.325	4.191	4.107	4.051	4.01	3.979	3.955	3.936	3.92	3.907	3.896	3.886	3.878	3.87	3.864	3.858	3.853	3.849	3.844	3.828	3.817	3.804	3.795	3.79	3.782	3.778	3.761
5	4.06	3.78	3.619	3.52	3.453	3.405	3.368	3.339	3.316	3.297	3.282	3.268	3.257	3.247	3.238	3.23	3.223	3.217	3.212	3.207	3.187	3.174	3.157	3.147	3.14	3.132	3.126	3.105
6	3.776	3.463	3.289	3.181	3.108	3.055	3.014	2.983	2.958	2.937	2.92	2.905	2.892	2.881	2.871	2.863	2.855	2.848	2.842	2.836	2.815	2.8	2.781	2.77	2.762	2.752	2.746	2.722
7	3.589	3.257	3.074	2.961	2.883	2.827	2.785	2.752	2.725	2.703	2.684	2.668	2.654	2.643	2.632	2.623	2.615	2.607	2.601	2.595	2.571	2.555	2.535	2.523	2.514	2.504	2.497	2.471
8	3.458	3.458	2.924	2.806	2.726	2.668	2.624	2.589	2.561	2.538	2.519	2.502	2.488	2.475	2.464	2.455	2.446	2.438	2.431	2.425	2.4	2.383	2.361	2.348	2.339	2.328	2.321	2.293
9	3.36	3.006	2.813	2.693	2.611	2.551	2.505	2.469	2.44	2.416	2.396	2.379	2.364	2.351	2.34	2.329	2.32	2.312	2.305	2.298	2.272	2.255	2.232	2.218	2.208	2.196	2.189	2.159
10	3.285	2.924	2.728	2.605	2.522	2.461	2.414	2.377	2.347	2.323	2.302	2.284	2.269	2.255	2.244	2.233	2.224	2.215	2.208	2.201	2.174	2.155	2.132	2.117	2.107	2.095	2.087	2.055
11	3.225	2.86	2.66	2.536	2.451	2.389	2.342	2.304	2.274	2.248	2.227	2.209	2.193	2.179	2.167	2.156	2.147	2.138	2.13	2.123	2.095	2.076	2.052	2.036	2.026	2.013	2.005	1.972
12	3.177	2.807	2.606	2.48	2.394	2.331	2.283	2.245	2.214	2.188	2.166	2.147	2.131	2.117	2.105	2.094	2.084	2.075	2.067	2.06	2.031	2.011	1.986	1.97	1.96	1.946	1.938	1.904
13	3.136	2.763	2.56	2.434	2.347	2.283	2.234	2.195	2.164	2.138	1.116	2.097	2.08	2.066	2.053	2.042	2.032	2.023	2.014	2.007	1.978	1.958	1.931	1.915	1.904	1.89	1.882	1.846
14	3.102	2.726	2.522	2.395	2.307	2.243	2.193	2.154	2.122	2.095	2.073	2.054	2.037	2.022	2.01	1.998	1.988	1.978	1.97	1.962	1.933	1.912	1.885	1.869	1.857	1.843	1.834	1.797
15	3.073	2.695	2.49	2.361	2.273	2.208	2.158	2.119	2.086	2.059	2.037	2.017	2	1.985	1.972	1.961	1.95	1.941	1.932	1.924	1.894	1.873	1.845	1.828	1.817	1.802	1.793	1.755
16	3.048	2.668	2.462	2.333	2.244	2.178	2.128	2.088	2.055	2.028	2.005	1.985	1.968	1.953	1.94	1.928	1.917	1.908	1.899	1.891	1.86	1.839	1.811	1.793	1.782	1.766	1.757	1.718
17	3.026	2.645	2.437	2.308	2.218	2.152	2.102	2.061	2.028	2.001	1.978	1.958	1.94	1.925	1.912	1.9	1.889	1.879	1.87	1.862	1.831	1.809	1.781	1.763	1.751	1.735	1.726	1.686
18	3.007	2.624	2.416	2.286	2.196	2.13	2.079	2.038	2.005	1.977	1.954	1.933	1.916	1.9	1.887	1.875	1.864	1.854	1.845	1.837	1.805	1.783	1.754	1.736	1.723	1.707	1.698	1.657
19	2.99	2.606	2.397	2.266	2.176	2.109	2.058	2.017	1.984	1.956	1.932	1.912	1.894	1.878	1.865	1.852	1.841	1.831	1.822	1.814	1.782	1.759	1.73	1.711	1.699	1.683	1.673	1.631
20	2.975	2.589	2.38	2.249	2.158	2.091	2.04	1.999	1.965	1.937	1.913	1.892	1.875	1.859	1.845	1.833	1.821	1.811	1.802	1.794	1.761	1.733	1.708	1.69	1.677	1.66	1.65	1.607
21	2.961	2.575	2.365	2.233	2.142	2.075	2.023	1.982	1.948	1.92	1.896	1.875	1.857	1.841	1.827	1.815	1.803	1.793	1.784	1.776	1.742	1.719	1.689	1.67	1.657	1.64	1.63	1.586
22	2.949	2.561	2.351	2.219	2.128	2.06	2.008	1.967	1.933	1.904	1.88	1.859	1.841	1.825	1.811	1.798	1.787	1.777	1.768	1.759	1.726	1.702	1.671	1.652	1.639	1.622	1.611	1.567
23	2.937	2.549	2.339	2.207	2.115	2.047	1.995	1.953	1.919	1.89	1.866	1.845	1.827	1.811	1.796	1.784	1.772	1.762	1.753	1.744	1.71	1.686	1.655	1.636	1.622	1.605	1.594	1.549
24	2.927	2.538	2.327	2.195	2.103	2.035	1.983	1.941	1.906	1.877	1.853	1.832	1.814	1.797	1.783	1.77	1.759	1.748	1.739	1.73	1.696	1.672	1.641	1.621	1.607	1.59	1.579	1.533
25	2.918	2.528	2.317	2.184	2.092	2.024	1.971	1.929	1.895	1.866	1.841	1.82	1.802	1.785	1.771	1.758	1.746	1.736	1.726	1.718	1.683	1.659	1.627	1.607	1.593	1.576	1.565	1.518
26	2.909	2.519	2.307	2.174	2.082	2.014	1.961	1.919	1.884	1.855	1.83	1.809	1.79	1.774	1.76	1.747	1.735	1.724	1.715	1.706	1.671	1.647	1.615	1.594	1.581	1.562	1.551	1.504
27	2.901	2.511	2.299	2.165	2.073	2.005	1.952	1.909	1.874	1.845	1.82	1.799	1.78	1.764	1.749	1.736	1.724	1.714	1.704	1.695	1.66	1.636	1.603	1.583	1.569	1.55	1.539	1.491
28	2.894	2.503	2.291	2.157	2.064	1.996	1.943	1.9	1.865	1.836	1.811	1.79	1.771	1.754	1.74	1.726	1.715	1.704	1.694	1.685	1.65	1.625	1.592	1.572	1.558	1.539	1.528	1.478
29	2.887	2.495	2.283	2.149	2.057	1.988	1.935	1.892	1.857	1.827	1.802	1.781	1.762	1.745	1.731	1.717	1.705	1.695	1.685	1.676	1.64	1.616	1.583	1.562	1.547	1.529	1.517	1.467
30	2.881	2.489	2.276	2.142	2.049	1.98	1.927	1.884	1.849	1.819	1.794	1.773	1.754	1.737	1.722	1.709	1.697	1.686	1.676	1.667	1.632	1.606	1.573	1.552	1.538	1.519	1.507	1.456
31	2.875	2.482	2.27	2.136	2.042	1.973	1.92	1.877	1.842	1.812	1.787	1.765	1.746	1.729	1.714	1.701	1.689	1.678	1.668	1.659	1.623	1.598	1.565	1.543	1.529	1.509	1.498	1.446

TABLE 13 *Contd...*

Degrees of freedom in denominator	Degrees of freedom in numerator																												
	1	2	3	4	5	6	7	8	9	10	11	12	13	14	15	16	17	18	19	20	25	30	40	50	60	80	100	Inf
32	2.869	2.477	2.263	2.129	2.036	1.967	1.913	1.87	1.835	1.805	1.78	1.758	1.739	1.722	1.707	1.694	1.682	1.671	1.661	1.652	1.616	1.59	1.556	1.535	1.52	1.501	1.489	1.437
33	2.864	2.471	2.258	2.123	2.03	1.961	1.907	1.864	1.828	1.799	1.773	1.751	1.732	1.715	1.7	1.687	1.675	1.664	1.654	1.645	1.608	1.563	1.549	1.527	1.512	1.493	1.48	1.428
34	2.859	2.466	2.252	2.118	2.024	1.955	1.901	1.858	1.822	1.798	1.767	1.745	1.726	1.709	1.694	1.68	1.668	1.657	1.647	1.638	1.601	1.576	1.541	1.52	1.505	1.485	1.473	1.419
35	2.855	2.461	2.247	2.113	2.019	1.95	1.896	1.852	1.817	1.787	1.761	1.739	1.72	1.703	1.688	1.674	1.662	1.651	1.641	1.632	1.595	1.569	1.535	1.513	1.497	1.478	1.465	1.411
36	2.85	2.456	2.243	2.108	2.014	1.945	1.891	1.847	1.811	1.781	1.756	1.734	1.715	1.697	1.682	1.669	1.656	1.645	1.635	1.626	1.589	1.563	1.528	1.506	1.491	1.471	1.458	1.404
37	2.846	2.452	2.238	2.103	2.009	1.94	1.886	1.842	1.806	1.776	1.751	1.729	1.709	1.692	1.677	1.663	1.651	1.64	1.63	1.62	1.583	1.557	1.522	1.5	1.484	1.464	1.452	1.397
38	2.842	2.448	2.234	2.099	2.005	1.935	1.881	1.838	1.802	1.772	1.746	1.724	1.704	1.687	1.672	1.658	1.646	1.635	1.624	1.615	1.578	1.551	1.516	1.494	1.478	1.458	1.445	1.39
39	2.839	2.444	2.23	2.095	2.001	1.931	1.877	1.833	1.797	1.767	1.741	1.719	1.7	1.682	1.667	1.653	1.641	1.63	1.619	1.61	1.573	1.546	1.511	1.488	1.473	1.452	1.439	1.383
40	2.835	2.44	2.226	2.091	1.997	1.927	1.873	1.829	1.793	1.763	1.737	1.715	1.695	1.678	1.662	1.649	1.636	1.625	1.615	1.605	1.568	1.541	1.506	1.483	1.467	1.447	1.434	1.377
50	2.809	2.412	2.197	2.061	1.966	1.895	1.84	1.796	1.76	1.729	1.703	1.68	1.66	1.643	1.627	1.613	1.6	1.588	1.578	1.568	1.529	1.502	1.465	1.441	1.424	1.402	1.388	1.327
60	2.791	2.393	2.177	2.041	1.946	1.875	1.819	1.775	1.738	1.707	1.68	1.657	1.637	1.619	1.603	1.589	1.576	1.564	1.553	1.543	1.504	1.476	1.437	1.413	1.395	1.372	1.358	1.291
80	2.769	2.37	2.154	2.016	1.921	1.849	1.793	1.748	1.711	1.68	1.653	1.629	1.609	1.59	1.574	1.559	1.546	1.534	1.523	1.513	1.472	1.443	1.403	1.377	1.358	1.334	1.318	1.245
100	2.756	2.329	2.139	2.002	1.906	1.834	1.778	1.732	1.695	1.663	1.636	1.612	1.592	1.573	1.557	1.542	1.528	1.516	1.505	1.494	1.453	1.423	1.382	1.355	1.336	1.31	1.293	1.214
200	2.731	2.329	2.111	1.973	1.876	1.804	1.747	1.701	1.663	1.631	1.603	1.579	1.558	1.539	1.522	1.507	1.493	1.48	1.468	1.458	1.414	1.383	1.339	1.31	1.289	1.261	1.242	1.144
Infinity	2.706	3.912	2.084	1.945	1.847	1.774	1.717	1.67	1.632	1.599	1.571	1.546	1.524	1.505	1.487	1.471	1.457	1.444	1.432	1.421	1.375	1.342	1.295	1.263	1.24	1.207	1.185	1

Annexure - II
SF-36v2® Health Survey Measurement Model

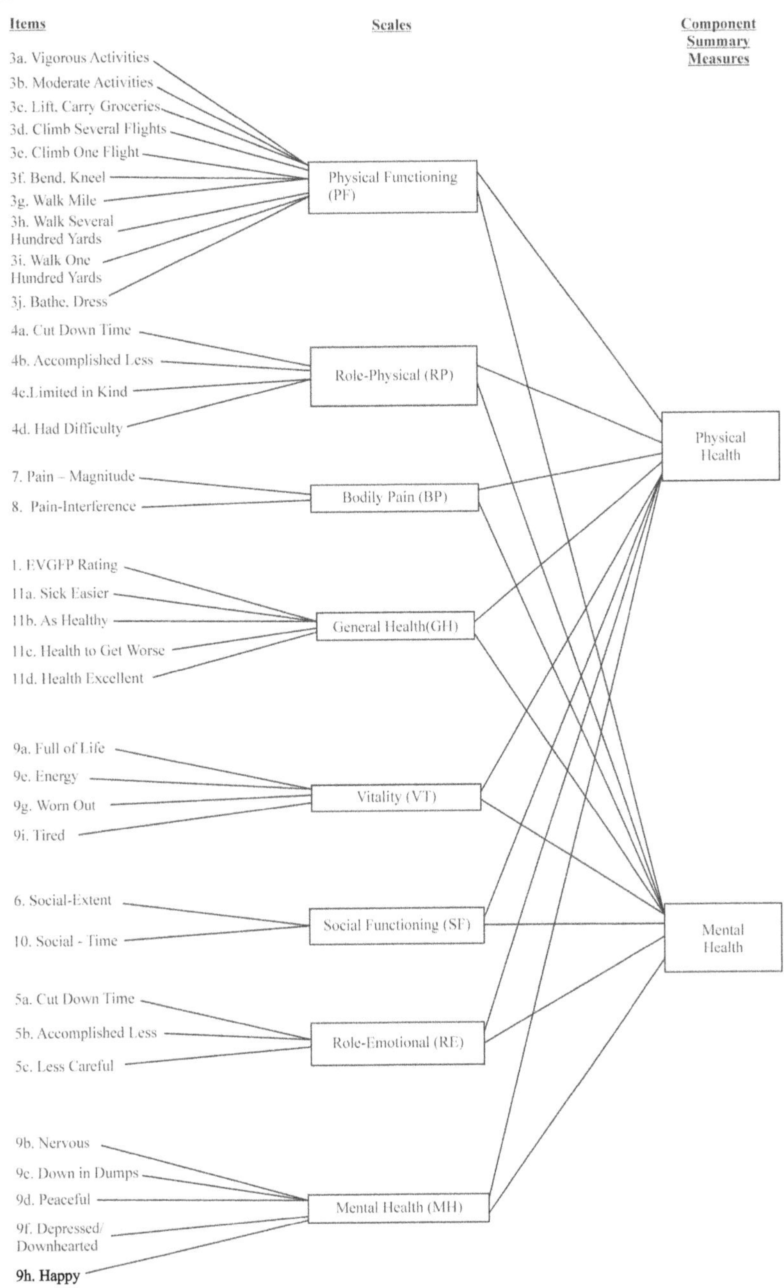

Note. All health domain scales contribute to the scoring of both the Physical and Mental Component Summary measures. Scales contributing most to the scoring of the summary measures are indica ted by a connecting solid line (—). Scales contributing to the scoring of the summary measures to a lesser degree are indicated by a dotted line (······).

SF-36v2® Health Survey Measurement Model

Annexure - III
The RAND 36-Item Health Survey

Introduction

The RAND 36-Item Health Survey (Version 1.0) laps eight concepts: physical functioning, bodily pain, role limitations due to physical health problems, role limitations due to personal or emotional problems, emotional well-being, social functioning, energy/fatigue, and general health perceptions. It also includes a single item that provides an indication of perceived change in health. These 36 items, presented here, are identical to the MOS SF-36 described in Ware and Sherbourne (1992). They were adapted from longer instruments completed by patients participating in the Medical Outcomes Study (MOS), an observational study of variation in physician practice styles and patient outcomes in different systems of health care delivery (Hays & Shapiro, 1992: Stewart, Sherbourne, Hays, et al., 1992).

A revised version of the RAND 36-Item Health Survey (Version 1.1) that differs slightly from version 1.0 in terms of item wording is currently in development.

SCORING RULES FOR THE RAND 36-ITEM HEALTH SURVEY (Version 1.0)

We recommend that responses be scored as described below. A somewhat different scoring procedure for the MOS SF-36 has been distributed by the International Resource Centre for Health Care Assessment (located in Boston, MA). Because the scoring method described here (a simpler and more straightforward procedure) differs from that of the MOS SF-36, persons using this scoring method should refer to the instrument as the RAND 36-Item Health Survey 1.0.

Scoring the RAND 36-Item Health Survey is a two-step process. First, precoded numeric values are recoded per the scoring key given in Table 1. Note that all items are scored so that a high score defines a more favourable health state. In addition, each item is scored on a 0 to 100 range so that the lowest and highest possible scores are set at 0 and 100, respectively. Scores represent the percentage of total possible score achieved. In step 2, items in the same scale are averaged together to create the 8 scale scores. Table 2 lists the items averaged together to create each scale. Items that are left blank (missing data) are not taken into account when calculating the scale scores. Hence, scale scores represent the average for all items in the scale that the respondent answered.

Example: Items 20 and 32 are used to score the measure of social functioning. Each of the two items has 5 response choices. However, a high score (response choice 5) on item 20 indicates extreme limitations in social functioning, while a high score (response choice 5) on item 32 indicates the absence of limitations in social functioning. To score both items in the same direction, Table 1 shows that responses 1 through 5 for item 20 should be recoded to values of 100, 75, 50, 25, and 0, respectively. Responses 1 through 5 for item 32 should be recoded to values of 0, 25, 50, 75, and 100, respectively. Table 2 shows that these two recoded items should be averaged together to form the social functioning scale. If the respondent is missing one of the two items, the person's score will be equal to that of the non missing item.

Table 3 presents information on the reliability, central tendency and variability of the scales scored using this method.

References

1. Ware, J.E., Jr., and Sherbourne, C. D. "The MOS 36-Item Short-Form Health Survey (SF-36): I. Conceptual Framework and item Selection," Medical Care, 30:473-483, 1992.
2. Hays, R.D., & Shapiro, M.F. "An Overview of Generic Health-Related Quality of Life Measures For HIV Research." Quality of Life Research, 1:91-97, 1992.
3. Stewart, A. L., Sherbourne, C., Hays, R. D., et al. "Summary and Discussion of MOS Measures," In A. L. Stewart & J. E. Ware (eds.), Measuring Functioning and Well-Being: The Medical Outcome Study Approach (pp. 345-371). Durham, NC: Duke University Press, 1992.

Please refer to **www.sf-36.org** for further information

Note: The Workplace Safety & Insurance Board (WSIB) acknowledges that the RAND-36-Short Form Health Survey (SF-36) was developed at RAND as part of the Medical Outcomes Study.

TABLE 1

STEP 1: RECORDING ITEMS

ITEM NUMBERS	Change original response category (a)	To recoded value of:
1,2,20,22,34,36	1---------->	100
	2---------->	75
	3---------->	50
	4---------->	25
	5---------->	0
3,4,5,6,7,8,9,10,11,12	1---------->	0
	2---------->	50
	3---------->	100
13,14,15,16,17,18,19	1---------->	0
	2---------->	100
21,23,26,27,30	1---------->	100
	2---------->	80
	3---------->	60
	4---------->	40
	5---------->	20
	6---------->	0
24,25,28,29,31	1---------->	0
	2---------->	20
	3---------->	40
	4---------->	60
	5---------->	80
	6---------->	100
32,33,35	1---------->	0
	2---------->	25
	3---------->	50
	4---------->	75
	5---------->	100

(a) Precoded response choices as printed in the questionnaire.

TABLE 2

STEP 2: AVERAGING ITEMS TO FORM SCALES

Scale	Number Of Items	After Recoding Per Table 1, Average The Following Items:
Physical functioning	10	3 4 5 6 7 8 9 10 11 12
Role limitations due to physical health	4	13 14 15 16
Role limitations due to emotional problems	3	17 18 19
Energy/fatigue	4	23 27 29 31
Emotional well-being	5	24 25 26 28 30
Social functioning	2	20 32
Pain	2	21 22
General health	5	1 33 34 35 36

TABLE 3 Reliability, Central Tendency and Variability of Scales in the Medical Outcomes Study

Scale	Items	Alpha	Mean	SD
Physical functioning	10	0.93	70.61	27.42
Role functioning/physical	4	0.84	52.97	40.78
Role functioning/emotional	3	0.83	65.78	40.71
Energy/fatigue	4	0.86	52.15	22.39
Emotional well-being	5	0.90	70.38	21.97
Social functioning	2	0.85	78.77	25.43
Pain	2	0.78	70.77	25.48
General health	5	0.78	56.99	21.11
Health change	1	——	59.14	23.12

Note: Data is from baseline of the Medical Outcomes Study (N – 2471), except for Health change, which was obtained one year later.

RAND 36-Item Health Survey 1.0 Questionnaire Items

1. In general, would you say your health is:	
Excellent	1
Very good	2
Good	3
Fair	4
Poor	5

2. **Compared to one year ago,** how would your rate your health in general **now**?	
Much better now than one year ago	1
Somewhat better now than one year ago	2
About the same	3
Somewhat worse now than one year ago	4
Much worse now than one year ago	5

Note: The WSIB acknowledges that the RAND 36-Item Short Form Health Survey was developed at RAND as part of the Medical Outcomes Study.

The following items are about activities you might do during a typical day. Does **your health now limit you** in these activities? If so, how much?

(Circle One Number on Each Line)

	Yes, Limited a Lot	Yes, Limited a Little	No, Not limited at All
3. **Vigorous activities,** such as running, lifting heavy objects, participating in strenuous sports	[1]	[2]	[3]
4. **Moderate activities,** such as moving a table, pushing a vacuum cleaner, bowling, or playing golf	[1]	[2]	[3]
5. Lifting or carrying groceries	[1]	[2]	[3]
6. Climbing **several** flights of stairs	[1]	[2]	[3]
7. Climbing **one** flight of stairs	[1]	[2]	[3]
8. Bending, kneeling, or stooping	[1]	[2]	[3]
9. Walking **more than a mile**	[1]	[2]	[3]
10. Walking **several blocks**	[1]	[2]	[3]
11. Walking **one block**	[1]	[2]	[3]
12. Bathing or dressing myself	[1]	[2]	[3]

Note: The WSIB acknowledges that the RAND 36-Item Short Form Health Survey was developed at RAND as part of the Medical Outcomes Study.

During the **past 4 weeks,** have you had any of the following problems with your work or other regular daily activities **as a result of your physical health?**
(Circle One Number on Each Line)

	Yes	No
13. Cut down the amount of time you spent on work or other activities	1	2
14. **Accomplished less** than you would like	1	2
15. Were limited in the **kind** of work or other activities	1	2
16. Had **difficulty** performing the work or other activities (for example, it took extra effort)	1	2

During the **past 4 weeks,** have you had any of the following problems with your work or other regular daily activities **as a result of any emotional problems** (such as feeling depressed or anxious)?
(Circle One Number on Each Line)

	Yes	No
17. Cut down the **amount of time** you spent on work or other activities	1	2
18. **Accomplished less** than you would like	1	2
19. Didn't do work or other activities as **carefully** as usual	1	2

20. During the **past 4 weeks,** to what extent has your physical health or emotional problems interfered with your normal social activities with family, friends, neighbours, or groups?

    (Circle One Number)

    Not at all 1

    Slightly 2

    Moderately 3

    Quite a bit 4

    Extremely 5

21. How much **bodily** pain have you had during the **past 4 weeks?**

    (Circle One Number)

    None 1

    Very mild 2

    Mild 3

    Moderate 4

    Severe 5

    Very severe 6

22. During the **past 4 weeks**, how much did **pain** interfere with your normal work (including both work outside the home and housework)?

    (Circle One Number)

    Not at all 1

    A little bit 2

    Moderately 3

    Quite a bit 4

    Extremely 5

These questions are about how you feel and how things have been with you **during the past 4 weeks**. For each question, please give the one answer that comes closest to the way you have been feeling.

How much of the time during the past 4 weeks . . .

(Circle One Number on Each Line)

	All of the Time	Most of the Time	A Good Bit of the Time	Some of the Time	A Little of the Time	None of the Time
23. Did you feel full of pep?	1	2	3	4	5	6
24. Have you been a very nervous person?	1	2	3	4	5	6
25. Have you felt so down in the dumps that nothing could cheer you up?	1	2	3	4	5	6
26. Have you felt calm and peaceful?	1	2	3	4	5	6
27. Did you have a lot of energy?	1	2	3	4	5	6
28. Have you felt downhearted and blue?	1	2	3	4	5	6
29. Did you feel worn out?	1	2	3	4	5	6
30. Have you been a happy person?	1	2	3	4	5	6
31. Did you feel tired?	1	2	3	4	5	6

32. During the **past 4 weeks**, how much of the time has your **physical health or emotional problems** interfered with your social activities (like visiting with friends, relatives, etc.)?

(Circle One Number)

All of the time 1

Most of the time 2

Some of the time 3

A little of the time 4

None of the time 5

How **TRUE** or **FALSE** is each of the following statements for you.

(Circle One Number on Each Line)

	Definitely True	Mostly True	Don't Know	Mostly False	Definitely False
33. I seem to get sick a little easier than other people	1	2	3	4	5
34. I am as healthy as anybody I know	1	2	3	4	5
35. I expect my health to get worse	1	2	3	4	5
36. My health is excellent	1	2	3	4	5

Question Bank
(for Theory, Practical and Viva-voce)

1. What is the role of Bio-Statistics in health care and pharmaceutical sectors?
2. What is the distinction feature of mathematical statistics and bio-statistics?
3. How to identify a research problem and initiate a research?
4. What are the various information sources?
5. How to conduct a systematic literature search?
6. How to conduct a patented literature search and plan for off-patent strategies?
7. What is Meta-Analysis? How to conduct a Meta-Analysis? What is its significance in research?
8. What are the various kinds of research documents? What are their roles and significance?
9. Write in detail the role of various parts of a research proposal, research report, research paper, patent document and synopsis.
10. How to conduct a clinical study?
11. How to design a clinical study?
12. Classify and explain in detail various clinical study designs.
13. What are the principles involved in experimental design?
14. Classify and explain in detail various approaches of experimental designs either pre-clinical, clinical or non-clinical relating to health or pharmaceutical sectors.
15. What is the role of sampling? What are the various techniques used for sampling?
16. What is a scale? What is a physical and abstract scale? Classify different types of measurement scales. What are the salient features of measurement scales?
17. What are the principles involved in developing an abstract scale?
18. How to develop a questionnaire or instrument or abstract scale?
19. What is the basis for developing a measurement scale/questionnaire/abstract scale?
20. Explain with a suitable well accepted questionnaire, the basis and principle involved in developing a questionnaire/instrument.
21. What is data relating to health or pharmaceutical sector? How data is processed and explain the various ways the data is presented? How to overcome with missing data?

22. What are the various distribution curves?

23. Explain in detail binomial, poisson, normal, chi-square, F distributions. How to interpret the kind of distribution, the data collected belong?

24. What is central tendency? What is its role? Explain the various measures of central tendency.

25. What is the difference between standard error and statistical error? How to calculate the statistical Power?

26. Write in detail about Type I and Type II Statistical errors. What is meant by Power of a test? What is the pharmaceutical permissible limit of type I and type II errors?

27. What is the significance of confidence level, confidence limit and confidence interval in research?

28. Explain with suitable example, how to establish confidence level, confidence limit and confidence interval for a clinical or non-clinical research attribute relating to health care or pharmaceutical sector?

29. What is Hypothesis? What is the rationale behind defining a null and alternate hypothesis?

30. Write from developing a hypothesis for a research problem, how you will step wise conclude a research problem after conducting a suitable statistical test?

31. What is parametric and non-parametric data? Whether for a parametric data, a non-parametric test can be conducted?

32. How to ensure whether the data obtained to be conducted with parametric or non-parametric test?

33.   When a binomial, passion, normal, chi-square, student 't', F-test is conducted? What are the distinguishing features?

34. Under what circumstances, a data is preferred for parametric test?

35. Under what circumstances, a data is preferred for non-parametric test?

36. Explain in detail Binomial distribution. Explain with a pharmaceutical related example, when a binomial test is conducted?

37. Explain in detail Poisson distribution. Explain with a pharmaceutical related example, when a poisson test is conducted?

38. Explain in detail Chi-square distribution. Explain with a pharmaceutical related example, when a chi-square test is conducted?

39. What is the rationale behind student 't' distribution. What are the two different types of student 't' tests?

40. Explain in detail paired and un-paired student 't' tests.

41. Compare and contrast paired and un-paired student 't' tests.

42. What is F-test? Explain with a suitable example, how an F-test is conducted?

43. What is ANOVA? Explain when an ANOVA test is conducted? How to conduct an ANOVA test?

44. What are the different types of ANOVA tests?

45. Explain the different types of parametric and non-parametric ANOVA tests.

46. What are one-way, two-way, cross over and three way ANOVA tests?

47. What is non-parametric test? What are the various statistical non-parametric tests?

48. Explain in detail Sign Test and its significance.

49. Explain in detail Signed Rank Test (also called as Wilcoxon Signed Rank test) and its significance.

50. Explain in detail Rank Sum Test (also called as Wilcoxon Rank Sum Test or Mann-Whitney U-test) and its significance.

51. What is non-parametric one-way ANOVA test (also called as Kruskal-Wallis Test)?

52. What is Friedman test (also called as non-parametric two-way ANOVA test)?

53. What is rationale behind sample size determination? What are the approaches in which sample size is determined?

54. What is epidemiology? What are the various terminology involved in epidemiology studies?

55. What are the various statistical softwares available? Explain their role.

56. Can we conduct statistical test in Microsoft Excel? Input data and conduct a statistical test in Microsoft Excel.

57. Explain in detail about SAS, SPSS, Epi info and Minitab softwares.

58. Explain step wise how to input and analyze data using various kinds of statistical softwares?

59. A researcher wishes to conduct a bio-equivalence study for two paracetamol tablet dosage form (innovator and generic). Explain how to calculate sample size? How to design experiment? how to define null and alternate hypothesis? How to collect data, what kind of statistical test to be conducted? how to say the test is significant or not? how to conclude the innovator and generic paracetamol tablets are bio-equivalent or not?

60. A researcher wants to design a questionnaire with abstract scaling for a disease condition. How to design a questionnaire based on abstract scaling? How to test the data collected and questionnaire is reliable?

61.   A pharmaceutical industry wishes to establish distribution curves for various attributes for the dosage forms available with them. How to plan, develop distribution curves, establish confidence limits, confidence level, confidence interval and set accepted standard levels for the attribute?

62.   A pharmaceutical industry wishes to establish distribution curves, establish confidence limits, confidence level, confidence interval on retrospective basis for various quality attributes of their different products? How to plan and establish based on past manufacturing and quality data?

63. A pharmaceutical company is manufacturing paracetamol 500 mg tablets on regular basis. How to plan and ensure statistically the batches of products produced are of significant quality?

64. Two lots of paracetamol 500 mg tablets are available in the quarantine area of a pharmaceutical industry for packing. Samples were drawn from the lots and assay values of the tablets were determined. How to plan a statistical test and ensure whether the two lots of tablets belong to same batch or not?

65. A pharmaceutical industry wishes to establish shelf life for a formulation? Explain the role of linear regression and correlation coefficient.

66. A researcher has obtained triplicate values of Absorbance vs. Concentration of a drug substance after dilutions. How to determine linear regression, correlation coefficient both mathematically and by using Microsoft Excel?

67. What is inventory system? What is the purpose of inventory system? Explain in detail various methods of establishing inventory in a hospital, in a pharmaceutical industry and in a pharmacy.

68. What is the role of Accountancy in health care sector?

69. Explain the principles, various kinds of book keeping. Explain, how to make entries in a journal and in a ledger?

70. Write in detail about Management report. What is the difference between management and research report?

71. What is the role of computers in health and pharmaceutical sectors?

72. Write a note on parenteral admixtures.

73. The sleep of 10 patients was observed during one night with the drug and one night with placebo. The results obtained are as mentioned in the table. The average number of additional hours slept with the drug compared with the placebo was x(bar)=1.78, the standard deviation s=1.77 hours. The standard error is $s/\sqrt{n}=1.77/\sqrt{10}=0.56$ hours. Conduct a suitable student 't' test and give conclusion.

Results of a placebo-controlled clinical trial to test the effectiveness of a sleeping drug										
Patient	1	2	3	4	5	6	7	8	9	10
Hours of Sleep	6.1	7.0	8.2	7.6	6.5	8.4	6.9	6.7	7.4	5.8
	5.2	7.9	3.9	4.7	5.3	5.4	4.2	6.1	3.8	6.3

74. Physicians from seven clinics in the United States were each asked to test a new drug on three patients. These physicians are considered to be among those who are expert in the disease being tested. The seventh physician tested the drug on only two patients. The physicians had a meeting prior to the experiment to standardize the procedure so that all measurements were uniform in the seven sites. The results were as follows:

Clinic						
1	2	3	4	5	6	7
9	11	6	10	5	7	12
8	9	9	10	3	7	10
7	13	9	7	4	7	---

Conduct an ANOVA test at 5% level and conclude.

75. Tablets were made on six different tablet presses during the course of a run (batch). Five tablets were assayed during the five-hour run, one tablet during each hour. The results are as follows:

Hour	Press					
	1	2	3	4	5	6
1	47	49	46	49	47	50
2	48	48	48	47	50	50
3	52	50	51	53	51	52
4	50	47	50	48	51	50
5	49	46	50	49	47	49

Conduct an ANOVA test and conclude.

76. Dissolution is compared for three experimental batches with the following results (each point is the time in minutes for 50% dissolution for a single tablet). Conduct a suitable test and conclude.

Batch 1	15	18	19	21	23	26
Batch 2	17	18	24	20	---	---
Batch 3	13	10	16	11	9	---

77. The birth weights of children born to 15 non-smokers with those of children born to 14 heavy smokers are mentioned in the table. Conduct a suitable test and draw conclusions.

Birth Weight (kg)	Non-smokers	3.99	3.79	3.6	3.73	3.21	3.6	4.08	3.61	3.83	3.31	4.13	3.26	3.54	3.51	2.71
	Heavy smokers	3.18	2.84	2.9	3.27	3.85	3.52	3.23	2.76	3.6	3.75	3.59	3.63	2.38	2.34	---

78. A drug is formulated to be dissolved more rapidly by substituting lactose for part of the lipoidal lubricant in the regular-release product. The formulator is convinced that this formulation change only could increase the rate of drug dissolution. A one-sided test at the 5% level is proposed when comparing the drug dissolution from the two products. The time to 50 % dissolution for six tablets of each product (minutes) is

Original Product	25	22	29	30	26	24
Modified Product	18	23	24	22	19	16

Conduct a suitable student 't' test and draw conclusions.

79. The following are the inhibition zone diameters (in mm) observed in a microbiological assay: 240, 295, 225, 250, 245, 260, 275, 245, 225, 260, 265, 240, 260, 275, 250. Compute sample mean, standard deviation (SD), sample variance, range, standard error of mean (SEM) and CV.

80. A medical investigation team claims that the average number of infections per number of 17.7 infections. The sample S.D is 1.8. Is there enough evidence to reject the investigator's claim at 5% significance level? (Given critical value: 2.262).

81. In a pharmacokinetics study the following Cmax (in mg/ml) were noted: 715, 728, 735, 716, 706, 715, 712, 717, 731, 709, 722, 701, 698, 741, 723, 718, 726, 716, 720, 721. Calculate mean, median and construct box plot.

82. Using linear regression model find out slope, intercept and correlation coefficient from the data:

Time (Months)	6	12	18	24	36	48
Assay (mg)	995	984	973	960	952	948

83. The following are the intensities of fluorescence for the corresponding concentrations of quinine sulphate using fluorimetry at 360 nm in 0.1 N sulphuric acid. Calculate the correlation coefficient, slope and intercept using the data and determine the concentration of the unknown for which intensity of fluorescence is given. Also plot a graph and compare the graphical concentration with the calculated concentration.

Concentration (ppm)	0.0	2	4	6	8	10	Unknown
Intensity of Fluorescence at 360 nm	0	22.0	43.3	62.6	82.4	100	77.0

84. The following are the absorbances of salicylic acid at various concentrations using ferric nitrate reagent at 540 nm. Calculate the correlation coefficient, slope and intercept using the standard solution data and determine the unknown concentration of salicylic acid for which absorbance is given. Also plot a graph and compare the graphical concentration with the calculated concentration.

Concentration (mcg/ml)	10	20	30	40	50	Unknown
Absorbance at 540nm	0.018	0.032	0.047	0.063	0.081	0.077

85. The absorbances of crystal violet at various concentrations at 544 nm are as follows. Calculate the correlation coefficient, slope and intercept using the data.

Concentration (mcg/ml)	1	2	4	8	16	32
Absorbance at 544 nm	0.097	0.108	0.191	0.339	0.674	1.34

86. The absorbances of sulphacetamide at various concentrations after adding hydrochloric acid, sodium nitrite and ammonium sulphamate using Bratten Marshall reagent at 540 nm are as follows. Calculate the correlation coefficient, slope and intercept using the data and calculate the unknown concentration by linear equation and by graph.

Concentration (mcg/ml)	2	4	6	8	10	Unknown
Absorbance (540 nm)	0.0757	0.1674	0.3872	0.5850	0.6777	0.3187

87. In order to find the fluorescence quenching, the intensities of fluorescence of various concentrations of quinine sulphate in sulphuric acid are as follows in 0.1 N sulphuric acid. Calculate the correlation coefficient, slope, intercept to achieve a straight line.

Concentration (ppm)	2	4	8	16	32	64
Intensity of Fluorescence	5.1	9.5	19.5	35.1	62.3	100.0

88. Bio-assay of acetylcholine by interpolation method was conducted. The following are the volume of injection of acetylcholine and its corresponding acetylcholine dose, log (dose) in mcg and height of the response (in cm) are as follows. (Concentration of standard acetylcholine = 10 mcg/ml)

Acetylcholine Volume		Dose in mcg	log (dose) in mcg	height of the response (cm)
Standard	0.1 ml	1	0.0000	1.1
	0.2 ml	2	0.3010	1.5
	0.4 ml	4	0.6020	2.0
	0.8 ml	8	0.9030	2.4
Test	0.1 ml	---	---	1.0
	0.2 ml	---	---	1.7
	0.4 ml	---	---	2.3

Calculate the correlation coefficient, slope, intercept using the standard response and later find the average concentration of test responses.

89. The surface (local) anesthetic activity on rabbit using procaine in left eye and xylocaine in right eye was conducted. The response of corneal refluxes was examined using a cotton fiber. The following are the responses.   Conduct an appropriate statistical test and judge whether there is any significant difference in the local anesthetic activity of the drugs and which drug has good surface anesthetic activity. [Hint: Procaine less lipid soluble and does not show surface anesthesia, whereas xylocaine shows surface anesthesia]

Time in minutes	Corneal Reflux	
	Left eye (Procaine)	Right eye (Xylocaine)
0	+	+
5	+	+
10	+	+
15	+	+
20	+	+
25	+	-
30	+	-

90. The nerve block anesthetic activity on pitted frog's gastrocnemius muscle-sciatic nerve was conducted by placing a cotton ball of local anesthesia (procaine). The withdrawal responses are at various hydrochloric acid strengths is as follows. Conduct appropriate statistical test and draw conclusions.

Drug	Time in minutes	Withdrawal response and HCl strength	
		0.1 N	0.2 N
Procaine	0	+	+
	1	+	+
	2	+	+
	3	+	+
	4	---	---
	5	---	---

91. The temperature readings of different students on different days during COVID-19 are as follows. Conduct appropriate statistical tests and conclude any difference within student and among students.

Student No	Temp 1	Temp 2	Temp 3	Temp 4	Student No	Temp 1	Temp 2	Temp 3	Temp 4
1	95.3	95.2	95	97.8	44	97.8	97.8	96.2	96.9
2	96.2	96.4	95.7	97.8	45	98.4	98.2	95	94
3	97.7	95.7	95.1	97.1	46	97.5	97.8	97.7	96.2
4	97.8	93.3		97.8	47	97.1	98	98	97.8
5	98	98.2	98	98.2	48	95.1	98.2	97.3	96.8
6	96.6	96.8	97.3	97.5	49	97.3	97.8	97.8	95.3
7	94.2	94.8	97.7	97.8	50	97.1	98.2	92.8	97.5
8	97.3	98.2	93.5	97.8	51	98.2	96.4	96.6	97.1
9	98.2	95.7	98	98.2	52	97.5	98	95.5	95.5
10	96.9	96.9	96.9	98.9	53	97.3	97.7	91.5	96
11	96.9	97.9	97.8	95.5	54	96.8	98.2	96.6	94.1
12	98.2	98.5	97.5	97.1	55	96.8	98.2	97.3	97.7
13	96.6	96.9	97.1	96.2	56	98	97.8	96.2	97.5
14	95	96.4	93.3	93.7	57	96.8	96.6	97.5	97.5
15	96.6	96.8	98	97.7	58	94.2	98	96.9	96.8
16	98.4	96	98	98	59	97.7	97.7	97.1	96.7
17	98.2	98	97.6	96.4	60	96	97.8	95.1	96.6
18	96.9	96.6	95.1	95.5	61	97.5			97.7
19	97.1	96.4	95.3	95.9	62	98.2	97.7	97.7	97.1
20	96.9	95.5	94.1	95.1	63	98.2	96.9		
21	98.2	96.9	98.1	98.2	64	97.5	95.7	96.2	96.6
22	96.9	94.1	97.3	97.5	65	97.5	97.8	96.6	96.2
23	97.5	96.6	96.9	98.2	66	98	97.3	96.8	96.8
24	97.1	96.9	97.8	98.2	67	96.4	97.1	96.9	96.8
25	98.2	95.7	96	98.2	68	96.7	96.9	97.7	
26	96.9	95	95	97.7	69	97.8	93.2	96.8	96.8
27	98.2	96.6	98	98.2	70		97.5		96.6
28	98.2	98.2	98	98.2	71	95.1	96.8	97.1	98.4
29	95.5	96.8	98	98.2	72	97.5	96.9	96.9	98.2
30		97.3	98.6		73	96.9	96.6	95.7	96.8
31	97.1		98	97.1	74		96.4	94.8	96.6
32	98	98	98	95.1	75	98	96.8	96.6	

Contd...

33	97.3	98	96.9		76	96.6	96.9	96.8	96.4
34	96.8		96.6	96.8	77	98	98	97.1	97.7
35	98.6	98	98	96.5	78	98	97.8	96.8	96.8
36	98.9	98.2	97.3	97.8	79		97.5	97.7	97.5
37	93.2	95.9	97.3		80	96.9	98	97.8	97.8
38	98		96.9	98	81	97.1	97.1	96	97.7
39	96.2	97.7	97	93.9	82		98.2		98.2
40	97.8		98		83	98	96	97.1	96.9
41	97.3	98	96.6		84	97.3	96.8	94.2	96.8
42	96.8		96.8		85		97.5		96.8
43	96.8	97.5	96.9	96.2					

92.   A three point bio-assay of acetylcholine was conducted on frog's rectus abdominal muscle. The concentration of standard acetylcholine is 10 mcg/ml. The following are the responses of standard and the test. After four dose response curves of standard and the test each with different volumes, the doses of the standard (s_1, s_2) and the test (t) are given in a sequence after washout period and tissue stabilization in the order s_1, t, s_2; t, s_1, s_2 and s_2, s_1, t. The following are the details of the doses and responses:

Acetylcholine	**Dose (ml)**	**log (dose)**
s_1	0.2 ml $\equiv$ 2 mcg	0.3010
s_2	0.4 ml $\equiv$ 4 mcg	0.6020
t (unknown)	0.2 ml (unknown)	

Height of Response in cms		
$s_1 = 1.6$	$t = 2.5$	$s_2 = 2.9$
$t = 2.1$	$s_1 = 1.3$	$s_2 = 2.5$
$s_2 = 2.3$	$s_1 = 1.6$	$t = 2.7$

Calculate the dose of the unknown acetylcholine solution both graphically and by correlation coefficient, slope and intercept and compare the concentration of the unknown (both graphically and by statistical calculation). [Hint: $y = mx + c$]

93.   An antacid product is reformulated with a new less expensive flavoring agent. Fifty subjects, users of this product, were randomly divided into two groups of 25 each, with each subject evaluating either the new or old formula. A specially designed thermometer scale [Superb (10), Excellent (9), Very good (8), Good (7), Fairly good (6), Fair (5), Fairly poor (4), Poor (3), Very poor (2), Terrible (1)] was used. Testing of the hypothesis of equality of means H_0: $\mu_1 = \mu_2$ was used and a two independent groups student 't' test was conducted at 5 % level. The standard 't' valued at df=47 is 2.01. The results are as follow. Give your conclusion. Hint: Use equation of parametric

independent student 't' test. The test is also called as Monadic or Single product test, even though the data is in the form of scores.

	Old Product	New Product
Number of Subjects	25	24
Average Score	7.44	6.88
Standard deviation	1.94	1.90

94. A preclinical study was performed to determine the carcinogenic potential of a new drug in which 100 control animals were compared to a group of 100 animals given the drug. At the end of the experiment, the animals were examined for tumors. Ten animals in the control group and eight in the drug group died of non-drug related caused before the experiment was completed, and these animals were not included in the final count. The results are as follows:

Actual and Expected Number of Animals with Tumors After Drug Treatment and Placebo			
	Number of Tumors	**Number without Tumors**	**Total**
Drug	18(16.18)	74 (75.82)	92
Placebo	14 (15.82)	76 (74.18)	90
Total	32	150	182

Conduct a chi-square statistic and come to conclusions.

95. A preclinical study, animals were treated with two antihypertensive experimental drugs and a control drug, with 12 animals randomly assigned to the three groups, four per group. One animal died from a non-drug related cause and was lost to the experiment. The results of blood pressure from baseline are as follows. Conduct a oneway ANOVA test and conclude.

Drug 1	Drug 2	Drug 3
15	8	---
12	14	16
19	13	20
11	6	22

96. A precision study during a method transfer from research laboratory to routine microbiologic laboratory for an erythromycin dosage form is illustrated below. Conduct suitable statistical tests and report within day, laboratory and between days, laboratories and report.

Claimed Level Erythromycin Conc. (%)	Sample Designation	Concentration of Erythromycin Potency Found			
		Routine Laboratory		Research Laboratory	
		Day 1	Day 2	Day 1	Day 2
80	a	77	79	79	84
80	b	85	77	85	86
80	c	80	86	70	86
80	d	78	80	80	80
80	e	83	84	78	84
80	f	81	79	79	87
100	a	102	108	94	120
100	b	105	103	108	92
100	c	97	110	108	102
100	d	101	107	115	102
100	e	104	102	97	106
100	f	98	108	105	115
120	a	130	135	115	147
120	b	132	118	110	140
120	c	133	130	124	120
120	d	128	127	111	140
120	e	131	133	117	133
120	f	130	130	122	126

97.   Anti-inflammatory activity of some selected compounds were evaluated using carrageenan (0.1 ml, 1 % w/v, injecting to sub-plantar region of rat's paw) induced rat hind paw oedema method. Each group consisting of six animals, the animals were grouped into control, standard and test groups. The control, standard and test groups were administered with Tween-80 (1 %) suspension, 20 mg/kg suspension of diclofenac sodium intra-peritoneally and 30 mg/kg of suspension of test compounds in Tween-80 respectively after half an hour after injecting carrageenan. The following are the results observed and conduct a suitable statistical test at 5 percent probability and conclude.

Chemical Compound No	Paw Volumes		
	After 1 hours	After 2 hours	After 3 hours
1	1.5	1.74	1.87
2	1.43	1.53	1.7
3	1.4	1.45	1.63
4	1.42	1.57	1.63
5	1.38	1.4	1.43
6	1.32	1.35	1.35
7	1.5	1.78	1.9
8	1.38	1.7	1.8

Contd...

9	1.3	1.65	1.75
10	1.48	1.57	1.65
11	1.45	1.53	1.63
12	1.28	1.42	1.48
Control	1.78	2.1	2.4
Diclofenac Sodium	0.99	1.11	1.11

98. For analgesic activity on animals, firstly the animals were selected based on their response within 2-3 seconds. The cut off time for determination of latent period was taken as 40 seconds to avoid the injury to the skin and based on pilot studies. Later the animals selected were divided into four groups of six animals each and the analgesic activity was observed after administration of test compounds, control, pentazocine HCl (standard). The control animals received only 1 % Tween -80, whereas test and control animals received individually test compounds in 1 % Tween-80 (intraperitonially) and pentazocine hydrochloride suspended in 1 % Tween-80 (vehicle) respectively. The average basal reaction time in seconds at pre-treatment (0 minutes), after treatment (15, 30, 45 and 60 minutes) are as follows:

Chemical Compound No	Pre-treatment '0' minutes (in seconds)	After treatment '15' minutes (in seconds)	After treatment '30' minutes (in seconds)	After treatment '45' minutes (in seconds)	After treatment '60' minutes (in seconds)
1	3.6	4.5	6.53	7.03	11.2
2	3.8	4.5	7.05	11.4	11.4
3	3.6	4.62	4.67	5.5	5.3
4	3.2	5.5	5.5	4.4	3.4
5	3.4	3.83	6.83	6.00	6.5
6	2.62	2.67	3.3333	4.67	4.0
7	3.6	4.17	5.17	8.0	9.83
8	3.2	4.00	5.5	6.17	6.67
9	3.5	5.33	8.83	5.67	5.33
10	3.1	7.17	11.17	10.67	9.67
11	3.6	6.33	7.76	10.33	9.25
12	3.6	3.67	3.83	4.33	4.33
Control	3.6	3.6	3.5	3.6	3.4
Diclofenac Sodium	3.6	4.93	8.9	10.1	12.5

99. Initially the animals were trained to remain on the rotating rod (moving at speed of 25 rpm) for 5 minutes and those animals that were able to remain on the rotating rod for 5 minutes and above were selected for conducting muscle relaxant activity. Three groups of animals as control, test and standard containing six animals each were divided. The test animals were administered with test compounds intraperitonially at a dose 30 mg/kg body weight in the form of suspension in 1 % Tween-80. The standard group animals received diazepam (standard drug) at a dose of 4 mg/kg body weight. After 30 minutes,

the mice were placed again on the rotating rod and animal's fall off time was recorded. Using the following data, conduct a suitable statistical test at 5 percent probability and conclude.

Chemical Compound No	Fall off Time before drug treatment	Fall off Time after drug treatment
1	43.00	15.50
2	23.50	14.17
3	26.17	16.00
4	38.50	22.50
5	26.83	20.67
6	34.83	16.67
7	44.00	33.67
8	35.67	30.62
9	42.33	38.17
10	32.67	15.33
11	26.17	10.83
12	30.17	12.00
Control	34.83	34.67
Diazepam	28.32	5.75